Oral Diseases for the General Dentist

Editors

ARVIND BABU RAJENDRA SANTOSH
ORRETT E. OGLE

DENTAL CLINICS OF NORTH AMERICA

www.dental.theclinics.com

January 2020 • Volume 64 • Number 1

ELSEVIER

1600 John F. Kennedy Boulevard • Suite 1800 • Philadelphia, Pennsylvania, 19103-2899

http://www.dental.theclinics.com

DENTAL CLINICS OF NORTH AMERICA Volume 64, Number 1
January 2020 ISSN 0011-8532, ISBN: 978-0-323-71211-8

Editor: John Vassallo; j.vassallo@elsevier.com
Developmental Editor: Laura Fisher

Dental Clinics of North America (ISSN 0011-8532) is published quarterly by Elsevier Inc., 360 Park Avenue South, New York, NY 10010-1710. Months of issue are January, April, July, and October. Business and Editorial Offices: 1600 John F. Kennedy Boulevard, Suite 1800, Philadelphia, PA 19103-2899. Periodicals postage paid at New York, NY and additional mailing offices. Subscription prices are $304.00 per year (domestic individuals), $633.00 per year (domestic institutions), $100.00 per year (domestic students/residents), $366.00 per year (Canadian individuals), $821.00 per year (Canadian institutions), $100.00 per year (Canadian students/residents) $424.00 per year (international individuals), $821.00 per year (international institutions), and $200.00 per year (international students/residents). International air speed delivery is included in all *Clinics* subscription prices. All prices are subject to change without notice. **POSTMASTER:** Send address changes to *Dental Clinics of North America*, Elsevier Health Sciences Division, Subscription Customer Service, 3251 Riverport Lane, Maryland Heights, MO 63043. **Customer Service (orders, claims, online, change of address): Elsevier Health Sciences Division, Subscription Customer Service, 3251 Riverport Lane, Maryland Heights, MO 63043. Tel: 1-800-654-2452 (U.S. and Canada). Fax: 314-447-8029. E-mail: journalscustomerservice-usa@elsevier.com (for print support); journalsonlinesupport-usa@elsevier. com (for online support).**

Reprints. For copies of 100 or more, of articles in this publication, please contact the Commercial Reprints Department, Elsevier Inc., 360 Park Avenue South, New York, NY 10010-1710. Tel.: 212-633-3874; Fax: 212-633-3820; E-mail: reprints@elsevier.com.

The Dental Clinics of North America is covered in *MEDLINE/PubMed (Index Medicus), Current Contents/Clinical Medicine, ISI/BIOMED* and *Clinahl.*

Contributors

EDITORS

ARVIND BABU RAJENDRA SANTOSH, BDS, MDS
Oral and Maxillofacial Pathologist, Senior Lecturer and Research Coordinator, School of Dentistry, Faculty of Medical Sciences, The University of the West Indies, Mona, Jamaica, West Indies

ORRETT E. OGLE, DDS
Former Chief and Program Director, Oral and Maxillofacial Surgery, Woodhull Hospital, Brooklyn, New York, USA; Visiting Lecturer, School of Dentistry, Faculty of Medical Sciences, The University of the West Indies, Mona, Jamaica, West Indies; Oral and Maxillofacial Surgeon, Douglasville, Georgia, USA

AUTHORS

NATASHA BHALLA, DDS
Resident, Oral and Maxillofacial Surgery, The Brooklyn Hospital Center, New York, New York, USA

DORYCK BOYD, DDS, FICD
Oral and Maxillofacial Pathologist, Part Time Lecturer, College of Oral Health Sciences, University of Technology, Kingston, Jamaica, West Indies

AVNEESH CHHABRA, MD
Associate Professor of Radiology, Chief of Musculoskeletal Imaging, The University of Texas Southwestern Medical Center, Dallas, Texas, USA

CODY J. CHRISTENSEN, DDS
Resident, Oral and Maxillofacial Surgery Department, San Antonio Military Health System, San Antonio, Texas, USA

EARL CLARKSON, DDS
Chairman of NYCHHC, Department of Dentistry/Oral and Maxillofacial Surgery, Woodhull Medical Center, Brooklyn, New York, USA

HARRY DYM, DDS
Chairman and Program Director, Oral and Maxillofacial Surgery, The Brooklyn Hospital Center, New York, New York, USA

SUMITRA S. GOLIKERI, DMD
Program Director, Woodhull Medical and Mental Health Center, Brooklyn, New York, USA

JESSICA GRENFELL, DDS
Pediatric Dentistry Resident, Woodhull Medical and Mental Health Center, Brooklyn, New York, USA

LESLIE R. HALPERN, DDS, MD, PhD, MPH, FACS, FICD
Professor, Section Head, Oral and Maxillofacial Surgery, University of Utah, School of
Dentistry, Salt Lake City, Utah, USA

EUNSU JUNG, DDS
Chief Resident of NYCHHC, Department of Dentistry/Oral and Maxillofacial Surgery,
Woodhull Medical Center, Brooklyn, New York, USA

KEITH H. KANER, DDS
Private Practice, Boca Raton, Florida, USA; Department of Oral and Maxillofacial
Surgery, Nova Southeastern University, College of Dental Medicine, Ft Lauderdale,
Florida, USA

DAVID KIM, DDS
Pediatric Dentistry Resident, Woodhull Medical and Mental Health Center, Brooklyn, New
York, USA

K. KIRAN KUMAR, BDS, MDS, PhD
Professor, Department of Oral and Maxillofacial Pathology, SIBAR Institute of Dental
Sciences, Guntur, Andhra Pradesh, India

EUGENE KO, DMD, MS
Assistant Professor, Department of Oral Medicine, Robert Schattner Center, University of
Pennsylvania School of Dental Medicine, Philadelphia, Pennsylvania, USA

MICHAL KUTEN-SHORRER, DMD, DMSc
Assistant Professor, Division of Oral Medicine, Department of Diagnostic Sciences, Tufts
University School of Dental Medicine, Boston, Massachusetts, USA

KUMARASWAMY KIKERI LAXMINARAYANA, BDS, MDS
Oral and Maxillofacial Pathologist, Professor and Head, Department of Oral and
Maxillofacial Pathology, Farooqia Dental College and Hospital, Rajiv Gandhi University of
Health Sciences, Mysore, Karnataka, India

MARK A. LERMAN, DMD
Associate Professor, Division of Oral Pathology, Department of Diagnostic Sciences,
Tufts University School of Dental Medicine, Boston, Massachusetts, USA

RESHMA S. MENON, BDS, DMSc
Lecturer, Department of Oral Medicine, Infection and Immunity, Harvard School of Dental
Medicine, Boston, Massachusetts, USA

MEL MUPPARAPU, DMD, MDS
Professor and Director of Radiology, Department of Oral Medicine, Robert Schattner
Center, University of Pennsylvania School of Dental Medicine, Philadelphia, Pennsylvania,
USA

YOAV NUDELL, DDS
Resident, Oral and Maxillofacial Surgery, The Brooklyn Hospital Center, New York, New
York, USA

ORRETT E. OGLE, DDS
Former Chief and Program Director, Oral and Maxillofacial Surgery, Woodhull Hospital,
Brooklyn, New York, USA; Visiting Lecturer, School of Dentistry, Faculty of Medical
Sciences, The University of the West Indies, Mona, Jamaica, West Indies; Oral and
Maxillofacial Surgeon, Douglasville, Georgia, USA

TEMITOPE T. OMOLEHINWA, DMD, DScD
Assistant Professor of Oral Medicine, University of Pennsylvania School of Dental Medicine, Philadelphia, Pennsylvania, USA

CHRISTOPHER PAE, DDS
Pediatric Dentistry Resident, Woodhull Medical and Mental Health Center, Brooklyn, New York, USA

RAWLE FABIAN PHILBERT, DDS, FACD
Chairman and Program Director, Oral and Maxillofacial Surgery, Lincoln Medical and Mental Health Center, Bronx, New York, USA; Clinical Associate Professor, Oral and Maxillofacial Surgery, Columbia University College of Dental Medicine, Assistant Professor of Clinical Surgery (Dentistry Oral and Maxillofacial Surgery), Weill Cornell Medical College, New York, New York, USA

ARVIND BABU RAJENDRA SANTOSH, BDS, MDS
Oral and Maxillofacial Pathologist, Senior Lecturer and Research Coordinator, School of Dentistry, Faculty of Medical Sciences, The University of the West Indies, Mona, Jamaica, West Indies

B.V. RAMANA REDDY, BDS, MDS
Professor and Head, Department of Oral and Maxillofacial Pathology, SIBAR Institute of Dental Sciences, Guntur, Andhra Pradesh, India

NAVRAJ SINGH SANDHU, BSc, DMD
Intern, Oral and Maxillofacial Surgery, Lincoln Medical and Mental Health Center, Bronx, New York, USA

KATHERINE JIE SHI, DMD
Department of Endodontics, Tufts University School of Dental Medicine, Boston, Massachusetts, USA

JAYKRISHNA THAKKAR, DDS
Resident, Oral and Maxillofacial Surgery, The Brooklyn Hospital Center, New York, New York, USA

TIBEBU M. TSEGGA, DDS
Attending, Oral and Maxillofacial Surgery Department, San Antonio Military Health System, San Antonio, Texas, USA

STEPHANIE L. WETZEL, DDS
Oral and Maxillofacial Pathologist, Atlanta Oral Pathology, Decatur, Georgia, USA

JESSICA WOLLENBERG, DMD
Oral and Maxillofacial Pathologist, Randolph Oral Pathology Associates, Randolph, New Jersey, USA

Contents

> Oral diseases are pathologic conditions that affect oral and maxillofacial tissues. Dental caries and periodontal diseases are the most common forms of oral diseases, but there are a wide variety of diseases that can occur in oral and maxillofacial tissues. These oral diseases range from metabolic, inflammatory, infectious, neoplastic, autoimmune, developmental, to idiopathic origin. Numerous oral conditions have overlapping clinical signs and symptoms, which make the diagnosis and management challenging for the dentist. However, a comprehensive understanding of clinical behavior will help in differentiating the various oral diseases and will provide a logical pathway to formulating a diagnosis.

> Deviations from anthropometric norms related to facial skeletal development are a relatively normal occurrence in the dental management of the vast majority of patients. A consideration for correction is usually warranted only when there is associated morbidity, functional impairment, or psychosocial detriment. The vast majority of jaw and dental abnormalities are developmental and present themselves within a continuum of clinically conspicuous to overtly obvious. This article highlights a variety of developmental abnormalities that present with structural disharmony of the maxillomandibular complex and secondarily associated dental structures.

> Oral potentially malignant disorders (OPMDs) are precursor lesions that may undergo malignant transformation to oral cancer. These lesions most commonly present clinically as white patches (leukoplakia). However, they may also be red (erythroplakia), or red and white (erythroleukoplakia). There are many risk factors associated with the development of an OPMD, and with the risk of malignant transformation of the lesion. A biopsy with subsequent microscopic examination from the lesional tissue is necessary in identification of OPMD. This article reviews the clinical appearance of OPMDs, associated risk factors, diagnosis and histologic appearance, and treatment.

Benign and malignant neoplasm of oral cavity is usually presented as swellings or ulcerations of affected tissue. The lesions are broadly categorized as potentially malignant disorders, benign and malignant neoplasm of epithelial and connective tissue origin for the convenience of learning. Neoplasm of oral cavity has a significantly lower incidence. Because of uncommon occurrence of oral neoplasm, retention of diagnostic skills is a challenging task. However, comprehensive understanding on clinical and pathologic details will help in correlating and presenting complaint and assisting in formulation of possible diagnosis. The key for successful therapeutic management depends on achieving right and timely diagnosis.

This article focuses on describing nonodontogenic cysts of the oral and maxillofacial region. The lesions described include nasopalatine duct canal cyst, nasolabial cyst, traumatic bone cyst, Stafne bone cyst, aneurysmal bone cyst, focal osteoporotic bone marrow defect, dermoid cyst, epidermoid cyst, pilar cyst, and sebaceous cyst. The intent of this article is to make general dentists aware and knowledgeable of the nonodontogenic cysts they may encounter in everyday practice, so they can adequately manage or make an appropriate referral to improve treatment outcomes and reduce patient morbidity.

A variety of diseases, including obstructions, infections, and benign and malignant tumors, occur in salivary glands. The most common problem is painful blockage of ducts by stones that prevents drainage of saliva. Sialadenitis can be due to either infectious or noninfectious factors. Bacterial or viral infections are the most common causes of acute sialadenitis. Staphylococcus is the usual bacterial cause, whereas paramyxovirus (mumps) is the common viral cause. Eighty percent of salivary tumors are benign, whereas about 20% are malignant. Most tumors occur in the parotid gland and on the hard palate. Classifications, imaging, and suggested treatment are described.

Odontogenic cysts are epithelial-lined pathologic cavities and surrounded by fibrous connective tissue that originate from odontogenic tissues that occur in tooth-bearing regions of maxilla and mandible. Cystic conditions of the jaw cause bony destruction and may cause resorption or displacement of adjacent teeth. Odontogenic cysts have developmental or inflammatory origins. More cases have been published in the adult age group than the pediatric population. Periapical cyst and dentigerous cysts are frequently reported conditions in dental practice. Histopathologic examination remains the gold standard investigation. Odontogenic cysts are managed with enucleation or marsupialization procedures. Early recognition and referral to oral surgery minimize the extent of jaw bone destruction.

antidepressants have proved effective and are considered the treatment choice for AFP.

Mel Mupparapu, Eugene Ko, Temitope T. Omolehinwa, and Avneesh Chhabra

The maxillofacial region is complex in its anatomy and in its variation in the presentation of neurologic disorders. The diagnosis and management of neurologic disorders in clinical practice remains a challenge. A good understanding of the neurologic disorder in its entirety helps dentists in the diagnosis and appropriate referral to a specialist for further investigations and management of the condition. Neurologic disorders described in this article are under broad categories of sensory and motor disturbances as well as movement disorders and infections. This article summarizes the most common maxillofacial neurologic disorders that dentists might encounter in clinical practice.

DENTAL CLINICS OF NORTH AMERICA

FORTHCOMING ISSUES

April 2020
Surgical and Medical Management of Common Oral Problems
Harry J. Dym, *Editor*

July 2020
Controlled Substance Risk Mitigation in the Dental Setting
Michael E. Schatman, Ronald J. Kulich, David A. Keith, *Editors*

October 2020
The Journey to Excellence in Esthetic Dentistry
Yair Whiteman and David Wagner, *Editors*

RECENT ISSUES

October 2019
Caries Management
Sandra Guzmán-Armstrong, Margherita Fontana, Marcelle M. Nascimento, and Andrea G. Ferreira Zandona, *Editors*

July 2019
Unanswered Questions in Implant Dentistry
Mohanad Al-Sabbagh, *Editor*

April 2019
Prosthodontics
Lisa A. Lang and Lily T. García, *Editors*

SERIES OF RELATED INTEREST

Atlas of the Oral and Maxillofacial Surgery Clinics
http://www.oralmaxsurgeryatlas.theclinics.com

Oral and Maxillofacial Surgery Clinics
http://www.oralmaxsurgery.theclinics.com

THE CLINICS ARE AVAILABLE ONLINE!
Access your subscription at:
www.theclinics.com

Preface

Oral Diseases for the General Dentist

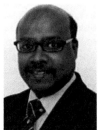
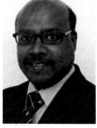

Arvind Babu Rajendra Santosh, BDS, MDS   Orrett E. Ogle, DDS

Editors

This issue of *Dental Clinics of North America* is geared to the dental and medical community as a refresher and an update on oral diseases. We believe that early detection, recognition, and referral to an oral disease specialist, oral surgeon, oral medicine, or oral pathologist, will greatly reduce the negative effects of chronic disease and the cost of clinical care. A major challenge in the diagnosis of oral disease is the need for memorizing long lists of oral lesions from oral pathology literature. This is made more difficult because many of these lesions are not frequently encountered by the dentist or medical practitioner. This current issue will highlight common and/or important oral conditions divided into various categories that a dentist may encounter in their practice. Pulpal, periapical, and periodontal diseases are intentionally not discussed in this issue since dentists are experienced in diagnosing and managing those conditions.

We trust that this issue, "Oral Diseases for the General Dentist," will serve as a tabletop reference in General Dental Practice. The discussion of the entire spectrum of oral diseases is beyond the scope of this issue; instead, we have selected what we believe to be common and/or fairly important oral conditions. Each article is written by an author well educated in the subject matter discussed. The information presented is primarily aimed to cover the diagnostic aspects and an overview of patient management. We recognize that the knowledge on best practices is continuously changing, and as such, we advise the readers to check the most current information available from updated sources.

The introductory article provides the dentist with an approach in formulating clinical diagnosis, various descriptive terms used in oral disease education, and preliminary information of various categories of oral diseases. Each article confers the most relevant information on the oral condition presented with emphasize on diagnostic information and management strategies. It is our hope that

Dent Clin N Am 64 (2020) xiii–xv
https://doi.org/10.1016/j.cden.2019.09.001
0011-8532/20/© 2019 Published by Elsevier Inc.   **dental.theclinics.com**

"Oral Diseases for the General Dentist" will integrate the principles of oral medicine and oral pathology into clinically applicable concepts that will enable the general dentist to develop clinical differential diagnosis, and participate in definitive diagnosis through a multidisciplinary approach with dental specialty teams.

No issue of the *Dental Clinics of North America* could come to a successful fruition without the contributions of well-qualified authors. We are extremely thankful to the authors who have taken their professional and personal time for their valuable contribution to this issue.

We are extremely pleased and thankful for the support received from the editorial staff of the *Dental Clinics of North America*. I would like to recognize and honor the support received from Mr John Vassallo, Editor, and Ms Laura Fisher, Developmental Editor, and other technical team members from the Elsevier family for bringing this issue to the dental and medical community. We believe that this issue of *Dental Clinics of North America* will be a valuable contribution to the dental literature.

ACKNOWLEDGMENTS

From Dr Santosh: I am privileged and pleased with Dr Orrett E. Ogle for his partnering editorial hand in guiding this issue to be a reality. He brought his enormous knowledge and support once again to every step of this issue publication. I would like to sincerely thank and respect his dedication and for helping me to develop this issue. I would like to recognize the fact that bringing out this issue would be challenging in his absence, and his support and endless efforts deserve my sincere respect with thanks.

I would like to express my special thanks and gratitude to School of Dentistry, Faculty of Medical Sciences, The University of the West Indies, Jamaica (West Indies) for granting me adequate time in writing and editing this issue. I take this opportunity to thank Dr Thaon Jones, Head of Dental School, and Dr Tomlin Paul, Dean-Faculty of Medical Sciences, University of the West Indies, Jamaica for allowing me to fulfill this golden opportunity. My special thanks to Mrs Faith McKoy-Johnson, Medical Branch Librarian, for accessing literature through both online and print channels of publication.

This issue is dedicated to my teacher, the late Prof Naresh Lingaraju, Professor of Oral Medicine, from my alma mater Farooquia Dental College and Hospital, Karnataka, India. I would like to express gratitude and appreciation of my teachers and mentors: Prof. Ramana Reddy BV, Prof. Kumaraswamy KL, Prof. Anuradha, Prof. Ratheesh Kumar Nandan and Prof. Chandrasekar Poosarla for all that they taught, recognizing skills, continued motivation, support, guidance and feedback for the way forward.

Thanks to my senior and junior colleagues, students, and patients from whom I have gained the experience of learning and teaching.

I also dedicate this issue to my parents, my wife, Ramyaa, and 2 children, Ryaan Santosh and Ayaan Santosh, sister, brother-in-law, and niece. I thank them for allowing me to take family time and for being patient supporters of this academic and professional contribution.

From Dr Ogle: I would like to thank all the authors for their valuable contribution to this issue and for meeting the set deadlines. From a surgeon's point of view, early diagnosis and referral will always produce successful surgical results. It's hopeful that this issue will serve as a good review for general practitioners and help in the early recognition of oral diseases. Like Dr Santosh, I'd like to thank my family and special friends for their continuous support and encouragement.

Arvind Babu Rajendra Santosh, BDS, MDS
School of Dentistry
The University of the West Indies
Mona campus, Kingston 7
Jamaica, West Indies

Orrett E. Ogle, DDS
Oral and Maxillofacial Surgery
Woodhull Hospital
Brooklyn, NY 11206, USA

School of Dentistry
The University of the West Indies
Mona Kingston-7
Jamaica, West Indies

4974 Golf Valley Court
Douglasville, GA 30135, USA

E-mail addresses:
arvindbabu2001@gmail.com (A.B. Rajendra Santosh)
oeogle@aol.com (O.E. Ogle)

Clinical Outline of Oral Diseases

Arvind Babu Rajendra Santosh, BDS, MDS[a],*, Doryck Boyd, DDS, FICD[b],
Kumaraswamy Kikeri Laxminarayana, BDS, MDS[c]

KEYWORDS

- Clinical diagnosis • Jaw cysts • Odontogenic tumors • Mucocutaneous disorders
- Salivary gland pathologic condition

KEY POINTS

- High-quality clinical examination skills are a key factor to achieving a correct diagnosis.
- Appropriate use of clinical descriptive terms is important in recognizing clinical characteristics of an oral condition.
- A diagnostic algorithm or decision-making tree is a useful tool in a clinical situation where critical thinking or logical answering is required.
- Correlating the clinical information with radiological and/or histopathologic interpretation is the correct approach for arriving a final diagnosis.
- Not all oral conditions require treatment, but all oral conditions must have a diagnosis.

INTRODUCTION

A clinical examination of the patient is essential to determine the nature of the pathologic condition and is significantly important in formulating a diagnosis. Dental surgeons possess an advantage in that they can see the part of the body that they are called upon to treat. The primary objective of routine clinical examination of the oral cavity is to distinguish between health and disease.[1] Common symptoms of oral diseases include swelling, ulcer, color change, surface/textural changes, tenderness/pain, and functional changes. Epidemiologic details of oral disease can guide the dental practitioner into understanding the relevance of clinical conditions in their setting and of the public health impact of early recognition, assessment, and prevention or treatment care.[2] Because of the low prevalence of oral diseases in the general dental practice, the general dentist has only a very low level of exposure to oral diseases, which makes diagnosis difficult. In addition, the shift in approach for disease

[a] School of Dentistry, Faculty of Medical Sciences, The University of the West Indies, Mona campus, Kingston 7, Jamaica, West Indies; [b] College of Oral Health Sciences, University of Technology, Arthur Wint Dr, Kingston 5, Jamaica, West Indies; [c] Department of Oral and Maxillofacial Pathology, Farooqia Dental College and Hospital, Rajiv Gandhi University of Health Sciences, Tilak Nagar, Mysore 570021, Karnataka, India
* Corresponding author.
E-mail address: arvindbabu2001@gmail.com

Dent Clin N Am 64 (2020) 1–10
https://doi.org/10.1016/j.cden.2019.08.001
0011-8532/20/© 2019 Elsevier Inc. All rights reserved.

diagnosis with an emphasis on imaging and laboratory technology has further reduced the skills and confidence in oral examination and clinical diagnosis. Despite the reliance on technology, recognition of abnormalities by the generalist is still required. A late recognition or poor examination skills can lead to incorrect diagnosis or a misdiagnosis, with delays in life-saving treatments.[3] The purpose of this article is to provide (i) an approach in formulating clinical diagnosis and (ii) an outline of the clinical nature of oral diseases. Although the presentation of detailed clinical information of oral diseases is beyond the scope of this article, basic information and an introductory clinical outline of the most commonly encountered categories of oral diseases are presented. For the convenience of the reader, the topics discussed are the common categories of oral diseases, which are given in **Box 1**.

Approach in Formulating Clinical Diagnosis

A step-by-step approach in gathering information on the pathologic condition presented and critical analysis of the findings are the most important elements in the logical formulation of diagnosis. Successful management of the pathologic condition is always preceded by the correct diagnosis. The steps in the diagnostic process are as follows: (1) patient communication, (2) structured extraoral and/or intraoral examination, (3) assessment and correlation of problem listing, (4) critical analysis of procured data, (5) formulation of differential and provisional diagnosis, (6) investigation, and (7) arriving at the definitive diagnosis.[4]

The predominance of dental caries, pulpal and periapical pathologic conditions, and gingival or periodontal problems is higher when comparing oral lesions.[5] Because of this, the dentist may often overlook oral lesions, although the lesions may not be so rare. Compounding the problem, dental patients may not complain to the dentist about their oral condition when there is no functional disturbance or pain or because of fear.

The clinical appearance of the oral lesion is very important in understanding the nature of the condition. The clinical description is the initial step in gathering examination details. The clinical presentation of various oral diseases may be similar, but the underlying cause of the diseases is different. The varied clinical presentations are white and red lesions, oral ulcerations, vesicle and blister, papillary, nodular, polypoid, macule, sessile, pedunculated, verrucous, erosion, or fissure. The descriptions of these terms are listed in **Table 1**. The dental surgeon should be familiar with these terms and apply them to clinical characters while describing the lesions and categorizing and formulating differential diagnosis.

Box 1
Common categories of oral diseases

1. Jaw and dental abnormalities
2. Precancerous lesions
3. Benign and malignant oral conditions
4. Salivary gland disorders
5. Jaw cysts
6. Odontogenic tumors
7. Mucocutaneous diseases
8. Neuralgic disorders

Table 1
Description of clinical terms used in oral diseases

Clinical Presentation	Description
White lesion	Lesion that appears as white patches
Red lesion	Lesion that appears as red patches
Oral ulceration	Lesion characterized by either loss of continuity of epithelium or total loss of surface epithelium
Blister	Superficial lesion characterized by clear fluid-filled swelling
Vesicle	Superficial blister with clear fluid-filled blister that is 5 or <5 mm in diameter
Bullae	Superficial blister with clear fluid-filled blister that is >5 mm in diameter
Pustule	Superficial blister filled with purulent exudate
Papillary	Growth of tumor or swelling showing numerous small fingerlike projections from the surface mucosa
Polypoid	Growth that resembles an intestinal polyp
Macule	Focal area of color change that is neither elevated nor depressed to adjacent mucosa
Papule	Raised solid lesion that is <5 mm in diameter
Nodular	Raised solid lesion that is >5 mm in diameter
Sessile	Base of the tumor or growth is the widest part of the lesion
Pedunculated	The base of the tumor or growth is narrow, and base appears similar to a stalk
Verrucous	Growth or tumor showing rough, irregular, and warty surface
Exophytic	Growth is characterized as protuberant or outward to the surface tissue
Endophytic	Growth is characterized as inward to the surface tissue
Erosion	Surface lesion is characterized by the partial or total loss of epithelium following rupture of blister (vesicle/bullae)
Fissure	Surface of the lesion that is either a narrow, slitlike ulceration or a groove
Petechia	Small, round, pinpoint-sized hemorrhage

The diagnosis of oral lesions requires critical and cognitive skills. The dentist needs to apply logical skills in a step-by-step approach to create a possible and closest clinical diagnosis. The approach for an oral condition is a step-by-step process; the first step is to recognize the symptom of the oral condition: swelling, ulcer, color change, surface or textural changes, functional alteration, tenderness, or pain. The next step is to identify whether the lesion is inflammatory, infected developing, benign, reactive, or of malignant origin. The dental surgeon should be knowledgeable on diagnostic, inclusion, and exclusion criteria of the common oral conditions under various categories.

An assumption of the best diagnosis without the appropriate diagnostic approach is dangerous because serious conditions could be ignored. Recently, a case report gave an account of a misdiagnosis of Bell palsy made in a patient who had an extensive acute embolic stroke secondary to infective endocarditis. Although this is a case from medical practice, it highlights the importance of thorough examination and history, the minimization of diagnostic errors, and early recognition of care.[6] Hence, it is important to organize the knowledge of oral diseases in a systematic manner, like a decision tree or a diagnostic algorithm, which places information in a step-by-step manner to arrive at a logical conclusion. Finkelstein and Hellstein[7] reported a guide to clinical differential diagnosis of oral mucosal lesions, which is a diagnostic algorithm that is very useful in structuring and in drawing a clinical decision through the clinical presentation. Similar to this report, other diagnostic decision trees were simulated for exophytic oral conditions (**Fig. 1**), oral erosions, and yellow oral lesions.[8–10] Having good background information on commonly encountered oral diseases will strengthen the diagnostic process. For the purpose of the general dentist, significant common laboratory tests and medication management (adult dose) of dental infections are presented in **Tables 2** and **3**.

Clinical Outline of Common Categories of Oral Diseases

Jaw and dental abnormalities
Abnormalities of the jaw bone and dental tissues are deformities of growth and development. Disturbances from the normal pattern of growth result in abnormal development of tissue and may predispose anatomic or functional variation. Disturbances of bone growth may lead to either increased or decreased jaw size, or even a lack of bone fusion, forming clefts. Disturbances in the teeth may lead to alteration of size, shape, number, or structure. These anatomic or functional variations of the teeth may cause disturbances in esthetics, occlusion, hygiene maintenance, or endodontic pathways, leading to diagnostic and operative challenges.[11–13]

Precancerous lesions
Precancerous lesions are the precursor of the pathologic condition of oral cancer. Recently, the term potentially malignant disorders (PMD) was given to precancerous lesions and conditions of the oral cavity.[14] PMD are the proportion of oral lesions that eventually become overtly malignant. The concept of oral precancer is derived from the following: (1) clinical alterations observed in precancer, that is, white and red patches, are seen to coexist at the margins of oral cancer (oral squamous cell carcinoma); (2) the proportion of PMD shares both morphologic and cytologic changes observed in oral cancer but without invasion of epithelium-connective tissue interface; (3) some of the alterations of chromosomes and genomic and molecular structures seen in oral cancer are also observed in PMD; (4) longitudinal studies stated that areas with PMD changes have shown malignant transformation during follow-up.[15,16] PMD of the oral cavity include leukoplakia, erythroplakia, palatal lesions in reverse smokers, oral submucus fibrosis, lichen planus, and discoid lupus erythematosus. Leukoplakia is the most common premalignant disorder observed in dental practice. PMDs are managed through habit cessation, surgical, or nonsurgical/medication management.[17]

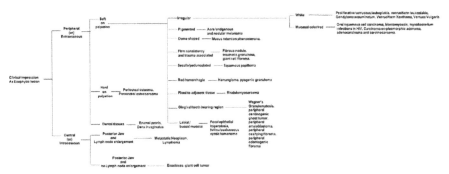

Fig. 1. Decision-making tree for oral exophytic lesions. (*From* Santosh AB, Boyd D, Laxminarayana KK. Proposed clinico-pathological classification for oral exophytic lesions. J Clin Diagn Res. 2015;9(9):ZE05; with permission.)

Table 2
Common clinical laboratory tests

Test	Normal Values	Function	Comment
HbA1c	Below 6%, that is, <42 mmol/mol	HbA1c refers to glycated hemoglobin, and the test measures average plasma glucose concentration	Prediabetes, 6%–6.4%, that is, 42–47 mmol/mol Diabetes, 6.5% or greater, that is, 48 mmol/mol or greater
International normalized ratio	Without anticoagulant therapy: 1	Measures extrinsic clotting function	With anticoagulant, therapeutic range: 2–3
Prothrombin time	12.7–15.4 s	Measures extrinsic clotting function	Prothrombin time is prolonged in liver disease and impaires vitamin K production
Hemoglobin	10.5–18 g/dL	Measures oxygen-carrying capacity of blood	Elevated in polycythemia vera and decreased in hemorrhage and anemia
Hematocrit	32%–52%	Measures relative volume of cells	Elevated in polycythemia and dehydration, levels are decreased in hemorrhage, anemia
Red blood cell	4–6 million/mm³	Measures oxygen-carrying capacity of blood	Elevated in polycythemia, heart disease, pulmonary disease, and reduced in hemorrhage and anemia
White blood cell	4000–11,000/mm³	Measures host defense against inflammation	Elevated in inflammation, trauma, toxicity, and leukemia Reduced in aplastic anemia, drug toxicity, and specific infections
Platelets	150,000–400,000/mL	Measures clotting potential	Elevated in polycythemia, leukemia, severe hemorrhage, and reduced in thrombocytopenia purpura

Benign and malignant tumors of oral cavity

A tumor is a swelling that is the result of a proliferation of underlying tissue. Benign and malignant conditions of the oral cavity usually present as swelling that can be easily detected in clinical examination. Benign tumors are characterized by slow-growing, circumscribed swelling, whereas malignant tumors are most likely to be fast growing and invade or infiltrate adjacent and deeper tissues like muscle, nerve, or connective

Table 3
Medication management (adult dosage) of common dental or oral diseases

Medication	Dosing	Type of Dental or Oral Diseases
Amoxicillin	500 mg, 3 times daily for 5–7 d	Useful against irreversible pulpitis, periapical abscess, apical periodontitis, localized and generalized aggressive periodontitis
Metronidazole	500 mg, 2 times daily for 10 d	May be useful in combination with amoxicillin or amoxicillin with clavulanate potassium (augmentin) against dental infection with abscess formation, gingival/periodontal abscess, or localized aggressive periodontitis
Clindamycin	150 mg, 3 times daily for 5 d or 300 mg, 2 times daily for 5 d	May be useful in combination with amoxicillin or amoxicillin with clavulanate potassium (augmentin) against dental infection with abscess formation, gingival/periodontal abscess, or localized aggressive periodontitis. Effective against periodontitis that is refractory to periodontitis
Azithromycin	500 mg, once daily for 4–7 d	Effective against odontogenic infections. Anaerobic/gram-negative bacilli infection. Odontogenic infections in the patient allergic to penicillin
Erythromycin	500 mg, 2 times daily for 10 d	Effective against odontogenic infections. Odontogenic infections in the patient allergic to penicillin
Cephalexin	250 mg, 4 times daily for 10 d	Drug of choice when penicillin is infective after 2 d
Ibuprofen	400 mg, 2 to 4 times daily for 3 to 5 d	Effective against mild to moderate dental pain
Acetaminophen	325 mg, 2 to 4 times daily for 3 to 5 d	Effective against mild to moderate dental pain
Diclofenac sodium	50 mg, 2 times daily for 3 to 5 d	Effective against mild to moderate dental pain
Diclofenac potassium	50 mg, 2 times daily for 3 to 5 d	Effective against mild to moderate dental pain
Nystatin ointment	30 g, apply to affected area 4 times daily	Denture-related candidiasis, angular cheilitis
Ketoconazole	200 mg, 1 tablet daily for 10 d	Oral candidiasis
Fluconazole	100 mg, 2 tablets initial dose, 1 tablet per day for 10 d	Oral candidiasis

tissue. Malignant lesions can cause ulcerations of overlying epithelium because of the excessive proliferation of neoplastic tissue. Benign and malignant tumors are classified into epithelial and connective tissues. Lymph node examination is a very important clinical marker in differentiating benign from malignant lesions. Palpable lymph nodes that are hard and fixed to the underlying structure usually represent an association of a malignant condition, whereas soft and movable, palpable lymph nodes represent a benign condition. Lymph node enlargement causes capsule stretching and may cause pain. Pain and tenderness of the lymph node is the result of an infection or underlying inflammation. Painful or painless lymph nodes cannot differentiate benign from malignant conditions.[18,19] Because of numerous lesions that are categorized under the entity of complex diagnosis, clinical judgment is highly essential when diagnosing these conditions. Knowledge of the clinical appearance, location, size, lymph node status, and habits of the patient will serve as an important factor in formulating clinical diagnosis.

Salivary gland disorders
Salivary gland disorders usually present with clinical swelling. The common causes of salivary gland swelling are a benign cause, or malignant neoplasm, cysts, salivary stones, and secondary to systemic diseases.[20] Tenderness and pain associated with salivary gland swelling are usually inflammatory. However, few malignant conditions of salivary gland disorders can produce painful swelling. Inflammatory salivary gland disorders are often more common than neoplastic conditions. Salivary gland conditions are more common in the submandibular, sublingual, and parotid regions. The complexity of diagnosis of salivary gland disorders increases with conditions such as xerostomia and excessive salivation, which are the result of multifactorial causes. Microscopy, cytology, imaging, and sialography methods are useful and reliable tools in the investigation of salivary gland diagnosis.[21]

Jaw cysts
Cysts are pathologic cavities that have fluid, semifluid, or gaseous content. Jaw cysts usually present with clinically visible swelling with normal-appearing overlying mucosa or sometimes a bony cavity that is detected on radiographic analysis. The jaw bone (maxilla and mandible) is reported to have a higher prevalence of cyst occurrence. Higher prevalence is probably due to the presence of epithelial remnants during development that may be triggered later in life. Based on the origin of tissue, cysts of the jaw are classified into odontogenic and nonodontogenic. Jaw cysts are predominantly intrabony; however, a few soft tissues are also noted.[22] Radiographic imaging methods play an important role in diagnosis. Radiographs help to interpret the cystic lesion in terms of (1) density of lesion, margin, locularity (unilocular/multilocular); (2) anatomic location, in relation to dentition; (3) cortical integrity, periosteal reaction, and soft tissue; and (4) effect on surrounding structures.[23] Challenges in radiographic interpretation are due to similar appearance; however, characters such as unilocular/multilocular, margin, location, density, proximity to tooth, presence or absence of calcification, and clinical data will help in achieving clinicoradiologic diagnosis. Microscopic examination of the lesional tissue is the only way to arrive at a definitive diagnosis. It is worth noting that few cysts have an aggressive potential and either recur or behave as a neoplasm.[24]

Odontogenic tumors
An odontogenic tumor is the specific term given to tumors of odontogenic tissue origin. Odontogenic tumors present as painless, slow, or rapidly growing swelling with or without lymph node changes. Odontogenic tumors are broadly classified

into benign, malignant, and hamartomatous lesions. Odontogenic tumors are usually derived from the tooth-forming apparatus.[25] Therefore, these tumors are exclusively observed in the jaw bone; however, a disseminated version of these tumors can be seen with malignant odontogenic conditions. Because of the occurrence of these tumors in the bone, the dentist possesses an advantage by viewing the changes in a radiograph. As with jaw cysts, radiographic examination of odontogenic tumors helps in the identification of density, location, size, relation to tooth and adjacent tissues, and cortical bone changes.[23] Although radiographs are very important and helpful in assisting diagnosis, it is worth reminding that the correlation of clinical, histologic, and radiographic interpretation will help in arriving at a definitive diagnosis.

Mucocutaneous diseases
Mucocutaneous diseases are mainly observed in dermatology practice, and symptoms of these conditions occur on the skin and the mucus membrane.[26] The mucus membrane component of mucocutaneous presentations can be observed on oral mucosal surfaces. The clinical manifestations of mucocutaneous diseases are usually fluid-filled blisters, that is, vesicle/bullae, erosions, or ulcerated areas. Oral mucosal manifestations may serve as an initial feature of disease, most important clinical sign or the only sign of such diseases. Muco-cutaneous conditions of autoimmune origin are usually benign in nature; however, late diagnosis may lead to a potentially fatal outcome.[27] Frequently encountered mucocutaneous conditions over the oral mucosa are pemphigus, pemphigoid, lichen planus, and lupus erythematosus.[28,29] A clinical correlation with microscopic and immunofluorescence investigations is helpful in arriving at a final diagnosis.[30]

Neuralgic disorders
Neuralgic disorders are diseases affecting the nerve that is characterized by the distribution of pain in the course of the nerve. Knowledge of neuralgia is very important for a general dentist not just for diagnosing underlying condition but also to differentiate from dental pain.[31,32] Comprehensive understanding of dental pain versus neuralgia is important because many patients may present their complaint of neuralgic pain as dental pain. The patient's thought on the relation of pain within the tooth region is probably owing to the site of pain, and scientifically, it is because of the proximity of the nerve to the tooth. Many reports have been published about extraction of teeth because of a misdiagnosis of trigeminal neuralgia with tooth pain. The most important and concerning neuralgias for the dentist are trigeminal neuralgia, glossopharyngeal neuralgia, cluster headache, and herpes zoster neuralgias. Trigeminal neuralgia is the most common type of neuralgia.[33,34] A complete understanding of the nature of dental and nondental pain is a very important tool in establishing a diagnosis, and for the referral of a patient at the right time for early and correct action.[35] Hence, diagnosis requires careful history taking and a thorough examination.

SUMMARY

High-quality clinical examination skills are the most important tool in arriving at a provisional clinical diagnosis. Knowledge and thorough understanding of clinical descriptive terms for various oral presentations will help to make the diagnosis much easier. The art of clinical examination skills can be improved by critical and logical thinking, utilization of the diagnostic algorithm, and strong theoretic knowledge. Although radiographic, microscopic, and/or advanced investigation will help in arriving at a final diagnosis, clinicopathologic correlation is a very important step in determining a final diagnosis. Thus, fusion of clinical examination skills with advanced technology can aid the dental surgeon in achieving diagnosis, but diagnosis cannot be achieved with just technology alone. The adage for this article is that "not all oral lesions require treatment but all oral lesions must be diagnosed."

REFERENCES

1. Ramirez-Amador VA, Esquivel-Pedraza L, Orozco-Topete R. Frequency of oral conditions in a dermatology clinic. Int J Dermatol 2000;39(7):501–5.
2. Rajendra Santosh AB, Ogle OE, Williams D, et al. Epidemiology of oral and maxillofacial infections. Dent Clin North Am 2017;61(2):217–33.
3. Oyedokun A, Adeloye D, Balogun O. Clinical history-taking and physical examination in medical practice in Africa: still relevant? Croat Med J 2016;57(6):605–7.
4. Eversole LR. Clinical outline of oral pathology. 4th edition. Connecticut: People's Medical Publishing House; 2011. p. 684.
5. Benjamin RM. Oral health: the silent epidemic. Public Health Rep 2010;125(2): 158–9.
6. Asif T, Mohiuddin A, Hasan B, et al. Importance of thorough physical examination: a lost art. Cureus 2017;9(5):e1212.
7. Michael W, Finkelstein EL, Hellstein JW. A guide to clinical differential diagnosis of oral mucosal lesions. 2017. Available at: Dentalcare.com. Accessed March 27, 2017.
8. Santosh ABR, Boyd D, Laxminarayana KK. Proposed clinico-pathological classification for oral exophytic lesions. J Clin Diagn Res 2015;9(9):ZE1–8.
9. Schafer DR, Glass SH. A guide to yellow oral mucosal entities: etiology and pathology. Head Neck Pathol 2019;13(1):33–46.
10. Benoit S, Hamm H. Differential diagnosis of oral mucosal erosions and ulcers in children. Hautarzt 2015;66(4):258–66 [in German].
11. Jälevik B, Szigyarto-Matei A, Robertson A. Difficulties in identifying developmental defects of the enamel: a BITA study. Eur Arch Paediatr Dent 2019. [Epub ahead of print].
12. Jafarzadeh H, Abbott PV. Dilaceration: review of an endodontic challenge. J Endod 2007;33(9):1025–30.
13. Bandaru B, Thankappan P, Kumar Nandan S, et al. The prevalence of developmental anomalies among school children in Southern district of Andhra Pradesh, India. J Oral Maxillofac Pathol 2019;23(1):160.
14. Warnakulasuriya S. Clinical features and presentation of oral potentially malignant disorders. Oral Surg Oral Med Oral Pathol Oral Radiol 2018;125(6):582–90.
15. Sarode SC, Sarode GS, Tupkari JV. Oral potentially malignant disorders: a proposal for terminology and definition with review of literature. J Oral Maxillofac Pathol 2014;18(Suppl 1):S77–80.
16. Warnakulasuriya S, Johnson NW, van der Waal I. Nomenclature and classification of potentially malignant disorders of the oral mucosa. J Oral Pathol Med 2007; 36(10):575–80.
17. Ogle OE, Santosh AB. Medication management of jaw lesions for dental patients. Dent Clin North Am 2016;60(2):483–95.
18. Ferrer R. Lymphadenopathy: differential diagnosis and evaluation. Am Fam Physician 1998;58(6):1313–20.
19. Fijten GH, Blijham GH. Unexplained lymphadenopathy in family practice. An evaluation of the probability of malignant causes and the effectiveness of physicians' workup. J Fam Pract 1988;27(4):373–6.

20. Mehanna H, McQueen A, Robinson M, et al. Salivary gland swellings. BMJ 2012; 345:e6794.
21. Rajendra Santosh A, Bakki S, Manthapuri S. A review of research on cytological approach in salivary gland masses. Indian J Dent Res 2018;29(1):93–106.
22. Imran A, Jayanthi P, Tanveer S, et al. Classification of odontogenic cysts and tumors–Antecedents. J Oral Maxillofac Pathol 2016;20(2):269–71.
23. Neyaz Z, Gadodia A, Gamanagatti S, et al. Radiographical approach to jaw lesions. Singapore Med J 2008;49(2):165–76 [quiz: 177].
24. Stoelinga PJW. The management of aggressive cysts of the jaws. J Maxillofac Oral Surg 2012;11(1):2–12.
25. Rajendra Santosh AB, Coard KCM, Williams EB, et al. Adenomatoid odontogenic tumor: clinical and radiological diagnostic challenges. J Pierre Fauchard Acad 2017;31(2–4):115–20.
26. Babu RA, Chandrashekar P, Kumar KK, et al. A study on oral mucosal lesions in 3500 patients with dermatological diseases in South India. Ann Med Health Sci Res 2014;4(Suppl 2):S84–93.
27. Koopaie M. A challenging in diagnosis of mucous membrane pemphigoid with desquamative gingivitis presentation: a case report. J Arch Mil Med 2018;6(1): e64548.
28. Rajendra Santosh AB, Reddy Baddam VR, Anuradha C, et al. Oral mucosal lesions in patients with pemphigus and pemphigoid skin diseases: a cross sectional study from southern India. Dentistry 3000 2017;5(1):7.
29. Chandra Sekhar P, Suvarna M, Arvind Babu RS, et al. Lupus erythematosus–a report of 3 cases. J Orofac Sci 2010;2(1):30–5.
30. Arvind Babu R, Chandrasekar P, Chandra K, et al. Immunofluorescence and its application in dermatopathology with oral manifestations: revisited. J Orofac Sci 2013;5(1):2–8.
31. Renton T. Dental (odontogenic) pain. Rev Pain 2011;5(1):2–7.
32. Cruccu G, Finnerup NB, Jensen TS, et al. Trigeminal neuralgia: new classification and diagnostic grading for practice and research. Neurology 2016;87(2):220–8.
33. Yadav YR, Nishtha Y, Sonjjay P, et al. Trigeminal neuralgia. Asian J Neurosurg 2017;12(4):585–97.
34. Burchiel KJ. A new classification for facial pain. Neurosurgery 2003;53(5):1164–6 [discussion: 1166–7].
35. Park H-O, Ha J-H, Jin M-U, et al. Diagnostic challenges of nonodontogenic toothache. Restor Dent Endod 2012;37(3):170–4.

Jaw and Dental Abnormalities

Tibebu M. Tsegga, DDS*, Cody J. Christensen, DDS

KEYWORDS

- Jaw abnormalities • Supernumerary teeth • Cleft lip and palate • Facial asymmetry

KEY POINTS

- Developmental disturbances in the maxillomandibular skeleton can produce aberrations in facial harmony and subsequent dental maldevelopment.
- Consideration for management relies on the prioritization of dysfunction, morbidity, and subjective psychosocial impact.
- Multidisciplinary care is often involved to correct the skeletal as well as dental aberrations.

INTRODUCTION

Observation of deviations from anthropometric norms related to facial skeletal development are a relatively normal occurrence in the dental management of the vast majority of patients. A consideration for correction is usually warranted only when there is associated morbidity, functional impairment, or psychosocial detriment. The vast majority of maxillomandibular and dental abnormalities are developmental and present themselves within a continuum of clinically conspicuous to overtly obvious. The main focus of this article was to highlight a variety of developmental abnormalities that present with structural disharmony of the maxillomandibular complex and secondarily associated dental structures. Case illustrations outline a general review focusing on identification/diagnosis, treatment dilemmas, and potential implication on the dental management of specified patients.

DISTURBANCES AFFECTING TEETH DEVELOPMENT
Cleidocranial Dysplasia

Cleidocranial dysplasia (CCD) is an autosomal dominant genetic disorder with variable expressivity that produces pathognomonic facial and physical features. The locus for CCD has been mapped to the RUNX2 gene located in chromosome 6p21, and any form of chromosomal translocations, deletions, insertions, and nonsense and

Disclosure Statement: The authors have nothing to disclose.
Oral and Maxillofacial Surgery Department, San Antonio Military Health System, 1100 Wilford Hall Loop, San Antonio, TX 78236, USA
* Corresponding author.
E-mail address: tibbs.tsegga@gmail.com

missense mutations can be present.[1,2] CCD is characterized by skeletal dysplasia in patent sutures, fontanels, and clavicles and results in wormian bone formation, shortened stature, supernumerary teeth, frontal bossing, and rudimentary or absent clavicles.[1,2,3] Other changes of the skull include absent or reduced frontal and paranasal sinuses, small or absent nasal bones, segmental calvarial thickening, underdeveloped maxilla, delayed union of the mandibular symphysis, and a small cranial base with reduced sagittal diameter and a large foramen magnum.[4] These skeletal changes result in characteristic facial and physical features that include a small, flat face with mandibular prognathism, hypertelorism, exorbitism, the ability of the patient to touch his or her shoulders together in the midline, a long neck with narrow, drooping shoulders, and a brachycephalic head with obvious frontal and parietal bossing. A metopic groove may be present in the midline of the forehead, and the scalp may have palpable soft areas due to open sutures.[4–5]

Oral examination will demonstrate over-retained primary teeth and absent permanent teeth, resulting in a malocclusion. The maxilla will be hypoplastic with a deep, narrow palate and the anteroposterior deficiency of the maxilla will create a pseudoprognathism.[5] Patients in the primary dentition stage will demonstrate normal eruption and formation of all 20 primary teeth on panoramic radiographs, whereas patients in the mixed and permanent dentition stage will demonstrate numerous unerupted and supernumerary teeth. The supernumerary teeth are morphologically similar to premolars even if they form in association with molars.[5] One hypothesis to explain the noneruption of permanent and supernumerary teeth is the lack of cellular cementum in the apical region of the impacted teeth.[6]

The classic triad of hypoplastic/missing clavicles, open fontanelles, and supernumerary teeth are diagnostic for CCD, and diagnosis is made by recognition of the components of this syndrome; however, the clinical presentation is variable. Treatment of CCD is aimed at correcting both the malocclusion and dentofacial deformity and requires a coordinated treatment plan with a restorative dentist, orthodontist, and oral surgeon. Treatment involves removing some, but not necessarily all supernumerary teeth. Supernumerary teeth that are associated with pathology or might interfere with orthodontic treatment are indicated for removal. Orthognathic surgery can be performed to correct the dentofacial deformity followed by orthodontic refinement to fine tune the final occlusion and implant placement to restore to a complete dentition.[5]

The case report shown in **Fig. 1** is of a 23-year-old man with a chief complaint of "I have multiple missing teeth and I have difficulty chewing." The patient had previously been diagnosed with CCD and had multiple unerupted teeth in the maxilla and mandible along with multiple supernumerary teeth. The proposed treatment plan was staged extraction of multiple supernumerary teeth in combination with autologous and allogeneic bone grafting. Because there is no associated metabolic impairment toward bone consolidation, once the bone graft has healed, the respective jaw bone can receive conventional dental implants with routine prosthetic rehabilitation.

Gardner Syndrome

Familial adenomatous polyposis (FAP) is a rare autosomal dominant form of intestinal polyposis and colorectal cancer caused by germ-line mutations in the adenomatous polyposis coli (APC) gene located on chromosome 5.[7] Gardner syndrome is a variant of FAP that is characterized by the triad of colonic polyposis, multiple osteomas, and mesenchymal tumors of the skin and soft tissue that was first described in 1951 by Eldon Gardner who reported the disease in a family from Utah.[7–9] Other findings in Gardner syndrome include dental abnormalities, such as supernumerary and

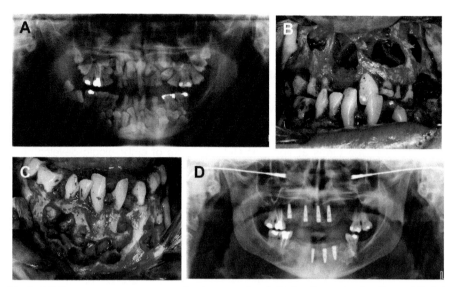

Fig. 1. (*A*) Numerous supernumerary teeth present on initial radiograph of patient with clei-docranial dysplasia. (*B*) Intraoperative picture of maxillae after removal of supernumerary teeth. (*C*) Intraoperative picture of mandible after removal of supernumerary teeth. Note the alveolar expansion and ensuing periodontal compromise of erupted teeth. (*D*) Postoperative imaging after bone graft consolidation and placement of endosseous implants.

impacted teeth, gastric and small intestine polyps, and congenital retinal pigmentation. Diagnosis is based on either genetic criteria or gastrointestinal endoscopy, and the presence of 100 or more colorectal adenomas or detection of a deleterious mutation in the APC gene provides a definitive diagnosis of Gardner syndrome.[10]

As dental practitioners it is important to note that the formation of osteomas and other oral signs typically precede the formation of other manifestations of this syndrome, including the formation of intestinal polyposis.[11] Osteomas are the hallmark extracolonic finding of Gardner syndrome, and will often be large, multilobulated masses found at the angle of the mandible and many will be confluent with adjacent osteomas. Radiographically, osteomas appear as round or oval radiopaque masses attached by a broad base.[5,12]

The presence of odontomas, supernumerary teeth, and impacted teeth occur 17% of the time.[5] Odontomas are benign odontogenic tumors associated with Gardner syndrome and they occur equally in the maxilla and mandible and are typically found in the incisor to premolar area. They are classified into 2 subcategories, complex or compound odontomas. Complex odontomas are unrecognizable as dental tissue, and appear as a mixed radiolucent-radiopaque lesion that cannot be diagnosed by radiographic appearance alone and requires histologic evaluation for definitive diagnosis. Compound odontomas, on the other hand, contain all 3 dental tissues and radiographically appear more organized so that the lesions contain many toothlike structures. These lesions often can be diagnosed from radiographic interpretation alone.

Gardner syndrome that is fully expressed will be easily distinguishable with clinical and radiographic data. Differential diagnosis for other conditions that may produce supernumerary teeth, odontomas, and radiodense masses include cleidocranial dysplasia, florid cemento-osseous dysplasia, and periapical cemento-osseous dysplasia. Turcot syndrome, Cowden syndrome, juvenile polyposis of the colon, and Peutz-Jeghers syndrome are all syndromes associated with intestinal polyposis.[5]

DISTURBANCES AFFECTING JAW AND TEETH DEVELOPMENT
Cleft Lip and Palate

Orofacial clefts are a group of developmental structural malformations that result in oral and facial deformities. Cleft lip and cleft palate are the main categories within this group and can occur in isolation, together, or in conjunction with syndromes. The primary palate forms at approximately 6 weeks of embryologic development when the median nasal prominence fuses with the lateral nasal prominences and maxillary prominences. The primary palate forms the base of the nose, nostrils, and upper lip, and when these components fail to fuse, a cleft of the lip and/or maxilla occurs.

At approximately 8 weeks of development, the palatal shelves elevate and fuse with the nasal septum to form the secondary palate. When one palatal shelf fails to fuse with the other components, a unilateral cleft of the secondary palate occurs. When both palatal shelves fail to fuse with each other and the nasal septum, a bilateral cleft of the secondary palate occurs. Clefts can be complete or incomplete depending on the degree of this failure of fusion. The etiology of clefts is thought to be multifactorial with genetics, maternal hypoxia, chemical exposure, teratogenic drugs, radiation, and nutritional deficiencies contributing to their development.[13]

Cleft lip with or without cleft palate is among the most common major congenital craniofacial malformations and occurs in approximately 1 in 700 live births.[14] The highest prevalence occurs in Native American individuals (3.6 per 1000 births) with lower prevalence among Asian (2.1 per 1000 births), White (1 per 1000 births), and African American (0.3 per 1000 births) individuals.[13,15] Unilateral cleft lips occur more commonly in male than female individuals and unilateral left-sided cleft lips are more common than unilateral right-sided cleft lips. In addition, unilateral cleft lips occur more frequently than bilateral cleft lips, and clefting of both the primary and secondary palates occurs more frequently when bilateral cleft lips are present.

Isolated cleft palate occurs in approximately 1 in 2000 live births with similar predilection across all racial ethnicities. Isolated cleft palate is more commonly seen in female individuals, which is the opposite of cleft lip and palate.[15] Most unilateral cleft lip and palate cases are isolated anomalies that are not associated with any syndromes or other major developmental abnormalities. In contrast, isolated cleft palate is often associated with syndromes such as Stickler, Van der Woude, Treacher Collins, and DiGeorge syndromes. Ocular abnormalities that can lead to severe myopia, glaucoma, and retinal detachment are associated with Stickler syndrome, thus patients with isolated cleft palates should be evaluated within the first year after birth by an experienced pediatric ophthalmologist.[13,16]

Ultrasound diagnosis of orofacial clefts is not feasible until approximately 15 weeks of gestation because of the position of the head and small size of the face.[17] Once an orofacial cleft has been diagnosed, the family receives a prenatal consultation to an experienced surgeon to explain the diagnosis and different stages of cleft lip and palate reconstruction that may be necessary. This important consultation helps prepare the family for practical considerations of the child, such as feeding, and gives them the opportunity to ask questions, calm fears, and learn about feeding techniques that will be important once the infant is born.[13,18]

Following birth, the family is referred to a cleft and craniofacial team for a thorough interdisciplinary approach to care. American Cleft Palate-Craniofacial

Association–approved teams are required to have a surgeon, orthodontist, speech-language pathologist, and a patient care coordinator. In addition, these teams must have access to an audiologist, geneticist, otolaryngologist, pediatrician, pediatric dentist or dental specialist, psychologist, and social worker. These teams foster a cohesive environment in which families can get the best information available to consider treatment decisions using an interdisciplinary care model that is patient and family oriented.[13]

Cleft lip and nasal repair is the first surgical step in reconstructing a cleft. The goals of initial repair include creation of an intact upper lip with appropriate vertical length and symmetry, repair of the underlying muscular structures producing normal function, and primary treatment of the associated nasal deformity.[19] Cleft palate repair usually occurs between 9 and 18 months of age, and the timing of repair is predicated on growth restriction following early surgery and speech development that requires an intact palate. If the cleft palate is repaired too soon, maxillary hypoplasia can occur later in life. The 2 main goals of cleft palate repair are watertight closure of the oronasal communication involving the hard and soft palates and the anatomic repair of the musculature within the soft palate that is critical for normal creation of speech.[13] Following repair of cleft palate, approximately 20% of patients will develop velopharyngeal insufficiency (VPI), which can produce hyper nasal speech. Diagnosis of VPI occurs between 3 and 5 years of age after a thorough examination by a speech pathologist who is familiar with clefts.[13]

Osseous reconstruction of the maxilla and alveolus can been performed during 3 different stages of development that are based off of the development of the dentition and not necessarily chronologic age. Primary reconstruction refers to osseous reconstruction during the deciduous dentition phase, secondary reconstruction occurs during the mixed dentition phase before eruption of the permanent canines, and tertiary reconstruction occurs during the permanent dentition stage. Timing of osseous reconstruction has been extensively studied in the literature and secondary repair of clefts has significant advantages over primary and tertiary repair and is currently considered the standard of care.[20]

The dental practitioner will most likely be involved in the care of the pediatric patient with cleft lip and palate during the mixed dentition phase (secondary reconstruction) in which these patients are leading up to the surgery that establishes bony continuity of the cleft within the maxillary alveolus. This age is usually between 8 and 11 years old and depends primarily on the prevailing philosophy within the regional craniofacial team. As a dental practitioner, the recognition of the mixed dentition phase, locality, and eruptive progression of the permanent canine and identification of missing permanent teeth would provide helpful guidance to the patient and the parents as they prepare mentally for the "next" surgery (**Fig. 2**).

In addition, and most importantly, one of the most significant measures toward alveolar grafting surgical success is preemptively addressing obstacles toward clinically acceptable oral hygiene and eliminating parafunctional or digit habits. An interesting nuance is that the cleft site provides an attractive region for tongue habits, and in some children an area for subconscious digit manipulation. In the primary author's experience, this has been one of the greatest contributors toward postoperative wound dehiscence and partial loss of the bone graft. Whether or not the general practitioner is active within a craniofacial team, paying attention to these details will pay dividends toward the optimization of these patients for treatment success.

Treating these patients is complex by nature and by systematically and methodically staging treatment to coincide with facial growth patterns, visceral function, and psychosocial needs brings clarity to each phase of treatment for both the clinician

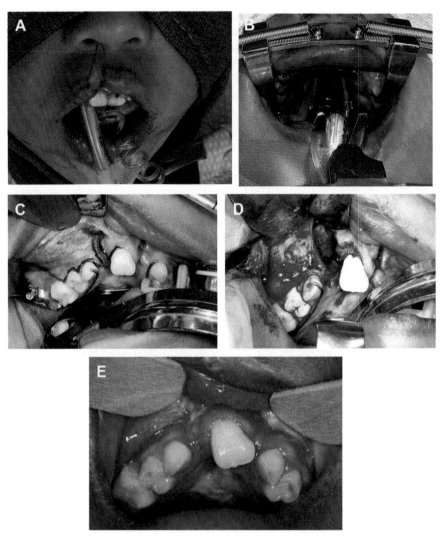

Fig. 2. (*A*) Primary noncomplete cleft lip. (*B*) Complete cleft palate. (*C*) Bilateral alveolar cleft with small primary segment retaining 1 adult incisor. (*D*) Surgical access to obtain bony continuity of alveolar cleft. (*E*) Continuity of maxillae after repair of bilateral alveolar cleft.

and family. Future management will likely be influenced by advances in genetic testing and tissue engineering. Meanwhile, continuing to evaluate and treat these patients using logical rationale for the timing, methods, and extent of surgical intervention and then objectively evaluating functional, morphologic (aesthetic), and psychosocial outcomes, the outlook for patients affected by this malformation will continue to improve.

Disturbances Leading to Jaw Asymmetry

The etiology of conditions that manifest as facial asymmetry are generally from 3 broad categories: developmental, neoplastic, or inflammatory. Oftentimes a detailed history of present illness, past medical history, focused head and neck examination, and cursory radiographic imaging will help to refine the list of possibilities to 1 of the 3 broad categories. For the focus of this article, we illustrate 3 developmental causes of facial asymmetry: hemifacial hyperplasia, fibrous dysplasia, and hemimandibular hyperplasia/elongation.

Hemifacial Hyperplasia

Hemifacial hyperplasia (HFH) was initially described by Merckel in 1882 and Wagner in 1839 as a sporadic congenital condition. The classic presentation is a unilateral overgrowth of the orofacial soft tissues, bone, and teeth. The right side of the face is affected more than the left side. HFH is more common in men than in women and in Caucasians compared with other racial groups.[21,22] Exact etiology of HFH is undetermined, but various theories have been postulated. Most of them fall in the category of developmental and/or metabolic and include endocrine imbalance, neural abnormalities, asymmetrical cell division and division of the twinning process, chromosomal abnormalities, alterations of intrauterine development, and vascular or lymphatic abnormalities.[23]

The following example (**Fig. 3**) is a 13-year-old patient with an unremarkable medical history and age-appropriate cognitive development. The parents attested to an uncomplicated pregnancy and birth. His primary complaint was with regard to the exaggerated facial asymmetry, malocclusion, and the concomitant psychosocial stigmata that has impacted his peer socialization. The medical-grade computed tomography

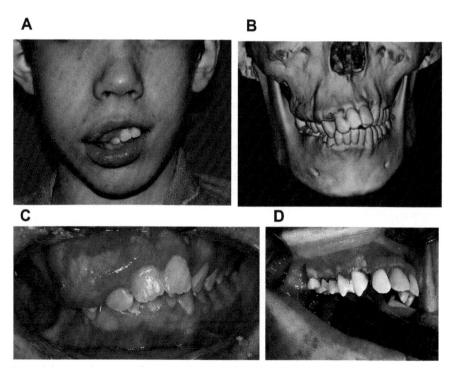

Fig. 3. (*A*) Frontal picture of patient with hemifacial hyperplasia, noted unilateral midfacial enlargement. (*B*) Skeletal view of patient. (*C*) Clinical view with pronounced alveolar enlargement, skeletal disharmony, and clinical crown submergence. (*D*) Surgical exposure of normal-appearing clinical crowns.

reconstruction demonstrates a volumetric segmental enlargement of the right maxillary bone, including the zygomatic buttress and the ipsilateral mandibular ramal/body unit. Further analysis of the radiograph demonstrates a contiguous cortical boundary with seemingly normal-appearing marrow content, which is usually altered in the setting of a neoplasm or bone-involving inflammatory process. The overlying skin was normal in thickness with no surface alteration. The ipsilateral ear has excessive conchal bowl cartilage giving it a more procumbent appearance. Intraorally, there was pronounced gingival coverage, which was overlying an exuberant amount of bone development coronal to the cemento-enamel junction of the respective teeth. This was within the confines of an expanded alveolus that was supra-erupted leading to a maxillary cant and concomitant transverse arch discrepancy in relationship to the mandible.

These particular clinical and radiographic findings are consistent with much of the reported case reports describing this entity.[24] Asymmetry in HFH is usually obvious at birth and accentuated at the end of adolescence. Uniquely, although the pseudo-submerged nature of the teeth are reminiscent of medication-induced gingival hypertrophy, this condition does not typically have exaggerated periodontal probing depths. Usually, there is a disharmony in chewing mechanics and jaw relationship, but the respective teeth can be maintained in good condition with diligent oral hygiene. Eventually, to achieve corrective jaw surgery, access to the respective teeth needs to occur with aggressive osseous recontouring and gingivectomy.

The dental management concerns include primarily an exclusion of other bone pathology, assessment of acquired and sometimes progressive malocclusion, and inadequate access to clinical crowns for hygiene or restorative care. Despite the concern for ongoing skeletal pathology, this presentation should not preclude these patients from being managed like any other routine nondysmorphic patient. Once a biopsy sample has confirmed normal bone architecture, and an underlying metabolic bone process has been excluded, these children can commence with routine care with a general practitioner. The exuberant hard and soft periodontal tissues causing a pseudo-impaction of the clinical crowns in the region of the HFH can be surgically excised without concern for recurrence. Oftentimes these patients are considered for corrective jaw surgery before standard skeletal maturity because of the overriding motivation of alleviating the stigmata associated with their facial dysmorphology. In addition, it is the author's impression that acquired developmental aberration of the craniofacial skeleton does not follow the standard maturation timeframe and using such criterion to pursue surgical correction is not overly useful.

Fibrous Dysplasia

Having a similar clinical presentation as HFH is craniofacial fibrous dysplasia (FD). Unlike HFH, craniofacial or monostotic FD is not only a cause for maxillomandibular asymmetry, but more importantly a gene mutation that affects both bone formation and resorption. Most isolated forms of FD are discovered incidentally on dental radiographic examination in the second decade of life.[25] The focus of this discussion is the singular variant known as monostotic craniofacial FD. Histologically it will not resemble normal bone architecture, but instead demonstrate an abnormal proliferation of immature, irregularly distributed fibro-osseous connective tissue.[26]

Because the etiology is categorically a genetic mutation, the timing of the mutation in relationship to the development of the fetus in utero seems to have a correlation with the degree of physical and organ-related aberrations that can be manifest with this pathologic process. For the dental practitioner, it is prudent to appreciate the diagnosis as being multifactorial and including some combination of clinical presentation, imaging, histologic description, biochemical data, and constitutional symptoms.[27] The most common maxillomandibular presentation is pronounced ipsilateral midfacial enlargement (**Fig. 4**A). The most common location of monostotic disease is the zygomatic-maxillary complex.[27] Oftentimes the imaging will be some ratio of a mixed radiopaque and radiolucent obliteration of affected craniofacial bones with volumetric enlargement compared with the contralateral unaffected side. FD has a tendency to undergo rapid progression during adolescent spectrum pubertal development. The dental practitioner's role in being aware of the subjective and objective changes can assist the patient in obtaining the necessary, and at times organ-saving, therapy. Progressive enlargement in proximity to the alveolus can manifest as alteration in chewing and speaking. The most reported dental anomaly in FD has been malocclusion and dental crowding or spacing (**Fig. 4**). This is secondary to the alveolar bone expanding at a rapid rate, causing improper positioning of the dentition.[28] Further mass effect near the paranasal region can at times cause nasal obstruction and at times challenge opening of the eyelid. After peak peripubertal enlargement or because of patient desires, systematic osseous recontouring can be used to establish facial symmetry. Similar to HFH, orthognathic surgery can be predictably used with good long-term stability.

Hemimandibular Hyperplasia

Asymmetric mandibular growth excess anomalies known as hemimandibular hyperplasia and hemimandibular elongation are specific patterns of dentofacial deformity

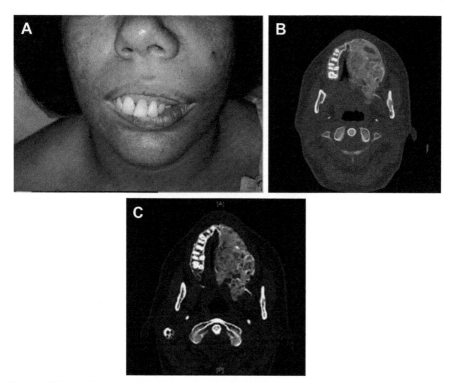

Fig. 4. (*A*) Frontal picture of patient with FD. (*B*) Axial slice computed tomography demonstrating the maxillary developmental abnormality and unilateral asymmetric enlargement. (*C*) After surgical recontouring, a more symmetric arch contour is reestablished in the maxilla.

that occur after birth. These conditions primarily affect the mandible; however, they also have a secondary effect on the morphology of the maxilla, nose, chin, position of the teeth, and overlying soft tissue drape.[29] The etiology is unknown, but there is a consensus that the growth of the affected condyle/mandible may be accelerated or prolonged after the end of general skeletal growth. Additional factors, such as hormonal influences, hypervascularity, trauma, infection, and genetics, also may play an undetermined role.[30]

Hemimandibular hyperplasia is a well-defined, asymmetric mandibular malformation that is characterized by 3-dimensional enlargement of the mandibular condyle, condylar neck, ramus, and body of one-half of the mandible that abruptly terminates at the symphysis. Clinically, patients will present with ipsilateral mandibular enlargement and asymmetry of the inferior border of the mandible without significant shifting of the chin or mandibular dental midline. Radiographically, a double contour is noticeable on a lateral cephalogram and an orthopantomogram reveals an increase in size of the mandibular body and ramus with a normal or acute gonial angle along with an increased distance from the apices of the teeth to the inferior border of the mandible.[31] This anomalous growth of the mandible typically occurs before or during puberty, which results in maxillary growth following the downward growth of the affected mandible. This results in the occlusal plane being tilted with varying types and degrees of malocclusion with a tendency toward a class III malocclusion and/or cross-bite on the affected side.[32,33]

Hemimandibular elongation differs from hemimandibular hyperplasia in that it results in excessive growth on one side of the mandible without an overall 3-dimensional increase in size of the affected mandible.[29] Clinically the chin and mandibular dental midline will deviate toward the unaffected side, a contralateral posterior cross-bite will be present and a class III molar relationship will be present on the ipsilateral side. Radiographically, hemimandibular elongation will demonstrate flattening of the gonial angle on the affected side but the mandibular body remains on the same level on both sides so no double contour is present on a lateral cephalogram. On orthopantomogram, hemimandibular elongation will not have an increased distance from the apices of the tooth roots to the inferior border of the mandible.[31]

The dental practitioner's role in identification of asymmetric overgrowth and monitoring of ongoing progression can assist in timing for corrective jaw surgery. Monitoring can simply be done by constructing a semirigid splint using either acrylic or a dense polyvinyl siloxane. The splint should capture the interdigitation of the upper and lower jaw in habitual occlusion at a defined temporal starting point. On subsequent dental visits, this baseline reference point can be used to provide an objective analysis of ongoing unilateral growth of the mandible. This rudimentary and simple tool can be valuable as an instructive guide for patients to understand the criterion for pursuing corrective jaw surgery. More enhanced imaging to quantify the enhanced metabolic (anabolic) activity of one condylar growth center over the other can be achieved with the application of PET (**Fig. 5**). This modality is quite expensive, requires radiopharmaceutical tracers, and is impractical to serially repeat for consecutive comparisons. Once cessation overgrowth is confirmed, then conventional corrective jaw surgery options can be considered. Final treatment usually includes orthognathic surgery and recontouring of the inferior border of the mandible. Oftentimes a segmental LeFort osteotomy must be performed to correct the cant and arch form of the maxilla.[33]

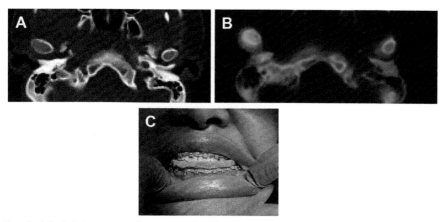

Fig. 5. (*A*) Axial computed tomography demonstrating unilateral enlargement of the temporomandibular joint in patient with hemimandibular (condylar) hyperplasia. (*B*) Corresponding hyperactive metabolic activity demonstrated as gradient of color intensity on nuclear medicine–enhanced imaging. (*C*) Clinical use of semirigid bite registration as baseline marker for evaluating ongoing asymmetric jaw growth.

SUMMARY

A general overview of acquired or developmental processes that afflict development of the craniofacial skeleton and primarily the maxillo-mandibular apparatus is inherent to being a comprehensive dental practitioner. Dental professionals have a vital role in observation, identification, and proper introductory education for patients who might be confronted with these ailments. Although some of the aforementioned developmental disturbances can be quite complex, a general understanding of how they divert the normal development of the jaw or related tooth structures will help to properly alleviate unnecessary patient fears and gently introduce a therapeutic plan that can be daunting and prolonged.

REFERENCES

1. Suda N, Hattori M, Kosaki K, et al. Correlation between genotype and supernumerary tooth formation in cleidocranial dysplasia. Orthod Craniofac Res 2010; 13:197–202.
2. Otto F, Kanegane H, Mundlos S. Mutations in the RUNX2 gene in patients with cleidocranial dysplasia. Hum Mutat 2002;19:209–16.
3. Suda N, Hamada T, Hattori M, et al. Diversity of supernumerary tooth formation in siblings with cleidocranial dysplasia having identical mutation in RUNX2: possible involvement of non-genetic or epigenetic regulation. Orthod Craniofac Res 2007;10:222–5.
4. Mundlos S. Cleidocranial dysplasia: clinical and molecular genetics. J Med Genet 1999;36:177–82.
5. Marx RE, Stern D. Oral and maxillofacial pathology: a rationale for diagnosis and treatment. Chicago: Quintessence Publishing Co; 2012.
6. Park T, Vargervik K, Oberoi S. Orthodontic and surgical management of cleidocranial dysplasia. Korean J Orthod 2013;43(5):248–60.
7. Gomez Garcia E, Knoers N. Gardner's syndrome (familial adenomatous polyposis): a cilia-related disorder. Lancet Oncol 2009;10:727–35.

8. Fotiadis C, Tsekouras DK, Antonakis P, et al. Gardner's syndrome: a case report and review of the literature. World J Gastroenterol 2005;11(34): 5408–11.

9. Gardner E, Stephens FE. Cancer of the lower digestive tract in one family group. Am J Hum Genet 1950;2:41–8.

10. Wijn MA, Keller JJ, Giardiello FM, et al. Oral and maxillofacial manifestations of familial adenomatous polyposis. Oral Diseases 2007;13:360–5.

11. Cahuana A, Palma C, Parri FJ. Oral manifestations of Gardner's syndrome in young patients: report of three cases. Eur J Paediatr Dent 2005;6(Suppl. 3):23–7.

12. Oner AY, Pocan S. Gardner's syndrome: a case report. Br Dent J 2006;200(12): 666–7.

13. Miloro M, Peterson LJ. Peterson's principles of oral and maxillofacial surgery. Shelton (CT): People's Medical Pub. House-USA; 2012.

14. Tolarova M, Cervenka J. Classification and birth prevalence of orofacial clefts. Am J Med Genet 1998;75:126–37.

15. Wyszynski DF, Beaty TH, Maestri NE. Genetics of non-syndromic and syndromic oral clefts revisted. Cleft Palate Craniofac J 1996;33:1640617.

16. Jones MC. Etiology of facial clefts: prospective evaluation of 428 patients. Cleft Palate J 1988;25:16–20.

17. Johnson N, Sandy J. Prenatal diagnosis of cleft lip and palate. Cleft Palate Craniofac J 2003;40(2):186–9.

18. Nahai F, Williams J, Burstein F, et al. The management of cleft lip and palate: pathways for treatment and longitudinal assessment. Semin Plast Surg 2005;19(4): 275–85.

19. Campbell A, Costello B, Ruiz R. Cleft lip and palate surgery: an update of clinical outcomes for primary repair. Oral Maxillofacial Surg Clin N Am 2010;22: 43–58.

20. Fahradyan A, Tsuha M, Wolfswinkel EM, et al. Optimal time of secondary alveolar bone grafting: a literature review. J Oral Maxillofac Surg 2019;77(4):843–9.

21. Pollock RA, Newman MH, Burdi AR, et al. Congenital hemifacial hyperplasia: an embryologic hypothesis and case report. Cleft Palate J 1985;22:173–84.

22. Islam MN, Bhattacharyya I, Ojha J, et al. Comparison between true and partial hemifacial hypertrophy. Oral Surg Oral Med Oral Pathol Oral Radiol Endod 2007;104:501–9.

23. Lee S, Sze R, Murakami C, et al. Hemifacial myohyperplasia: description of a new syndrome. Am J Med Genet 2001;103:326–33.

24. Miranda RT, Barros LM, Santos LA, et al. Clinical and imaging features in a patient with hemifacial hyperplasia. J Oral Sci 2010;52(No.3):509–12.

25. Grabias SL, Cambell CJ. Fibrous dysplasia. Orthop Clin North Am 1977;8:771.

26. Couturier A, Aumaître O, Gilain L, et al. Craniofacial fibrous dysplasia: a 10-case series. Eur Ann Otorhinolaryngol Head Neck Dis 2017;134:229–35.

27. Valentini V, Cassoni A, Marianetti TM, et al. Craniomaxillofacial fibrous dysplasia: conservative treatment or radical surgery? A retrospective study on 68 patients. Plast Reconstr Surg 2009;123:653–60.

28. Burke A, Collins MT, Boyce AM. Fibrous dysplasia of bone: craniofacial and dental implications. Oral Dis 2017;23(6):697–708.

29. Posnick JC. Orthognathic surgery: principles & practice. St Louis (MO): Elsevier Saunders; 2014.

30. Lippold C, Kruse-Losler B, Danesh G, et al. Treatment of hemimandibular hyperplasia: the biological basis of condylectomy. Br J Oral Maxillofac Surg 2007;45:353–60.

31. Deleurant Y, Zimmermann A, Peltomäki T. Hemimandibular elongation: treatment and long-term follow-up. Orthod Craniofac Res 2008;11:172–9.
32. Martchetti C, Cocchi R, Gentile L, et al. Hemimandibular hyperplasia: treatment strategies. J Craniofac Surg 2000;11:46–53.
33. Xu M, Chan FC, Jin X, et al. Hemimandibular hyperplasia: classification and treatment algorithm revisited. J Craniofac Surg 2014;25:355–8.

Oral Potentially Malignant Disorders

Stephanie L. Wetzel, DDS[a],*,[1], Jessica Wollenberg, DMD[b],[1]

KEYWORDS

- Premalignant • Leukoplakia • Erythroplakia • Risk factors • Epithelial dysplasia

KEY POINTS

- Oral potentially malignant disorders are epithelial lesions that may present clinically as white (leukoplakia), red (erythroplakia), or red and white (erythroleukoplakia) patches.
- There are many factors that increase patients' risk for developing a potentially malignant lesion.
- A biopsy of the lesion is the gold standard to differentiate between a potentially malignant lesion and other entities, and to diagnosis and grade epithelial dysplasia.
- After the diagnosis of a premalignant lesion is made, many patient-related and lesion-related factors influence the type and extent of treatment of the lesion.

INTRODUCTION

Oral potentially malignant disorder (OPMD) is defined as an epithelial lesion or disorder that has an increased risk for malignant transformation. The diagnosis of OMPD begins with a clinical examination, and, when present, it is most commonly described as a white lesion (leukoplakia) or less often as a red lesion (erythroplakia). These diagnoses are only clinical, and a definitive diagnosis must be determined through biopsy and histopathologic examination. Once the diagnosis of an OPMD is made, the patient's risk factors must be evaluated to determine the risk for malignant transformation and appropriate treatment. This article reviews the clinical presentation of OMPDs, including leukoplakia and erythroplakia; the risk factors, including tobacco, alcohol, actinic damage, and human papilloma virus (HPV); the necessary microscopic features to make the diagnosis; and the treatment and management of these lesions.

LEUKOPLAKIA

Oral leukoplakia is the most frequently seen potentially malignant disorder in the oral cavity. Leukoplakias were first reported in the literature in 1877, when the

Disclosure: The authors have nothing to disclose.
[a] Atlanta Oral Pathology, 2701 North Decatur Road, Decatur, GA 30022, USA; [b] Randolph Oral Pathology Associates, 447 Route 10, Suite 5, Randolph, NJ 07869, USA
[1] Co-first author.
* Corresponding author.
E-mail address: wetzeldds@gmail.com

Dent Clin N Am 64 (2020) 25–37
https://doi.org/10.1016/j.cden.2019.08.004
0011-8532/20/© 2019 Elsevier Inc. All rights reserved.

term was applied to any white lesion occurring in the oral cavity.[1] Leukoplakias are now defined as white, irreversible, and nonscrapable plaques that carry a questionable risk to transform into cancer.[1,2] More specifically, these lesions cannot be associated with any chemical, physical, or infectious causative agents except for tobacco, alcohol, or betel quid. In the general population the overall prevalence is approximately 2%, with increasing prevalence for older populations.[2] Leukoplakia has a male predilection and is usually seen in the fifth to sixth decades of life. One prospective study on leukoplakia found the incidence rates to be 1.1 to 2.4 per 1000 patients per year for men and 0.2 to 1.3 per 1000 patients per year for women.[1]

Clinically, leukoplakias can be classified according to their surface and morphologic features. Leukoplakias can be homogeneous in appearance and have a smooth, white, flat surface, with well-demarcated borders (**Figs. 1** and **2**). Nonhomogeneous leukoplakia is classified into 3 clinical categories:

1. Speckled leukoplakia
2. Nodular leukoplakia
3. Verrucous leukoplakia

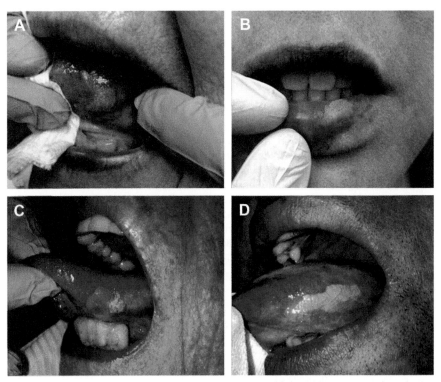

Fig. 1. (*A*) Granular leukoplakia featured on the left lateral border and ventral surface of the tongue. This lesion was diagnosed via biopsy as mild epithelial dysplasia. (*B*) Flat leukoplakia of the lower lip in a 50-year-old woman. Tissue biopsy showed features of actinic cheilitis. (*C*) Flat and verrucous leukoplakia of the ventral and lateral border of the tongue in an 85-year-old woman. (*D*) Corrugated leukoplakia of the left lateral border of the tongue in a 30-year-old man showing features of mild epithelial dysplasia.

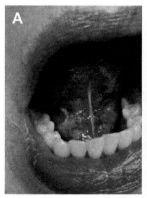 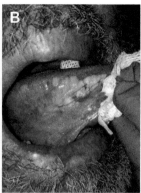 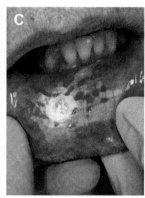

Fig. 2. (A) Leukoplakia with irregular borders of the floor of the mouth in a 48-year-old woman. The lesion showed features of moderate dysplasia. (B) Flat leukoplakia of the right ventral and lateral surfaces of the tongue in a 63-year-old man diagnosed via tissue biopsy as moderate epithelial dysplasia. (C) Flat and verrucous leukoplakia of the lower labial mucosa in a 71-year-old woman diagnosed as severe epithelial dysplasia.

Speckled leukoplakia is defined as a predominately leukoplakic lesion with areas of erythema appearing as small, dotlike spots, or larger, irregular patches. Speckled leukoplakia is now termed erythroleukoplakia and is discussed in more detail later. Nodular leukoplakia presents as an exophytic polypoid structure that is rounded and composed of both erythematous and leukoplakic surfaces. Verrucous leukoplakia has an elevated, proliferative, wrinkled, or corrugated surface[3] Most importantly, nonhomogeneous leukoplakia presents a higher risk for malignant transformation than homogeneous leukoplakia. There is an overall malignant transformation rate of 1.5% to 34% for oral leukoplakic lesions. This rate can be further broken down to a transformation rate of 3% for homogeneous lesions and 13.4% to 14.5% for nonhomogeneous lesions. Furthermore, 1 study showed that verrucous leukoplakia has a transformation rate of 4.6%, with erosive lesions having a 28% risk of malignant transformation.[2]

Leukoplakic lesions can occur at any site in the oral cavity. The most common sites include the lateral border of the tongue and the floor of the mouth, followed by buccal mucosa, hard and soft palate, and gingival/alveolar mucosa. Oral leukoplakia may be localized to 1 site or present as diffuse and widespread oral mucosal disease.

Proliferative verrucous leukoplakia (PVL) is a rare but high-risk form of leukoplakia. PVL most commonly presents in women more than 60 years of age who lack a clinical history of tobacco or alcohol use. An ethnic predilection is not seen. A strong female predilection of 4:1 has been reported with PVL. Initially, lesions of PVL present as asymptomatic, small, well-defined white patches or plaques with or without surface thickening. As the disease progresses, the lesions slowly enlarge and involve diffuse surfaces along multiple sites of the oral mucosa. Lesions of PVL evolve from flat patches to become increasingly exophytic and verrucous (**Figs. 3** and **4**).[4,5] PVL may involve multiple sites of the oral cavity, including the gingiva, alveolar mucosa, tongue, palate, and buccal mucosa. The gingiva is the most commonly affected area. Furthermore, gingival and palatal lesions are the most commonly affected sites to undergo malignant transformation. The reported malignant transformation rate for lesions of PVL is 63.3% to 100%.[2] Even with ablative treatment, PVL has a recurrence rate of up to 85%.[6] Therefore, close surveillance of patients with PVL is of the utmost

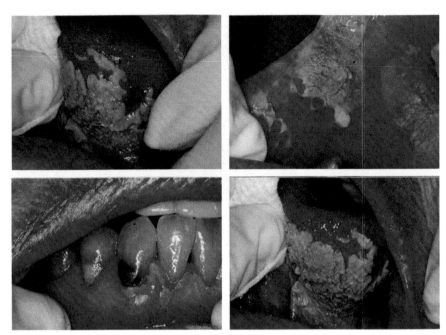

Fig. 3. PVL in an 83-year-old woman. The gingival lesion showed features of mild epithelial dysplasia. (*Courtesy of* Donna Thomas Moses, DMD, Carrollton, GA).

importance. Because of the serious nature of PVL, making the correct diagnosis is critical for the health of the patient. Criteria for the diagnosis of PVL include:

1. Existence of a verrucous area
2. Involvement of more than 2 sites
3. Lesions that have increased in size and spread to other sites during the development of the disease over at least 5 years
4. Recurrence in a previously treated area
5. Representative biopsy samples of lesional tissue have been microscopically examined, and the presence of an invasive squamous cell carcinoma has been ruled out[2,3]

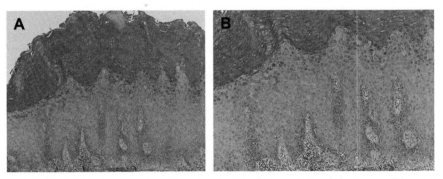

Fig. 4. (*A*) PVL featuring verrucous hyperkeratosis and hyperplasia of the basal cell layer. Lichenoid inflammation is also identified (hematoxylin-eosin, original magnification ×10). (*B*) PVL with chevron keratinization and orthokeratinization with a prominent granular cell layer (hematoxylin-eosin, original magnification ×40).

Despite these criteria, all lesions of PVL do not have a verrucous surface. A more inclusive term for this condition, proliferative multifocal leukoplakia, has been suggested.[3]

The differential diagnosis for leukoplakic lesions can be separated into the broad categories of congenital, infectious, inflammatory, and mucosal injury. Common congenital white lesions include leukoedema, which disappears after stretching of the mucosa, and white sponge nevus (also known as Cannon disease or familial white folded dysplasia), which typically affects the buccal mucosa bilaterally. White lesions of infectious cause include pseudomembranous candidiasis and oral hairy leukoplakia. However, pseudomembranous candidiasis presents as a white membrane that can be physically wiped away leaving a raw erythematous mucosal base. Oral hairy leukoplakia occurs as a secondary manifestation in patients with compromised immune systems and infected with the Epstein Barr virus and is also known as human herpesvirus 4. Leukoplakic lesions of inflammatory cause present with a lichenoid appearance and include lichen planus, lichenoid mucositis as a result of medication side effects and contact hypersensitivities, oral lesions of systemic lupus erythematosus, and graft-versus-host disease in patients with a history of bone marrow transplant. A detailed clinical history aids in differentiation of inflammatory lesions from true leukoplakia. Chemical and thermal mucosal burns, morsicatio, linea alba, and frictional keratoses all present as white areas as a result of mucosal injury. The diagnosis of a mucosal injury can be reached by determining the location of the injury and detailed questioning of the patient.[6]

ERYTHROPLAKIA

Erythroplakia is defined as a potentially malignant disorder of the oral cavity that presents as a red patch of the oral mucosa that cannot be diagnosed as any other definable lesion. The lesion cannot have traumatic, vascular, or inflammatory causes. Erythroplakia occurs in middle-aged and elderly patients, most commonly in the sixth and seventh decades of life. It occurs with equal frequency in both genders. Erythroplakia has a prevalence range from 0.02% to 0.83%, with a mean prevalence of 0.11% in the general population.[7,8] Although erythroplakia is rare, it has a much higher rate of malignant transformation than other premalignant conditions, such as leukoplakia and submucous fibrosis. The reported transformation rates range from 14% to 50%,[8] 4 times greater than the malignant transformation rates of leukoplakic lesions.[9] Systematic reviews have shown a range of 1.3% to 34% of malignant transformation in erythroplakic lesions in the global population.[5]

Clinically, erythroplakia presents as an erythematous mucosal lesion that is often smooth in appearance (**Fig. 5**). Erosive, granular, or nodular changes can be seen in long-standing lesions.[7] Rarely, lesions can be depressed below the mucosal surface, alluding to their atrophic nature. Typically, these lesions are asymptomatic. Visually, a well-defined margin can be appreciated between the lesional tissue and adjacent normal mucosa. Most commonly, erythroplakia presents as a solitary lesion. However, examples of multicentric lesions and lesions involving extensive portions of oral mucosa have been reported.[3,7] When palpated, erythroplakias are typically soft. Indurated areas or lesions that are firm to palpation occur when malignant transformation and invasion are present.[2] The soft palate is the most common site for erythroplakia to occur. Other common sites include ventral tongue, floor of mouth, and tonsillar pillars.[2] Other areas of the tongue are rarely affected.[2] A diagnostic biopsy is required to differentiate between a true erythroplakia and other pathologic entities of the oral

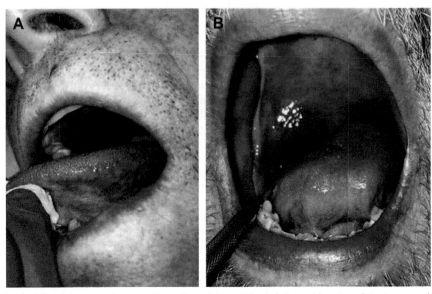

Fig. 5. (A) A 74-year-old man with erythroplakia of the left lateral border of the tongue. (B) Erythroplakia soft palate.

cavity. Microscopic examination of affected tissue aids in distinguishing a true erythroplakia from erythematous candidiasis and lichenoid lesions, including lichen planus, lichenoid mucositis, and oral lesions of lupus erythematosus, which can have similar clinical appearances. In addition, a biopsy can also rule out hemangiomas and other vascular anomalies, Kaposi sarcoma, median rhomboid glossitis, lesions secondary to local irritation, and erythema migrans. Disorders manifesting as desquamative gingivitis present as erythema of the gingiva, and include lichen planus, pemphigus vulgaris, and mucous membrane (cicatricial) pemphigoid.[7,8]

Erythroleukoplakia has a mixed red and white appearance. Unlike erythroplakia, which is well demarcated, erythroleukoplakia often has a blended or ill-defined margin. Clinically, erythroleukoplakia, previously termed speckled leukoplakia, presents in 2 general patterns (**Fig. 6**): either numerous small and irregular leukoplakic areas within a red patch, or as an erythroplakia adjacent to a leukoplakia. Unlike leukoplakia and erythroplakia, patients with erythroleukoplakia often present with symptoms such as pain or soreness. Age, gender, and commonly affected sites for erythroleukoplakia are the same as erythroplakia.[7]

RISK FACTORS
Tobacco

Smoking tobacco poses the greatest increase in risk to develop precancerous lesions in the oral cavity. Heavy cigarette smoking is the strongest predictor, with 1 study showing that smoking more than 20 cigarettes per day led to an increased risk of oral leukoplakia by 2.4 to 15 times that of nonsmokers. The cumulative effect of smoking is more important than current smoking status, which suggests that chronic long-term tobacco smoking plays a role in premalignant changes. Benzopyrene, a by-product of tobacco smoking, has been shown to be both mutagenic and carcinogenic. In addition to cigarettes, cigar and pipe smoking produce similar risks.[10]

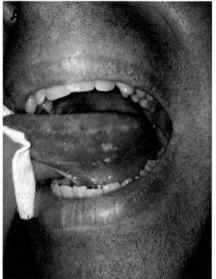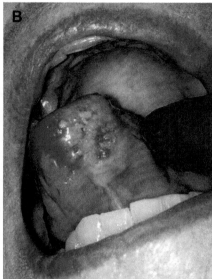

Fig. 6. (*A*) Erythroleukoplakia on the left lateral border of tongue in a 46-year-old man. (*B*) Erythroleukoplakia of the ventral tongue in an 85-year-old woman with exophytic areas of leukoplakia.

In some populations, the habit of placing the lit end of a cigarette into the oral cavity is practiced, and is known as reverse smoking. The mucosal changes observed with this practice manifest as leukoplakic plaques of the palate, mucosal nodularity, and thickening of the mucosa surrounding salivary gland ducts. The leukoplakia associated with reverse smoking has a higher risk of malignant transformation compared with lesions in regular cigarette smokers.[3]

Smokeless Tobacco

Smokeless tobacco was brought to popularity by Native Americans in North America in the early 1900s. Smokeless tobacco saw a slight decline with the invention of cigarettes, but smokeless tobacco usage has continued to surge at a steady pace since. Forms of smokeless tobacco include loose-leaf chewing tobacco, moist snuff, and dry snuff. It is estimated that from 6 million to 22 million Americans use some form of smokeless tobacco.

Clinically, lesions associated with smokeless tobacco use appear in the oral cavity as inflammatory gingival and periodontal lesions, and as leukoplakia, some of which are diagnosed as epithelial dysplasia. Squamous cell carcinoma has also been reported in patients who use smokeless tobacco products. However, some studies fail to account for risk factors such as alcohol and cigarettes. Regardless, most reports have found clinical changes in the oral mucosa as a result of smokeless tobacco use. The mucosal change is commonly referred to as smokeless tobacco keratosis and can be seen at the site where the quid is placed as soon as 6 months after initial use. The affected mucosa becomes leathery, grey-white to white, and fissured. The risk of smokeless tobacco keratosis transforming into premalignancy or squamous cell carcinoma is a topic of contention. In general, most studies have found low transformation rates. High-risk sites for epithelial dysplasia seen in conjunction with smokeless tobacco use are the buccal/vestibular mucosa and the gingiva, which are the locations where the tobacco comes into direct contact with the mucosa. One study by Boffetta and colleagues[11] estimated that up to 4% of oral cancers in men in the United States are associated with the use of smokeless tobacco products.

Alcohol

Approximately 65% of adults in the United States consume alcoholic beverages.[12] Regardless of frequency of drinking, consuming alcohol with meals, or the type of beverage, alcohol consumption is consistently linked to an increase risk of oral prema-lignant lesions. One study showed that ever having alcohol increases the risk devel-oping a leukoplakic lesion 1.5 times compared with nondrinkers.[12] It has also been shown that patients who regularly drink alcohol are at increased risk of developing recurrent disease after an initial oral precancerous lesion has been treated. The floor of mouth and ventral-lateral tongue are the sites most closely associated with alcohol as a risk factor, possibly because of prolonged contact with the offending substance. Acetaldehyde, a metabolite of ethanol produced by the liver, is carcinogenic. In addi-tion, alcohol may increase oral mucosal permeability to other carcinogens seen in as-sociation with tobacco use, which alters epithelial proliferation. This process exponentially increases the risk to develop oral precancerous lesions.[13]

Actinic Damage

Excessive sun exposure has been shown to cause actinic cheilitis, which is an inflammatory-associated precancerous lesion of the lower lip. It presents as a white lesion with crusting, flaking, or dryness. Blurring of the vermillion border is a common finding seen with this condition. People who are at risk to develop actinic cheilitis include men, fair-skinned individuals, and patients who spend extended periods participating in outdoor activities.[14]

Oral Submucous Fibrosis

Oral submucous fibrosis (OSF) is associated with the long-term use of betel quid. Typically, the quid consists of areca nut, slaked lime, tobacco, and sometimes other additives such as spices, wrapped in a betel leaf. The quid is then placed in the vestibule and causes a sense of euphoria for the user. OSF is most commonly seen in patients of southeast Asian and south Asian descent.[3] OSF is a chronic disorder of the mucosa in which fibroelasticity of the affected tissue is lost.[9] OSF is characterized by palpable fibrous bands leading to limited mouth opening and tongue rigidity. Early in the disease process, blanching of the mucosa is seen. Rate of malignant transformation seen in submucous fibrosis is 9.13% and patients with OSF have a risk of developing oral cancer 29.26 times that of patients without oral submucous fibrosis.[15] A predominant male predilection is seen in OSF. Affected sites include buccal mucosa, which is the most commonly affected, fol-lowed by tongue, lip, palate, and gingiva.[15] Areca nut contains arecoline, which stimulates fibroblasts. The slaked lime promotes penetration of arecoline into the mucosa, leading to fibrosis of the lamina propria. The mucosal lesion most often associated with OSF is oral leukoplakia. Increased duration of use of areca nut is directly proportional to an increased risk of oral leukoplakia and oral squamous cell carcinoma associated with OSF.

Human Papilloma Virus

HPV is a well-known cause of squamous cell carcinoma. HPV has been detected in the oral cavity at a rate of up to 12% and high-risk types have shown a prevalence of up to 3%. Histopathologic evidence has been seen in some instances of oral epithelial dysplasia. These lesions most commonly present as leukoplakia, but erythroplakias and erythroleukoplakias have also been described. There is a male predilection, and the most common sites for HPV-associated oral epithelial dysplasia to occur are the tongue and floor of mouth. The most common subtype of HPV seen in these lesions is HPV-16, followed by HPV-33 and HPV-58. Immunohistochemical staining for p16 serves as a surrogate marker for HPV infection. However, the standard to confirm the presence of HPV in dysplastic oral lesions is through in situ hybridization.[5,16]

MICROSCOPIC DESCRIPTION

Because oral epithelial dysplasias (OEDs) are a precursor to malignant transformation, creating a grading system for these lesions is of utmost importance.[17] Many attempts have been made to produce a grading system for oral epithelial dysplasia that is both reproducible and can serve as a reliable predictor of malignant transformation. However, assessing the degree of dysplasia in order to predict the prognosis and management of OED remains challenging. The current 2017 World Health Organization (WHO) 3-tiered grading system remains the gold standard in classification of these lesions.[18,19] Pathologists use this system to classify lesions into mild, moderate, and severe epithelial dysplasia using diagnostic criteria for both architectural and cytologic changes. Carcinoma in situ is considered synonymous with severe epithelial dysplasia.[18] The recent WHO update also mentions a binary system that was proposed by Kujan and colleagues.[20] This system uses similar diagnostic criteria to the WHO 2017 system but classifies the lesions as either low-grade or high-grade dysplasias, thus eliminating the in-between category of moderately dysplastic lesions. Binary systems are used for precursor lesions at other sites throughout the body, including the larynx, and are considered to be more reproducible and clinically relevant systems compared with the 3-tiered approach.[19–21] However, a binary system has yet to be validated for use in the oral cavity.[19,22] Regardless, the aim of both classification systems is to ensure standardization in reporting and therapeutic treatments of OED.[21]

Epithelial dysplasia is defined as an abnormal growth pattern that affects the normal maturation sequence of the surface mucosa. It includes both architectural and cytologic alterations, which can only be seen histologically. However, these changes can manifest as a clinically visible lesion. The 2005 WHO diagnostic criteria classify the lesion as mild dysplasia if alterations of the epithelial maturation sequence are seen only in the lower one-third of the surface mucosa (**Fig. 7**). Moderate dysplastic lesions have changes that encompass two-thirds of the epithelium (**Fig. 8**). Greater

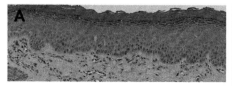
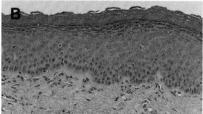

Fig. 7. (A) Mild epithelial dysplasia showing atypical features confined to the lower one-third of the epithelium (hematoxylin-eosin, original magnification ×10). (B) Mild maturational alterations include nuclear hyperchromatism, increased nuclear to cytoplasmic ratio, and hyperplasia of the basal cell layer (hematoxylin-eosin, original magnification ×40).

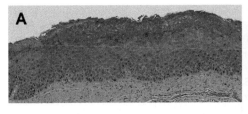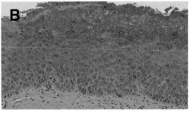

Fig. 8. (A) Moderate epithelial dysplasia in which the atypia extends beyond the lower one-third of the surface mucosa, but does not extend the full thickness of the epithelium (hematoxylin-eosin, original magnification ×10). (B) Dyskeratosis, increased mitotic activity, hyperplasia of the basal cell layer, and nuclear hyperchromatism are identified (hematoxylin-eosin, original magnification ×40).

than two-thirds of the epithelium showing atypical features is severe dysplasia and full-thickness changes are classified as carcinoma in situ (**Fig. 9**).[18,23] The 2005 diagnostic criteria are similar to the newly updated 2017 version.[23]

The 2017 WHO diagnostic criteria are listed as follows:

Architectural Changes

1. Irregular epithelial stratification
2. Loss of polarity of basal cells
3. Drop-shaped rete ridges
4. Increased number of mitotic figures
5. Abnormal superficial mitosis
6. Premature keratinization in single cells (dyskeratosis)
7. Keratin pearls within rete ridges
8. Loss of epithelial cohesion

Cytologic Changes

1. Abnormal variation in nuclear size
2. Abnormal variation in nuclear shape
3. Abnormal variation in cell size
4. Abnormal variation in cell shape
5. Increased nuclear-cytoplasmic ratio
6. Atypical mitotic figures
7. Increased number and size of nucleoli

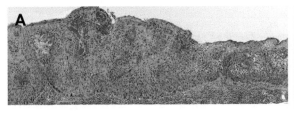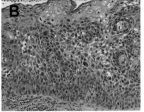

Fig. 9. (A) Severe epithelial dysplasia of the oral cavity showing dysplastic features throughout the surface mucosa (hematoxylin-eosin, original magnification ×10). (B) The dysplastic features seen in this case of severe epithelial dysplasia include increased nuclear to cytoplasmic ratio, drop-shaped rete ridges, and abnormal variation in nuclear size and shape. Increased mitotic activity and irregular stratification are also seen (hematoxylin-eosin, original magnification ×40).

8. Hyperchromasia

Included in the 2017 WHO Classification of Head and Neck Tumors.

Minor modifications have been made from the previously adapted 2005 WHO classification system. These changes include elimination of basal cell hyperplasia and the addition of loss of epithelial cohesion in the architectural change category. Furthermore, increase in nuclear size is no longer included as a cytologic feature of dysplasia.[18,23]

TREATMENT AND MANAGEMENT OF ORAL PREMALIGNANT LESIONS

Over the past 3 decades there has been little improvement in the 5-year survival rate for patients with oral cancer.[24] The current 5-year survival rate has been reported to be approximately 57% (https://oralcancerfoundation.org/facts/). It is crucial that clinicians embrace the importance of early detection and treatment of premalignant lesions.

Clinical examination and biopsy are the gold standard for the detection and diagnosis of oral premalignant lesions. There are many adjunctive aids available on the market to help detect these lesions, including autofluorescence, vital staining, and brush cytology/biopsy. These tests are minimally invasive; however, they have considerable false-positive and false-negative results.[24] Screening examinations for oral cancer, as part of a comprehensive head and neck examination, are recommended at all new patient visits, recall appointments, and emergency visits.[4]

The patient evaluation must begin with the collection of a detailed history from the patient. The following information should be discussed with the patient and documented:

- Demographic data
- History of chief complaint, including onset, progression, and symptoms
- Medical history and review of systems
- Social history, including alcohol, tobacco, and areca nut use
- Other risk factors, such as family history of cancer, and any environmental exposures[4]

The clinical examination begins with an extraoral examination. Examination should look for any head and neck asymmetry, and cutaneous lesions, followed by palpation of the midline and lateral neck and of the major salivary glands. The intraoral examination must include visualization and palpation of all sites of the oral cavity[4]; this is especially important because leukoplakia is often multifocal.[1] If a lesion is noted, its characteristics, including location, size, color, surface texture, and texture and symptoms on palpation, must be assessed. An irritative cause of the lesion should also be sought out. If irritation is suspected as the cause of the lesion, the cause of the irritation must be removed, and the lesion then be reevaluated in 1 to 2 months. Photographs of the lesions aid in the reevaluation process. If there is no change, or if no irritative factor is present, a biopsy of the lesion is mandatory.[1] Histopathology is the most important factor in the diagnosis of oral premalignant lesions.[4]

Risk factors associated with an increased risk of malignant transformation of a premalignant lesion must also be assessed. Factors that increase risk of malignant transformation that are patient related include female gender, patients 45 years of age or older, and nonsmoking status (so-called idiopathic leukoplakia).[5] Factors associated with the premalignant lesion that increase the risk of malignant transformation include site (floor of the mouth, ventral-lateral tongue, soft palate, and retromolar pad), size

($>$200 mm^2), clinical appearance (nonhomogeneous lesions, presence of multiple lesions), and higher grade of dysplasia.[4,25]

Treatment and management of patients with oral precancerous lesions are determined by evaluating their risk for malignant progression. The most important factors used to stratify patients include the clinical factors discussed earlier and histologic grade. Treatment of low-risk lesions that show mild dysplasia on biopsy may include habit cessation, surveillance, or surgical intervention.[4] One study has shown that there was a 44% rate of clinical improvement in lesions of mild dysplasia in smokers who discontinued tobacco use. The decision whether to treat a lesion of mild dysplasia should take into account the extent of the lesion, whether the lesion is multifocal, risk factors, and the patient's preference.[1]

High-risk lesions, and lesions that show moderate or severe dysplasia on biopsy, should be treated. The goal of treatment is to remove all the epithelium affected by the oral precancerous lesion.[1] Surgical removal with cold-blade scalpel excision or electrocautery excision significantly reduces the risk of transformation of the lesion. The lesion may also be treated by laser ablation. Most commonly a CO_2 laser is used to vaporize the affected epithelium. Regardless of how the lesion is to be treated, a 1-mm to 2-mm margin of normal mucosa is recommended.[4]

After appropriate treatment of an oral precancerous lesion, close, long-term surveillance is imperative. The interval between reevaluation visits varies depending on the patient's risk factors. It has been recommended that a complete extraoral and intraoral examination be done every 3 to 6 months. If any changes or new lesions are noted, a biopsy is required.[1] Regardless of the patient's risk factors and previous treatments, lifelong monitoring is suggested.[4]

SUMMARY

Identifying OPMDs in the oral cavity begins with thorough clinical examination of the soft tissue in the oral cavity and assessment of the patient's risk factors. Presence of an OPMD is confirmed via biopsy and microscopic examination of the lesional tissue. The treatment of OPMDs depends on the definitive diagnosis rendered from the biopsy specimen. Low-risk epithelial dysplasias should be closely monitored and biopsied when any changes to the lesion occur. High-risk dysplastic lesions need to be excised surgically with close and long-term follow-up of the patient. Adherence to this protocol for OPMD remains the standard of care in prevention of transformation to malignancy.

REFERENCES

1. Bewley AF, Farwell DG. Oral leukoplakia and oral cavity squamous cell carcinoma. Clin Dermatol 2017;35(5):461–7.
2. Maymone MB, Greer RO, Kesecker J, et al. Premalignant and malignant mucosal lesions: clinical and pathological findings part II. Premalignant and malignant mucosal lesions. J Am Acad Dermatol 2018. https://doi.org/10.1016/j.jaad.2018.09.060.
3. Warnakulasuriya S. Clinical features and presentation of oral potentially malignant disorders. Oral Surg Oral Med Oral Pathol Oral Radiol 2018;125(6):582–90.
4. Nadeau C, Kerr AR. Evaluation and management of oral potentially malignant disorders. Dent Clin North Am 2018;62(1):1–27.
5. Speight PM, Khurram SA, Kujan O. Oral potentially malignant disorders: risk of progression to malignancy. Oral Surg Oral Med Oral Pathol Oral Radiol 2018;125(6):612–27.

6. Mortazavi H, Safi Y, Baharvand M, et al. Oral white lesions: an updated clinical diagnostic decision tree. Dentistry J 2019;7(1):15.
7. Reichart P. S2.4 Erythroplakia — clinical markers. Oral Oncol Suppl 2005;1(1):47.
8. Villa A, Villa C, Abati S. Oral cancer and oral erythroplakia: an update and implication for clinicians. Aust Dent J 2011;56(3):253–6.
9. Rhodus NL, Kerr AR, Patel K. Oral Cancer. Dent Clin North Am 2014;58(2): 315–40.
10. Dietrich T, Reichart PA, Scheifele C. Clinical risk factors of oral leukoplakia in a representative sample of the US population. Oral Oncol 2004;40(2):158–63.
11. Greer RO. Oral manifestations of smokeless tobacco use. Otolaryngol Clin North Am 2011;44(1):31–56.
12. Maserejian NN, Giovannucci E, Rosner B, et al. Prospective study of fruits and vegetables and risk of oral premalignant lesions in men. Am J Epidemiol 2006; 164(6):556–66.
13. Goodson M, Hamadah O, Thomson P. The role of alcohol in oral precancer: observations from a North-East England population. Br J Oral Maxillofac Surg 2010; 48(7):507–10.
14. Neville BW, Damm DD, Allen CM, et al. Oral and maxillofacial pathology. St Louis (MO): Elsevier; 2016.
15. Cai X, Yao Z, Liu G, et al. Oral submucous fibrosis: a clinicopathological study of 674 cases in china. J Oral Pathol Med 2019;48(4):321–5.
16. Lerman MA, Almazrooa S, Lindeman N, et al. HPV-16 in a distinct subset of oral epithelial dysplasia. Mod Pathol 2017;30(12):1646–54.
17. Thomson P, Mccaul J, Ridout F, et al. To treat…or not to treat? Clinicians' views on the management of oral potentially malignant disorders. Br J Oral Maxillofac Surg 2015;53(10):1027–31.
18. Raganathan K, Kavitha L. Oral epithelial dysplasia: classification and clinical relevance in risk assessment of oral potentially malignant disorders. J Oral Maxillofac Pathol 2019;23(1):19–27.
19. Müller S, Thompson LDR. An update on salivary gland pathology. Head Neck Pathol 2013;7(S1):1–2.
20. Kujan O, Oliver RJ, Khattab A, et al. Evaluation of a new binary system of grading oral epithelial dysplasia for prediction of malignant transformation. Oral Oncol 2006;42(10):987–93.
21. Dost F, Cao KL, Ford P, et al. Malignant transformation of oral epithelial dysplasia: a real-world evaluation of histopathologic grading. Oral Surg Oral Med Oral Pathol Oral Radiol 2014;117(3):343–52.
22. Cho K-J, Song JS. Recent changes of classification for squamous intraepithelial lesions of the head and neck. Arch Pathol Lab Med 2018;142(7):829–32.
23. Chan JKC, El-Naggar AK, Grandis JR, et al. WHO classification of head and neck tumours. Lyon (France): International Agency for Research on Cancer; 2017.
24. Awadallah M, Idle M, Patel K, et al. Management update of potentially premalignant oral epithelial lesions. Oral Surg Oral Med Oral Pathol Oral Radiol 2018; 125(6):628–36.
25. Ho M, Risk J, Woolgar J, et al. The clinical determinants of malignant transformation in oral epithelial dysplasia. Oral Oncol 2012;48(10):969–76.

Benign and Malignant Lesions of Jaw

B.V. Ramana Reddy, BDS, MDS[a],*, K. Kiran Kumar, BDS, MDS, PhD[a],
Arvind Babu Rajendra Santosh, BDS, MDS[b]

KEYWORDS

- Potentially malignant disorders • Benign • Malignant • Reactive • Oral lesions
- Child abuse

KEY POINTS

- Swelling of oral cavity may arise from surface epithelium or alternatively arise from pathology of underlying connective tissue structures.
- Most oral neoplasms are benign. Fibroma is the most common soft tissue tumor of oral cavity.
- Leukoplakia is the most common precancerous condition of oral cavity. Leukoplakia is strongly associated with smoking.
- Cancer of the head and neck is the fifth most common type of cancer in the world. Oral squamous cell carcinoma is the most common type of oral cancer.
- Benign/malignant lesion of jaw associated with child abuse is discussed.

INTRODUCTION

Benign, malignant, and reactive lesions of oral cavity present clinically as swelling/growth or an ulcerated swelling. Academically swelling is termed as tumors and growth of tumor is called as tumefaction, and hence many of the lesions described in this article are suffixed with "oma" (fibroma), which represents tumor.[1] Oral tissues are vulnerable for benign or malignant growth due to factors such as trauma, infection (bacterial/viral/fungal), local irritation, smoking, alcohol misuse, or genetic damage. Tumors of oral cavity constitute to a small number of cases identified in a clinical practice and therefore challenges dentist in their office for diagnosis and/or management. Hence dentists are required to be more academically familiar, and continuously educating them on these conditions, especially on common type of oral conditions of this category, will enable dentists either to institute appropriate management or refer their patient to oral disease expert and oral surgeon at a right time. Although

[a] Department of Oral and Maxillofacial Pathology, SIBAR Institute of Dental Sciences, Takkellapadu, Guntur, Andhra Pradesh 522 509, India; [b] School of Dentistry, Faculty of Medical Sciences, The University of the West Indies, Mona campus, Kingston 7, West Indies
* Corresponding author.
E-mail address: drramanabv@gmail.com

Dent Clin N Am 64 (2020) 39–61
https://doi.org/10.1016/j.cden.2019.08.005
0011-8532/20/© 2019 Elsevier Inc. All rights reserved.

clinical and/or radiological details provide a clue in diagnosis, biopsy is required for arriving to a final definitive diagnosis, because some of the swellings may be associated with dysplastic features that may require an intensive surgical management.

This article discusses potentially malignant disorders and reactive lesions, benign, malignant conditions of oral cavity. In addition, oral lesions of abovesaid category that are associated with child abuse are also discussed. For the convenience of the reader, commonly encountered oral conditions on this category are listed in **Table 1**. The oral conditions discussed will provide information on diagnosis, investigation, and outline on management.

DIAGNOSTIC APPROACH FOR SWELLING

The tumors can originate from epithelial or mesenchymal tissue and may be the result of inflammatory, neoplastic, developmental, or systemic diseases. The differential diagnosis on swelling from oral tissue must be formulated on parameters of surface appearance of swelling, location, consistency, and the presence or absence of pain. The first step in diagnostic approach for oral swelling is to check whether the swelling is arising from surface epithelium or, alternatively, arising from pathologic changes from the underlying soft tissue (ie, fibrous, fat tissue, blood vessels, lymphatic vessels, nerves, cartilage, or bone), resulting in secondary elevation of surface epithelium/tissue. The second step is to categorize them into benign, malignant, inflammatory, or reactive growth. The swellings that are movable, firm, and not indurated are in the benign category. The swellings that are fixed, indurated, ulcerated, or ulceroproliferative are likely to be malignant type.[2] The swellings that are either tender or painful with or without sinus/fistulation are probably of an inflammatory origin. The swellings that occur secondary to injury are reactive lesions and may be associated with or without pain. Third step is to evaluate clinical parameters such as surface appearance of swelling, location, consistency, and the presence or absence of pain. The swelling observed on oral tissues may be a regular swelling or one of the following types: papillary, verrucous, dome-shaped, papule, polypoid, diffuse, or multifocal (**Table 2**). Fourth step is evaluating status of lymph nodes. Lymph nodes that are palpable and hard and fixed to underlying structure are likely to be an association of malignant condition. Lymph nodes that are palpable and soft and movable favor benign growth association. Tenderness/pain associated with lymph node palpable is the characteristic of inflammation.[3,4] The presence and absence of lymph node cannot differentiate benign from malignant conditions.

The fifth step is to formulate differential diagnosis based on clinical details and plan for investigation for arriving at a final diagnosis through microscopic examination, that is, biopsy (**Fig. 1**).

Potentially Malignant Disorders

Potentially malignant disorders convey that "not all lesions and conditions described under this term may transform to cancer, rather there is a family of morphologic alterations among which some may have an increased potential for malignant transformation." Potentially malignant disorders serve as a clinical marker for future malignancy in oral mucosa.[5] The risk factors for oral cancer and precancer are broadly categorized as established, strongly suggestive, possible, and speculative factors[6] (**Table 3**).

Oral lichen planus

Lichen planus affects both skin and oral mucosa due to multiple factors (**Box 1**), with prevalence of 0.5% to 1%. Lichen planus is characterized by symmetric appearance

Table 1
List of benign and malignant oral lesions

Potentially Malignant Disorders	Reactive Lesions	Epithelial Tumors	Connective Tissue Tumors	Oral Lesions Associated with Child Abuse
Leukoplakia	Pyogenic granuloma	Benign tumors	Benign tumors	Herpes simplex,
Erythroplakia	Peripheral giant cell	Squamous papilloma	Fibroma	Epstein–Barr Virus,
Oral submucous	granuloma	Verruca vulgaris (common wart)	Lipoma	cytomegalovirus, gonorrhea
fibrosis	Perpheral ossifying	Focal melanosis (oral melanotic	Neurofibroma	Molluscumcontagiosum
Lichen planus	fibroma	macules)	Neurilemoma	Condyloma Accuminatum
	Epulisfissuratum (inflammatory	Mole (aquired melanocytic nevus)	Hemangioma	
	fibrous hyperplasia)	Keratoacanthoma	Lymphangioma	
	Inflammatory papillary	Malignant tumors:	Osteoma	
	hyperplasia	Oral squamous cell carcinoma	Malignant tumors:	
		Verrucous carcinoma	Fibro sarcoma	
		Basal cell carcinoma	Osteosarcoma	
		Melanoma		

Table 2
Description on the various appearances of swelling

Appearance of Swelling	Description
Papillary	The swellings that appear as fingerlike surface projections.
Verrucous	The swellings that have multiple fingerlike appearance but characterized by more irregular surface.
Dome-shaped	These are oval-shaped swellings with rolled margin and a central pit that may or may not be plugged with keratinaceous material.
Papules	These are small swellings that are <0.5 cms and are usually multiple in number.
Polypoid	These are similar to papules but exceed 1 cm in growth size and tend to be multifocal.
Nodular	These are raised solid lesions that are >5 mm in diameter.
Macule	Focal area of color change, which is neither elevated nor depressed to adjacent mucosa.
Diffuse	Swellings that are characterized by their multifocal appearance.

of bilateral white/white-grey striations or plaque.[7] The lesion is predominantly observed on buccal mucosa, tongue, and gingival. The lesion tends to show erythematous, erosion- or blister-like appearance.

Clinical features The lesion is characterized by bilateral symmetric radiating white or greyish white striae, small angular, flat-topped papules only 0.5 mm to 2 cm with slight female predilection. The striae have lacelike appearance, which is termed as "Wickham striae."[8] The clinical types of lichen planus are reticular (**Fig. 2**), atrophic, papular, bullous, plaque, erosive, or ulcerative.[9] Erosive type has potential for malignant transformation to oral squamous cell carcinoma (OSCC).[10]

Diagnosis Clinical appearance is diagnostic; however, microscopic examination is necessary for securing final diagnosis.

| Step 1 | PRELIMINARY INFORMATION |

• Whether swelling is arising from surface epithelium or secondary elevation of surface epithelium from underlying connective tissue.

| Step 2 | CATEGORIZATION |

• Categorize the swelling as benign, malignant, inflammatory or reactive growth.

| Step 3 | CLINICAL DETAILS |

• Evaluate: appearence of swelling, location, consistency and association of tender and pain.

| Step 4 | LYMPH NODE EVALUATION |

• Lymphnode evaluation for differentiation of benign, malignant or inflammatory origin of swelling.

| Step 5 | DIFFERENTIAL DIAGNOSIS |

• Formulation of differential diagnosis and planning investigation. Securing final diagnosis through microscopic examination.

Fig. 1. Steps in diagnostic approach of swellings.

Table 3				
Risk factors for oral cancer and precancer				
Established	**Strongly Suggested**	**Possible**	**Speculative**
Smoking	Sunlight (lip)	Viruses	Mouthwashes
Chewing tobacco	Radiation	Immune deficiency	Mate drinking
Snuff dipping		Dentition?	Periodontal disease
Alcohol misuse		Ethnicity?	Familial
Betel quid syphilis			

Adapted from Warnakulasuriya S. Global epidemiology of oral and oropharyngeal cancer. Oral Oncol. 2009;45(5):309–16; with permission.

Management Corticosteroids and topical retinoid are helpful in relieving symptoms. Associated causative factors require elimination.

Erythroplakia

Erythroplakia is an uncommon potentially malignant disorder characterized by red patch that cannot be clinically or pathologically diagnosed as any other condition with a prevalence of 0.001% to 0.83%, whereas most of the erythroplakia diagnosed is 1.2 per 100,000 population in the United States. The causative factors for erythroplakia are tobacco, alcohol, candidial infection, hematinic deficiency, and chronic trauma.

Clinical features Erythroplakia is characterized by well-defined erythematous patch or plaque with soft and velvety texture. Intermixed red and white patch is termed as erythroleukoplakia. Erythroplakia is predominantly observed in geriatric population (65–75 years) with no gender predilection. Frequently reported locations are floor of the mouth, tongue, and soft palate. Microscopic examination is usually indicated to rule out OSCC.[11]

Management Cessation of habit is the most important strategy in the patient management. Surgical excision is used due to association of dysplastic features in the tissue. The recurrence rate is lesser than 5% and postoperative follow-up is required.

Leukoplakia

Leukoplakia is a white patch or plaque that cannot be characterized clinically or pathologically as any other diseases. Tobacco smoking is the most common cause, with prevalence of leukoplakia ranging from 1.5% to 4.3%.[12]

Box 1
Causative factors for oral lichen planus
Tobacco smoking and chewing
Stress
Dental materials
Drugs
Infectious components
Autoimmunity
Food allergies
Immunologic alterations

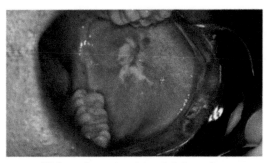

Fig. 2. Reticular pattern of lichen planus involving left buccal mucosa and left commissure of lip. (*From* Olson MA, Rogers RS, Bruce AJ. Oral lichen planus. Clin Dermatol 2016;34(4):495–504; with permission.)

Clinical features Leukoplakia is characterized by flat to slighted elevated, nonscrapable white or gray patches that are usually seen among midaged adult men with smoking habit. Leukoplakia can be seen at vermillion border of the lip, buccal mucosa, floor of the mouth, gingiva, or tongue. Causes of leukoplakia include tobacco smoking or chewing; betel quid; alcohol; trauma; infections such as syphilis and Candida albicans; chemicals such as Sanguinaria; ultraviolet radiation; iron-deficiency anemia; immune deficiency state; human papillomavirus (HPV) 16 and 18; and deficiency of vitamin A, B12, and C. Various clinical forms of leukoplakia are thin, thick, homogenous, granular, nodular, verrucous, verruciform, speckled, or proliferative verrucous leukoplakia. Intermixed white-red patches are called as erythroleukoplakia. Speckled leukoplakia has a higher potential of malignant transformation to OSCC.[13]

Diagnosis Differential diagnosis of leukoplakia include aspirin burn, candidiasis, frictional keratosis, leukoedema, linea alba, lupus erythematosus, cheek bite, syphilis, smoker's palate, and white sponge nevus.[5] History and clinical details are adequate for ruling out differential diagnosis. Microscopic examination should be done to confirm diagnosis of leukoplakia and evaluate the association of dysplasia. Biopsy is also important to rule out squamous cell carcinoma.

Management Cessation of habit is the most important strategy in the patient management. Surgical excision is used due to association of dysplastic features in the tissue. An approach for management of leukoplakia depend on elimination of cause and biopsy report[14,15] (**Fig. 3**).

Reactive Lesions

Reactive lesions are growths resulting from trauma or irritation and characterized by slow-growing, painless, pedunculated or sessile mass with or without bleeding tendency. The surface of the growth may vary from smooth to ulcerated tissue. Lymph node may be palpable and tender due to inflammatory origin.[16]

Pyogenic granuloma

Pyogenic granuloma is a tumorlike growth exuberant resulting from tissue response to local irritation or trauma.

Clinical features Pyogenic granuloma is characterized by painless, smooth, lobulated, pedunculated mass with bleeding tendency. However, cases have been reported with sessile growth or without bleeding tendency. Lesion appears red to pink with

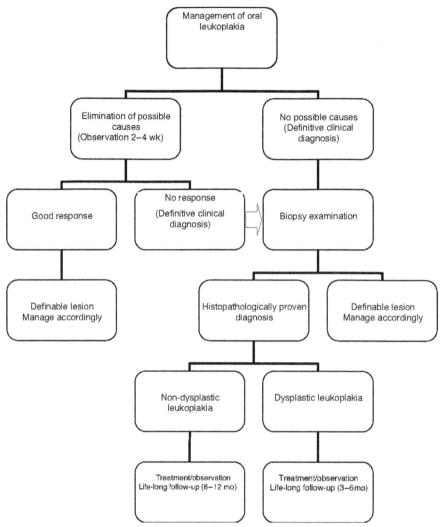

Fig. 3. Management of leukoplakia. (*From* Kumar A, Cascarini L, McCaul JA, et al. How should we manage oral leukoplakia? Br J Oral Maxillofac Surg. 2013;51(5):377–83; with permission.)

varying size (**Fig. 4**). The lesion occurs due to trauma, calculus, plaque, overhanging restoration, implantitis, pregnancy or hormonal change. Rapid growth of tissue alarms with malignant appearance. Lesion is predominantly seen as gingival swelling more commonly from labial side.[17]

Diagnosis and management Microscopic examination is usually done to rule out malignancy. The treatment options include surgical excision, curettage, cryotherapy, chemical and electric cauterization, lasers, and intralesional corticosteroids.[18]

Peripheral ossifying fibroma
Peripheral ossifying fibroma is one of the common reactive growths of soft tissues, and mineralized component of the lesion possibly originates from periosteum or

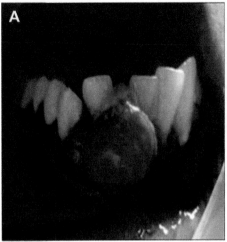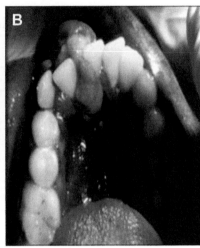

Fig. 4. Exophytic growth extending labiolingually through interdental space. (*A*) Labial view. (*B*) Lingual view. (*From* Deore GD, Gurav AN, Patil R, et al. Sclerotherapy: a novel bloodless approach to treat recurrent oral pyogenic granuloma associated with port-wine stain. Ann Vas Surg. 2014;28(6):1564; with permission.)

periodontal ligament. This lesion is considered to be a resultant of reparative response to intrabony hemorrhage and inflammation.[19]

Clinical features Peripheral ossifying fibroma is characterized by nodular, red/pink, pedunculated/sessile mass occurring at papilla of the gingiva with surface ulceration. The lesion mimics pyogenic granuloma and is predominantly seen among teenagers and women. Most of the cases were reported in incisor and canine region of maxillae.[20]

Diagnosis Radiographic examination of the tissue shows minimal cortical plate expansion with or without severe root resorption. Microscopic examination is usually indicated to rule out pyogenic granuloma and peripheral giant cell granuloma.

Management Conservative surgical excision with curettage to prevent recurrence. Approximately 8% to 10% of cases show recurrence.

Peripheral giant cell granuloma
Peripheral giant cell granuloma is another reactive lesion that is categorized as tumor-like growth. Trauma is the most common cause for occurrence and seen predominantly in root canal–treated tooth. Radiographic changes are helpful in recognition.[21]

Clinical features Peripheral giant cell granuloma is a red or blue, nodular gingival or alveolar sessile/pedunculated mass that measures less than 2 cm. There is no specific age predilection and is frequently reported on women. Mandibular anterior is the most common region of occurrence.[22]

Diagnosis and management Radiologically the lesion shows cupping resorption of alveolar bone. The cupping effect is reflection of base of the lesion. Microscopic examination is required to rule out peripheral ossifying fibroma and pyogenic granuloma. Conservative surgical excision with thorough oral prophylaxis, scaling, and root planning are used for removal of source irritation that is, supra/sub-gingival calculus. Approximately 10% to 18% of cases showed recurrence.

Inflammatory papillary hyperplasia

This is a hyperplastic connective tissue growth that is seen among edentulous patients with ill-fitting partial or complete dentures. Ill-fitting denture, sharp edges, trauma, and poor denture hygiene are the most common causes.[23]

Clinical features Papillary hyperplasia is characterized by asymptomatic papillary/fingerlike growth of tissue beneath denture (**Fig. 5**) predominantly seen in hard palate surface and remains asymptomatic until secondary infection.[24] The secondary infection can cause redness, soreness, pain, or burning sensation.

Diagnosis and management Clinical appearance of the lesion is diagnostic. The growth is usually removed surgically. Denture hygiene instructions must be followed to prevent recurrence.

Inflammatory fibrous hyperplasia

Inflammatory fibrous hyperplasia is a reactive growth resulting from poor denture hygiene practices and chronic injury/irritation from the denture. Concurrent occurrence of candidiasis may be observed.

Clinical features The lesion is characterized by painless, pink to red, nodular, circumscribed polypoid mass with bleeding tendency. The lesion may be symptomatic, that is, pain when associated with irritation or erythematous changes. Female predilection is observed. Hard palate is the most common site and occasionally seen over mandibular alveolar ridge. Few cases of inflammatory fibrous hyperplasia have been reported with candidiasis and human immunodeficiency virus infection.[25,26]

Diagnosis and management Clinical appearance is diagnostic. Surgical removal of hyperplastic tissue and fabrication of new denture is advised. Individuals with candidiasis are managed with antifungal medications.

Tumors of Epithelial Tissue Origin

The tumors of this origin are characterized by the swelling that arises from surface epithelium. The recognition of tumors as epithelial versus mesenchymal

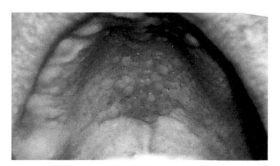

Fig. 5. Inflammatory papillary hyperplasia of the palate. (*From* Infante-Cossio P, Martinez-de-Fuentes R, Torres-Carranza E, Gutierrez-Perez JL. Inflammatory papillary hyperplasia of the palate: treatment with carbon dioxide laser, followed by restoration with an implant-supported prosthesis. Br J Oral Maxillofac Surg. 2007;45(8):658–60; with permission.)

tissue origin is not just academic importance but to understand relevance of clinical, histologic behavior, aggressiveness and prognosis. The relevance of abovementioned areas greatly varies in malignant neoplasms. Hence the topics covered here are discussed under 2 headings: benign and malignant lesions.

Benign epithelial tumors of oral mucosa

Squamous papilloma Squamous papilloma is a viral-induced benign proliferation of stratified squamous epithelium of oral tissue. The swelling is characterized by solitary occurrence of finger-like projection of surface epithelium. The occurrence of this lesion is presumably associated with low-risk type of HPV (types 6 and 11). The mode of transmission of HPV for inducing this lesion is not clear.[27]

Clinical presentation Squamous papilloma is characterized by painless, slow-growing, fingerlike projection of surface epithelium that are either sessile or pedunculated with normal-appearing color or whitish change. Soft palate is the most commonly encountered site involvement; however, it can occur on tongue, lips, or buccal mucosa. No specific gender predominance is observed. The dimension of the lesion is often varying with their size being less than 0.5 mm to 3 cm. Lymph nodes are not affected in this condition.[28]

Diagnosis Microscopic examination of biopsied tissue is helpful in achieving final diagnosis. The differential diagnosis of this condition can include verruca vulgaris when the lesion appears rougher and irregular surface tissue growth; condyloma accuminatum should be considered when the lesion is associated with whitish appearance and blunt surface projections.

Management Surgical excision of lesion along with base of the surface tissue will provide good prognosis. Recurrence of lesion is uncommon.

Verruca vulgaris Verruca vulgaris is characterized by white papillary growth of surface epithelium that is either sessile or pedunculated. The condition is predominantly observed in cutaneous surfaces, whereas in oral cavity it is observed in vermilion border of lip. Because of higher predilection on epidermis (skin) the condition is often noted as common/cutaneous wart. The lesion is often associated with low-risk type of HPV (HPV 2, 4, 6, and 40). The mode of transmission of HPV for inducing this lesion is autoinoculation of virus from affected skin or mucous membrane.[29]

Clinical presentation Verruca vulgaris is characterized by painless, white papillary growth of surface epithelium that is either sessile or pedunculated. Although it is uncommon in oral mucosal surfaces, the cases have been reported on labial mucosa and anterior tongue. The lesion appears in small size and grows rapidly to attain its maximum size. Multiple lesions can occur in oral cavity.

Diagnosis Microscopic examination of biopsied tissue is necessary for arriving final diagnosis. Differential diagnosis of squamous papilloma may be considered when the lesion has less white color.

Management Surgical excision of the lesion should include base of the lesion. Very few cases have reported with recurrence.

Focal melanosis Benign pigmented lesion is characterized by well-circumscribed, painless, flat, brown mucosal discoloration with increase in pigmentation possibly due to increase in number of melanocytes at basal cell layer of epithelium. Focal melanosis is frequently observed on lips. The lesion is managed by surgical excision specially to rule out malignant melanoma.

Clinical presentation Focal melanosis is a painless, slow-growing pigmented macule that is a predominantly brown change of oral mucosa on the affected region. However, cases with blue, brown, or black have been reported. Female predilection is observed and can be seen in any age group. Although lip is the most commonly encountered site, the lesion can be seen on gingiva, buccal mucosa, or palate (**Fig. 6**).[30,31]

Diagnosis Although clinical appearance of the lesion is adequate for diagnosis, incisional biopsy should be done to rule out malignant melanoma. Hence microscopic examination of biopsied tissue is necessary for final diagnosis.

Management The lesion undergoes spontaneous resolution after incisional biopsy; hence surgical management is not required. Surgery may be planned based on aesthetic needs of patients. Lesion has less tendency for recurrence. Reports mentioned that focal melanosis has no malignant transformation potential.[32]

Acquired melanocytic nevus This is a common malformation of the skin and mucosa and generally termed as "mole." Acquired melanocytic nevus is a benign, localized proliferation of cells from neural crest called as nevus cells. Acquired melanocytic nevus is the most common benign cutaneous tumor but uncommon intraoral lesion.[33]

Clinical presentation Acquired melanocytic nevus is a most common pigmentation that occurs in cutaneous surface, frequently reported in childhood with slight female predilection. Intraoral occurrence is uncommon, mostly observed in palate, gingiva, tongue, or other areas of oral mucosa.[34]

Diagnosis Clinical appearance of the lesion is characteristic and does not require biopsy and microscopic examination unless if acquired melanocytic nevus shows secondary characters such as rapid growth and ulceration.

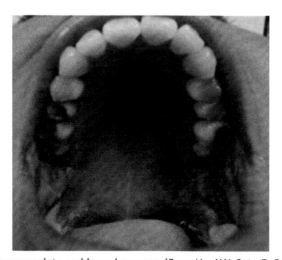

Fig. 6. Melanosis over palate and buccal mucosa. (*From* Ho AW, Sato R, Ramsdell A. JAAD grand rounds quiz. A case of oral melanosis. J Am Acad Dermatol. 2014;71(5):1030–3; with permission.)

Management Treatment is usually not required unless patient has aesthetic demands. When treatment is planned, conservative surgical excision is the treatment of choice. Recurrence is unlikely to occur and tends to regress with age.

Keratoacanthoma Keratoacanthoma is a relatively common benign epithelial proliferation of pilosebaceous glands with a self-healing potential. The lesion is considered as low grade and a variant of squamous cell carcinoma. The exact cause for appearance of this lesion is unclear but sunlight damage and HPV are possible reasons. Intraoral occurrence of this lesion is rare.[35]

Clinical presentation Keratoacanthoma is characterized by painless, slow-growing, well-demarcated, firm, sessile, dome-shaped swelling with keratin plugging in center. The central plug could be yellowish, brown, or black. A predominant number of cases were reported on lips. The lesion commonly occurs on a sun-exposed area and reported more frequently among midaged men. The progression of this lesion is divided into 3 phases: (1) growth, (2) stationary, and (3) involution phase. The lesion has a tendency for resolution and hence it is termed as "self-healing carcinoma." Regression usually occurs in 6 to 12 months from the time of onset.

Diagnosis Age, location, and clinical presentation are helpful in achieving provisional clinical diagnosis. However, keratoacanthoma must be differentiated with OSCC. Hence biopsy is usually required to rule out malignancy. Microscopic examination of biopsied tissue is necessary for arriving final diagnosis.

Management Excisional biopsy is usually indicated due to size of lesion. The lesion has a tendency for spontaneous regression and rarely recurs.

Malignant epithelial tumors of oral mucosa

Oral squamous cell carcinoma OSCC is the malignant neoplasm of oral epithelium. It is the most common oral cancer arising from oral mucosa. Smoking and smokeless tobacco are the most common causes for OSCC. Tongue and lips are the frequently affected areas. It can also affect the lips, cheek mucosa, tongue, palate or teeth-bearing alveolar segment, and gums.[36] Microscopic examination of the affected region is the key for diagnosis. Staging and grading are the most important steps in assessing the cancer. OSCC requires both surgery and radiotherapy.[37]

Clinical presentation The clinical presentation of OSCC is varying and can present as simple as white patch or can present with complex features such as swelling, ulcer, or ulceroproliferative swelling. Tobacco smoking, smokeless tobacco, sunlight damage, alcohol, betel quid, iron deficiency, radiation, phenolic agents, syphilis, vitamin A deficiency, oral candidiasis, oncogenic viruses (HPV), immunosuppression, and chronic injury are considered as risk factors for developing OSCC.[38] The lesion is predominantly characterized by exophytic and ulcerated growth. Ulceration varies in size with indurated margin and fixed to adjacent soft tissues. Metastasis of the malignant lesion can be observed in regional lymph nodes. Palpable regional lymph nodes may be identified with one or few of the characters: increase in size, number, and hard in consistency and immobile while palpation.[39]

Diagnosis OSCC is a clinically recognizable condition because it affects surface mucosa. Although the lesion is affecting oral mucosa, it can perforate bone and manifest in osseous tissue. Hence changes in bone can be observed in radiographs. Radiologically, the lesion shows multilocular appearance with radiolucent changes. Small-sized multiloculation shows honeycomb appearance, whereas large-sized multiloculation shows soap bubble appearance. Microscopic examination of incisional biopsy is mandatory for arriving final diagnosis. Histopathologic examination is helpful in grading the malignancy into well, moderate, or poorly differentiated OSCC based on dysplastic features, keratin pearls, and parental cell resemblance.

Management OSCC must be treated to achieve favorable prognosis. Cases diagnosed with OSCC are managed both surgically and by radiation therapy. OSCC has a tendency to recur.[40] Depending on the stage and grade of OSCC, neck dissection procedure is performed. Patient requires routine postoperative follow-up to monitor and prevent recurrence. Referral of the patient to Oncosurgeons and Faciomaxillary Surgeons at right time is very important in the patient management.

Verrucous carcinoma Verrucous carcinoma is a low-grade variant of squamous cell carcinoma. This condition is often associated with the use of smokeless tobacco, chewing tobacco, or snuff users. However, cases have been reported among nonusers of above-stated tobacco products. The lesion has least tendency to metastasis and hence surgical excision without neck dissection is a choice.

Clinical presentation Verrucous carcinoma is characterized by diffuse, painless, well-demarcated, exophytic proliferative growth of oral mucosa predominantly observed on vestibular space and midaged men. The lesion shows papillary or verruciform surface projections giving rough surface texture and appears white due to excessive keratin deposits. Gingiva, buccal mucosa, hard palate, and tongue are also reported as sites of occurrence. Site of verrucous carcinoma in oral cavity corresponds to the site of tobacco placement. Long-standing untreated cases of verrucous carcinoma can destroy underlying connective tissue structures such as cartilage, bone, muscle, or salivary glands. Lymph node enlargement is secondary to inflammatory changes and not due to metastatic deposits.[41]

Diagnosis Clinical appearance of the lesion is characteristic for achieving provisional diagnosis. However, microscopic examination is necessary for arriving final diagnosis. Microscopic examination of biopsied tissue is necessary to differentiate between verrucous carcinoma and verrucoid variant of oral squamous carcinoma. Differential diagnosis of verrucous carcinoma includes papillary hyperplasia and squamous cell carcinoma.

Management Verrucous carcinoma is managed through wide surgical excision. The lesion has a tendency for recurrence. Chemotherapy is used as a temporary management of verrucous carcinoma for inoperable cases.

Basal cell carcinoma Basal cell carcinoma (BCC) is a common malignancy of skin that is slow-growing, locally invasive neoplasm originating from basal cell layer of skin. BCC occurs on sun-exposed surface of the face, skin, and scalp of elderly persons. The lesion is managed through surgical procedures.

Clinical presentation BCC is characterized by solitary ulcer or nodular growth. The lesion may seem as solitary or multiple. Early lesions may show a pigmentation or nodular appearance. The ulcer tends to show rolled-out and indurated margins. The ulcer is locally invasive and shows furrowing appearance, hence the name "rodent ulcer." The lesion shows predilection for middle-aged men. This malignant neoplasm has a unique aggressive behavior but does not have metastatic property. Few cases are associated with nevoid BCC syndrome where the concurrence of this lesion with odontogenickeratocysts.[42]

Diagnosis Nonulcerated BCC must be differentiated from nevi, sebaceous cyst, or mesenchymal dermal tumors. Ulcerated lesions must be differentiated from squamous cell carcinoma. Hence microscopic examination of biopsied tissue is usually indicated to rule out differential diagnosis and arriving at a definitive diagnosis.

Management Small lesions are treated by surgical excision with laser or electrodessication and curettage. Large lesions require wide excision, and radiation/chemotherapy is required for aggressive lesions. During surgical procedure, normal-appearing adjacent mucosa is also excised for about 1 cm to avoid recurrences. Because of local invasion property of BCC, microscopic examination of excised tissue is important for evaluation of cancer-free cells at surgical margins.

Melanoma Malignant melanoma is a neoplasm of melanocytes that has unpredictable biological behavior. Melanoma is the third common malignancy of skin and occurs where melanocytes are present. Intraoral melanomas are reported. Ultraviolet radiation is a major risk factor for initiation of this malignancy. Surgical excision is the mainstay of treatment, and prognosis of melanoma is poor.

Clinical presentation Melanoma is characterized by pigmented (black, bluish black, or dark brown) lesions that begin as a focal area of macule. The lesion is rapidly progressive causing diffuse pigmentation with or without induration. Ulcerations may or may not be seen. Cases have been reported with nonpigmented appearance, which mimics inflammatory lesion or other benign neoplasm. Sun exposure, ultraviolet radiation, and xeroderma pigmentosum are the known risk factors.[42]

Diagnosis Differential diagnosis of pigmented lesions is important due to clinicopathologic similarity with other conditions. Differential diagnosis of melanoma includes traumatized nevus, pigmented variant of BCC, blue nevus, lentigo, traumatic hematoma, and pigmented actinic keratosis. The ABCDE diagnostic criteria for melanoma are instrumental in achieving a clinical diagnosis[43] (**Box 2**). Microscopic examination is indicated to rule out other conditions and arriving at a definitive diagnosis.

Management Malignant melanomas are treated by surgical procedure. Chemotherapy, radiotherapy, and immunotherapy have been used in the management of melanoma. Survival rate for melanomas is very low.

Connective Tissue Tumors

Benign connective tissue tumors of oral mucosa
Fibroma Fibroma is a benign proliferation of fibroblast resulting from trauma or irritation. Trauma from occlusal forces and irritation from dental materials are the most common reason for invitation of fibroma.

Box 2
ABCDE diagnostic criteria for melanoma

A—Asymmetry (one-half of the lesion does not symmetrically match with another half)

B—Border irregularity (borders of melanoma are blurred, notched, or ragged)

C—Color irregularity (pigmentation shows varied appearance, ie, brown, black, tan, red, white, and blue; all can be seen in the lesion)

D—Diameter (greatest diameter of the lesion is larger than 6 mm)

E—Elevation (surface of the lesion is elevated)

Clinical features Fibroma is characterized by painless, slow-growing nodular mass that is either sessile or pedunculated.[44] The size of the lesion is usually less than 1 or 2 cm. The surface may be ulcerated due to trauma. However, surface ulceration is not a consistent feature. The lesion has no specific location predominance but is seen frequently at the line of occlusion, that is, buccal mucosa or at the area of chronic trauma.[45]

Diagnosis and Management Clinical presentation is generally diagnostic. Conservative surgical excision is the treatment of choice with elimination of causative factor. Recurrences are uncommon.

Lipoma Lipoma is a benign tumor of adipose tissue and predominantly observed in trunk and proximities. Intraoral lipomas were reported in buccal mucosa. The exact cause remains unclear; however, few studies reported genetic influence in their occurrence.

Clinical features Lipoma is characterized by painless, slow-growing, smooth surface, sessile or pedunculated lobular mass. Superficial lipomaappears in yellow color, lipoma in deeper tissue appears normal mucosal color. The lesion is predominantly reported in adult population.[46]

Diagnosis and management Clinical appearance is generally diagnostic. Conservative surgical excision is the treatment of choice. Biopsied tissue usually floats in the fixative solution due to density of adipose tissue. Recurrences are uncommon.

Neurofibroma Neurofibroma is a benign peripheral nerve neoplasm that consists of 2 elements namely Schwann cells and fibroblasts. Neurofibromas can occur as multiple or solitary lesions. Intraoral lesions are predominantly solitary lesions.

Clinical features Neurofibroma is characterized by painless, slow-growing, small, and soft to firm nodules. Intraoral neurofibromas are often rare. However, when it occurs it is predominantly seen over tongue or buccal mucosa as solitary lesions. Intraosseous neurofibromas arise from central portion of bone.[47]

Diagnosis and management Radiological appearance of intraosseous neurofibromas are either well demarcated or poorly demarcated and uni- or multilocular. Surgical excision is the treatment of choice. Recurrence is not common. Individuals with solitary neurofibromas should be evaluated periodically for the multiple lesions.

Schwannoma (neurilemmoma) Neurilemmoma is a benign encapsulated neoplasm of nerve sheath that arises from Schwann cell origin. Approximately 25% to 48% neurilemmomas are from head and neck region.

Clinical features Neurilemmoma is a painless, slow-growing, encapsulated tumor that typically arises in association with nerve trunk.[48] Size of the swelling may range from few millimeters to centimeters. It is most commonly seen in young and middle-aged adults. Tongue is the most common site (**Fig. 7**).[49] Intrabony neurilemmomas are commonly reported in posterior mandible. Pain and paresthesia are not unusual for intrabony lesions.

Diagnosis and management Intrabony neurilemmomas radiologically appear as either unilocular or multilocular radiolucencies. Solitary lesions are managed by surgical excision. Recurrence is uncommon.[50]

Hemangioma Hemangioma is a developmental vascular anomaly or hamartoma rather than benign neoplasm. It occurs due to rapid growth of endothelial cells lining blood vessels and is frequently reported on infants and manifest within the first month of life.

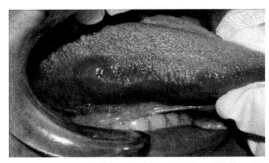

Fig. 7. Exophytic growth on the ride lateral surface of the tongue. (*From* López-Jornet P, Bermejo-Fenoll A. Neurilemmoma of the tongue. Oral Oncol Extra 2005;41(7):154–7; with permission.)

Clinical features Hemangioma is characterized by small, raised, brick red areas with firm and rubbery consistency. Superficial hemangiomas appear mucosal color, whereas deep lesions appear bluish. Approximately 4% to 5% of children younger than 1 year are affected. Female predilection is reported. They are frequently seen on white than other ethnic groups. Eighty percent of hemangiomas occur as solitary lesions, and 20% cases have concurrent occurrence with other tumors. Syndromes associated with hemangioma are given in **Box 3**.[43] Four variants of hemangiomas are capillary, cavernous, lobular, and arterial. Hemangiomas tend to regress.[51]

Diagnosis and management Clinical appearance is generally diagnostic. Management is employed based on aesthetic or functional needs of patient. Treatment options of hemangioma include surgery, radiotherapy, injection of sclerosing agents, cryotherapy, carbondioxide snow, and intralesional corticosteroids.[52]

Lymphangioma Lymphangioma is a benign hamartoma of lymphatic vessel than a true tumor. It arises due to developmental disturbance causing sequestration of lymphatic vessels. It is frequently in head and neck region. Intraoral lesions are reported on tongue.

Clinical features Lymphangiomas are predominantly reported on tongue. The tongue is enlarged, that is, macroglossia. Superficial lymphangioma is characterized by pebbled surface with numerous translucent vesicles of varying size. Men are commonly affected.[53] Three variants of lymphangioma are macro, microcystic, and mixed type (**Box 4**).

| Box 3 |
Syndromes associated with hemangiomas
Rendu-Osler-Weber syndrome
Struge-Weber-Dimitri syndrome
Kasabach-Merritt syndrome
Maffucci syndrome
Von Hippel-Lindau syndrome
Klippel-Trenaunay-Weber syndrome

| Box 4 |
Variants of lymphangioma
Macrocystic lymphangioma: cysticlike spaces more than 2 cm (eg, Cystic hygroma)
Microcystic lymphangioma: smaller vascular channels less than 2 cm in size
Mixed lymphangioma: combination of both macrocystic and microcystic

Diagnosis and management Clinical appearance is generally diagnostic. Management is employed based on aesthetic or functional needs of patient. Recurrences are common in lymphangioma. Treatment options include sclerosant, sodium tetradecyl sulfate and bleomycin. Head and neck lymphangiomas have a potential to cause obstruction to respiratory channel leading to death.

Osteoma Osteoma is a benign neoplasm of mature compact or cancellous bone. Cases have been reported on craniofacial and skeletal bones. Osteomas may arise from periosteal, endosteal, or extra-skeletal region. Osteomas result from injury, inflammation, or hamartomatous growth. Multiple osteomas are associated with Gardner syndrome.[54]

Clinical features Osteoma is characterized by slow-growing, well-defined, hard and asymptomatic swelling. Facial deformities are seen in unusually large osteomas. They are predominantly seen in adults. Condyle and body of mandible are common locations; other areas are angle of mandible, coronoid process, and ramus region. Lingual surface adjacent to premolars and molars are frequently observed with osteomas.

Diagnosis and management Radiologically osteoma appeared as well-defined and uniform-appearing radiopaque mass. Small and asymptomatic osteomas do not require any treatment, but periodic watch is important. Surgery is preferred when functional and aesthetic needs are important. Mouth opening and movement may be restricted due to osteomas at condyle or coronoid process.

Fibrosarcoma Fibrosarcoma is a malignant neoplasm of fibroblasts. Fibrosarcoma frequently occurs in extremities, and approximately 10% cases have been reported in head and neck region.

Clinical features Fibrosarcoma is characterized by slow-growing mass but reaches considerable size to cause disfigurement and pain. This lesion is common among young adults and children. Paranasal sinuses are common site in head and neck region. Intraoral lesions are uncommon.[55]

Diagnosis and management Microscopic examination of biopsied tissue is essential for final diagnosis. Wide surgical excision is the treatment of choice. Recurrence is seen in almost 50% of cases. The survival rate is approximately 5 years.

Osteosarcoma Osteosarcoma is a malignant neoplasm of mesenchymal with the ability to produce mineralized tissue. Osteosarcomas are the second common malignancy to arise from bone. Cause of osteosarcoma remains unclear; however, strong association was reported on genetics, radiation exposure, alkylating agents, and Paget disease. Distal femoral and proximal tibia metaphyses are commonly affected. Approximately 6% of cases constitute to gnathic osteosarcomas with predilection to mandible.

Table 4
Criteria for suspecting child abuse

	Yes	No
Physical findings: are there:		
Fresh bruises? Unusual locations or shapes?		
Old scars? Unusual locations or shapes?		
Past or current bums? Unusual locations or shapes?		
Signs of rectal, genital, or oral injury or infection?		
Medical experience:		
Is abuse or neglect suggested by:		
Current medical problems?		
Prior medical problems?		
Prior emergency visits—ingestions or trauma?		
Prior hospitalizations?		
Prior surgical interventions?		
Current or past venereal disease or pregnancy?		
Poor compliance with prior medical care or treatment?		
Incomplete immunizations for age?		
Poor mental or physical growth and development for age?		
Behavioral abnormalities: is there evidence of:		
Withdrawal or hyperactivity?		
Over compliance with physical examination?		
"Compliant posturing"?		
Phobias?		
Sleeping problems?		
Recent onset of enuresis or encopresis?		
"Sexualized play?"		
Excessive interest in genitalia?		
Psychosocial conditions: is there evidence of:		
Disturbed parent-child interaction?		
Violent interaction between parents?		
Violent interaction between siblings?		
Violent interaction with friends and relatives?		
Parents being abused as children?		
Parents being victims of sexual abuse?		
Extra stresses on the family?		
Marital discord?		
Unemployment?		
Alcoholism?		
Substance abuse?		
Recent death or illness in the family?		
Inappropriate custodial care of the child?		
Daytime?		
After school?		
Evening?		

(continued on next page)

Table 4 (continued)		
	Yes	No
Nights?		
Weekends?		
Inappropriate responsibilities for a child?		
Heavy chores such as cooking and housekeeping?		
Care of siblings?		
Family isolation?		
Lack of telephone?		
Lack of supportive relatives, friends, or neighbors to whom they can turn in a crisis situation?		
Previous referrals for abuse or neglect?		

From Schachner L, Hankin DE. Assessing child abuse in childhood condylomaacuminatum. J Am Acad Dermatol. 1985;12(1 Pt 1):157-60; with permission.

Clinical features Osteosarcomas are seen in both young and elderly age range. Osteosarcoma is characterized by swelling, pain, loosening of teeth, nasal obstruction, or paresthesia. Osteosarcomas of maxillae may be seen on alveolar ridge, sinus floor, palate.[56]

Diagnosis and management Radiologically osteosarcomas are recognized by radiopaque, mixed radiolucency with ill-defined borders. The elevation of the periosteum may give sun-ray or sun-burst appearance. Root resorption with symmetric generalized widening of the periodontal ligament space is a diagnostic clue for osteosarcoma. Management includes surgery, chemotherapy, and radiotherapy. Approximately 60% to 80% cases showed 5-year survival rate. Prognosis is somewhat better in gnathic osteosarcomas. Metastasis is frequently reported.

Oral Lesions Associated with Child Abuse

Child abuse is a one of the major social and health problems and often results from physical, sexual, and emotional abuses or neglect. It affects physical, cognitive, or emotion growth of child that may extend into adulthood. Child abuse is a wide topic for discussion; however, the context of explanation in this article is to recognize oral lesions that serve as possible markers for child abuse. Oral lesions associated with child abuse are herpes simplex, Epstein–Barr virus, cytomegalovirus, gonorrhea, molluscum contagiosum, and condyloma accuminatum. The discussion of condyloma accuminatum is made here due to linkage with benign neoplasm of oral cavity.

Condyloma accuminatum

Condyloma accuminatum is a benign epithelial neoplasm that is associated with HPV types 2, 6, 11, 53, and 54 often seen predominantly in genital, perianal region. HPV types 16, 18, and 31 are associated with anal lesions. The lesion can be seen in oral and laryngeal mucosa. The lesion is a sexually transmitted disease with development of lesion at the area of sexual contact.[57] Lawrence and colleagues stated that "Childhood condyloma accuminatum may often, but not always, be a manifestation of sexual abuse." They had provided a check-list criterion for suspecting child abuse, which cover 4 main areas: physical findings, medical experience, behavioral abnormalities, and psychosocial conditions. Any "yes" response to the checklist (**Table 4**) mandates a Child Protective Services consultation.[58] Condyloma accuminatum is diagnosed in young adults and frequently observed in labial mucosa, soft palate, and labial frenum.[43] Condyloma accuminatum is characterized by painless, slow-growing, well-demarcated, nontender, sessile, pink-colored exophytic growth with short and blunt surface projects. The size of the lesion varies between 0.5 and 2.0 cm. Microscopic examination is required for arriving final diagnosis. Immunohistochemical analysis of biopsied tissue is necessary for identification of HPV types in the pathology specimen. The lesion is managed by conservative surgical excision. The lesions associated with HPV types 16 and 18 have a potential for malignant transformation to OSCC.[59]

SUMMARY

General dentist has the training to identify a wide variety of oral conditions. Unfortunately, diagnostic skills are likely to fade due to uncommon prevalence of these conditions. The important step in approaching patients with these conditions is to provide critical insight to signs and symptoms presented. Comprehensive clinical examination will enable the dentist to identify whether the condition is reactive, benign, or malignant oral disease. The dentist should take a special initiative while handling oral disease cases for diagnosis and management. In doubt, or when the lesions are challenging, the patient must be referred timely to oral medicine, oral pathologists, or oral surgeon for further evaluation and management.

REFERENCES

1. Scully C, Porter S. Oral cancer. West J Med 2001;174(5):348–51.
2. Rivera C. Essentials of oral cancer. Int J ClinExpPathol 2015;8(9):11884–94.
3. Bryson TC, Shah GV, Srinivasan A, et al. Cervical lymph node evaluation and diagnosis. Otolaryngol Clin North Am 2012;45(6):1363–83.
4. Gaddey HL, Riegel AM. Unexplained lymphadenopathy: evaluation and differential diagnosis. Am Fam Physician 2016;94(11):896–903.
5. Warnakulasuriya S, Johnson NW, van der Waal I. Nomenclature and classification of potentially malignant disorders of the oral mucosa. J Oral Pathol Med 2007; 36(10):575–80.
6. Warnakulasuriya S. Global epidemiology of oral and oropharyngeal cancer. Oral Oncol 2009;45(4–5):309–16.
7. Chigurupati A, Poosarla C, Reddy GS, et al. Oral mucosal lichen planus in children – Report of three cases. J Orofac Sci 2011;3(1):20–3.
8. Olson MA, Rogers RS 3rd, Bruce AJ. Oral lichen planus. Clin Dermatol 2016; 34(4):495–504.
9. Babu RA, Chandrashekar P, Kumar KK, et al. A study on oral mucosal lesions in 3500 patients with dermatological diseases in South India. Ann Med Health Sci Res 2014;4(Suppl 2):S84–93.
10. Giuliani M, Troiano G. Rate of malignant transformation of oral lichen planus: a systematic review. Oral Dis 2019;25(3):693–709.
11. Villa A, Villa C, Abati S. Oral cancer and oral erythroplakia: an update and implication for clinicians. Aust Dent J 2011;56(3):253–6.
12. Warnakulasuriya S. Clinical features and presentation of oral potentially malignant disorders. Oral Surg Oral Med Oral Pathol Oral Radiol 2018;125(6):582–90.

13. Masthan KMK, Babu NA, Sankari SL, et al. Leukoplakia: a short review on malignant potential. J Pharm BioalliedSci 2015;7(Suppl 1):S165–6.

14. Kumar A, Cascarini L, McCaul JA, et al. How should we manage oral leukoplakia? Br J Oral Maxillofac Surg 2013;51(5):377–83.

15. van der Waal I, Axell T. Oral leukoplakia: a proposal for uniform reporting. Oral Oncol 2002;38(6):521–6.

16. Babu B, Hallikeri K. Reactive lesions of oral cavity: a retrospective study of 659 cases. J Indian Soc Periodontol 2017;21(4):258–63.

17. Punde PA, Malik SA, Malik NA, et al. Idiopathic huge pyogenic granuloma in young and old: An unusually large lesion in two cases. J Oral Maxillofac Pathol 2013;17(3):463–6.

18. Deore GD, Gurav AN, Patil R, et al. Sclerotherapy: a novel bloodless approach to treat recurrent oral pyogenic granuloma associated with port-wine stain. Ann Vasc Surg 2014;28(6):1564.e9-14.

19. Prasanth T, Chundru NS, ArvindBabu RS, et al. Peripheral ossifying fibroma: report of 2 cases. Dentaires Revista 2012;4(2):22–5.

20. Mishra MB, Bhishen KA, Mishra S. Peripheral ossifying fibroma. J Oral MaxillofacPathol 2011;15(1):65–8.

21. Abu Gharbyah AZ, Assaf M. Management of a peripheral giant cell granuloma in the esthetic area of upper jaw: a case report. Int J Surg Case Rep 2014;5(11):779–82.

22. Tandon PN, Gupta SK, Gupta DS, et al. Peripheral giant cell granuloma. Contemp Clin Dent 2012;3(Suppl 1):S118–21.

23. Gual-Vaqués P, Jané-Salas E, Egido-Moreno S, et al. Inflammatory papillary hyperplasia: a systematic review. Med Oral Patol Oral Cir Bucal 2016;22(1):e36–42.

24. Infante-Cossio P, Martinez-de-Fuentes R, Torres-Carranza E, et al. Inflammatory papillary hyperplasia of the palate: treatment with carbon dioxide laser, followed by restoration with an implant-supported prosthesis. Br J Oral Maxillofac Surg 2007;45(8):658–60.

25. Shukla P, Dahiya V, Kataria P, et al. Inflammatory hyperplasia: from diagnosis to treatment. J Indian Soc Periodontol 2014;18(1):92–4.

26. Jaimes M, Munante J, Olate S, et al. Inflammatory fibrous hyperplasia treated with a modified vestibuloplasty: a case report. J Contemp Dent Pract 2008;9(3):135–41.

27. Chaitanya P, Martha S, Punithvathy R, et al. Squamous papilloma on hard palate: case report and literature review. Int J Clin Pediatr Dent 2018;11(3):244–6.

28. Carneiro TE, Marinho SA, Verli FD, et al. Oral squamous papilloma: clinical, histologic and immunohistochemical analyses. J Oral Sci 2009;51(3):367–72.

29. Mattoo A, Bhatia M. Verruca vulgaris of the buccal mucosa: a case report. J Cancer Res Ther 2018;14(2):454–6.

30. Alawi F. Pigmented lesions of the oral cavity: an update. Dent Clin North Am 2013;57(4):699–710.

31. Ho AW, Sato R, Ramsdell A. JAAD grand rounds quiz. A case of oral melanosis. J Am Acad Dermatol 2014;71(5):1030–3.

32. Gondak R-O, da Silva-Jorge R, Jorge J, et al. Oral pigmented lesions: clinicopathologicfeatures and review of the literature. Med Oral Patol Oral Cir Bucal 2012;17(6):e919–24.

33. MarangonJúnior H, Souza PEA, Soares RV, et al. Oral congenital melanocytic nevus: a rare case report and review of the literature. Head Neck Pathol 2015; 9(4):481–7.

34. Gombra V, Kaur M, Sircar K, et al. Pigmented oral compound nevus of retromolar area - a rare case report. Singapore Dent J 2016;37:33–5.

35. Ramos LMA, Cardoso SV, Loyola AM, et al. Keratoacanthoma of the inferior lip: review and report of case with spontaneous regression. J Appl Oral Sci 2009; 17(3):262–5.

36. RajendraSantosh AB, Cumberbatch K, Jones T. Post-glossectomy in lingual carcinomas: a scope for sign language in rehabilitation. Contemp Oncol (Pozn) 2017;21(2):123–30.

37. Pires FR, Ramos AB, Oliveira JB, et al. Oral squamous cell carcinoma: clinico-pathological features from 346 cases from a single oral pathology service during an 8-year period. J Appl Oral Sci 2013;21(5):460–7.

38. Gudiseva S, Santosh ABR, Chitturi R, et al. The role of mast cells in oral squamous cell carcinoma. Contemp Oncol (Pozn) 2017;21(1):21–9.

39. Norling R, Buron BMD, Therkildsen MH, et al. Staging of cervical lymph nodes in oral squamous cell carcinoma: adding ultrasound in clinically lymph node negative patients may improve diagnostic work-up. PLoS One 2014;9(3): e90360.

40. Poosarla C, RajendraSantosh AB, Gudiseva S, et al. Histomolecularstructural aspects of high endothelial vessels in lymph node and its significance in oral cancer and metastasis. North Am J Med Sci 2015;7(12):540–6.

41. Alkan A, Bulut E, Gunhan O, et al. Oral verrucous carcinoma: a study of 12 cases. Eur J Dent 2010;4(2):202–7.

42. Feller L, Khammissa RAG, Kramer B, et al. Basal cell carcinoma, squamous cell carcinoma and melanoma of the head and face. Head Face Med 2016;12:11.

43. Neville BW, Damm DD, Allen CM. Textbook of oral and maxillofacial pathology. 2nd edition. Saunder's Company; 2002.

44. Santosh ABR, Boyd D, Laxminarayana KK. Proposed clinico-pathological classification for oral exophytic lesions. J Clin Diagn Res 2015;9(9):ZE01–8.

45. Kolte AP, Kolte RA, Shrirao TS. Focal fibrous overgrowths: a case series and review of literature. Contemp Clin Dent 2010;1(4):271–4.

46. Hoseini AT, Razavi SM, Khabazian A. Lipoma in oral mucosa: two case reports. Dent Res J (Isfahan) 2010;7(1):41–3.

47. Bharath TS, Krishna YR, Nalabolu GR, et al. Neurofibroma of the palate. Case Rep Dent 2014;2014:898505.

48. Babu RSA, Reddy BVR, Chigurupati A. Histogenetic concepts, terminology and categorization of biphasic tumours of the oral and maxillofacial region. J ClinDiagn Res 2014;8(2):266–70.

49. PíaLópez-Jornet A-F. Neurilemmoma of the tongue. Oral Oncology Extra 2005; 41(7):154–7.

50. Shim S-K, Myoung H. Neurilemmoma in the floor of the mouth: a case report. J Korean Assoc Oral Maxillofac Surg 2016;42(1):60–4.

51. Agarwal S. Treatment of oral hemangioma with 3% sodium tetradecyl sulfate: study of 20 cases. Indian J Otolaryngol Head Neck Surg 2012;64(3):205–7.

52. Ogle OE, Santosh AB. Medication management of jaw lesions for dental patients. Dent Clin North Am 2016;60(2):483–95.

53. da Silva WB, Ribeiro AL, de Menezes SA, et al. Oral capillary hemangioma: a clinical protocol of diagnosis and treatment in adults. Oral Maxillofac Surg 2014; 18(4):431–7.

54. Koh K-J, Park H-N, Kim K-A. Gardner syndrome associated with multiple oste-omas, intestinal polyposis, and epidermoid cysts. Imaging Sci Dent 2016;46(4): 267–72.
55. Reddy AVS, Prakash AR, Ram VS, et al. Intra oral fibrosarcoma with various his-topathological patterns: a rare case report. J Clin Diagn Res 2015;9(7):ED04–6.
56. Chaudhary M, Chaudhary SD. Osteosarcoma of jaws. J Oral Maxillofac Pathol 2012;16(2):233–8.
57. Percinoto ACC, Danelon M, Crivelini MM, et al. Condylomaacuminata in the tongue and palate of a sexually abused child: a case report. BMC Res Notes 2014;7:467.
58. Schachner L, Hankin DE. Assessing child abuse in childhood condylomaacumi-natum. J Am Acad Dermatol 1985;12(1 Pt 1):157–60.
59. Kui LL, Xiu HZ, Ning LY. Condylomaacuminatum and human papilloma virus infection in the oral mucosa of children. Pediatr Dent 2003;25(2):149–53.

Nonodontogenic Cysts

Rawle Fabian Philbert, DDS*, Navraj Singh Sandhu, BSc, DMD

KEYWORDS

- Nonodontogenic • Cyst • Pseudocyst • Jaws • Oral • Maxillofacial

KEY POINTS

- Nonodontogenic cysts of the jaws are not a common occurrence and occur much less frequently than odontogenic cysts of the jaws.
- Nonodontogenic cysts of the jaws most commonly encountered are the nasopalatine duct canal cyst, nasolabial cyst, traumatic bone cyst, Stafne bone cyst, aneurysmal bone cyst, and focal osteoporotic bone marrow defect.
- Nonodontogenic cysts of the oral and maxillofacial complex (excluding the jaws) commonly seen are the dermoid cyst, epidermoid cyst, pilar cyst, and sebaceous cyst.
- It is important that general dentists are able to recognize these nonodontogenic cysts of the oral and maxillofacial complex to adequately manage or make an appropriate referral to reduce patient morbidity.

INTRODUCTION

A cyst is a pathologic cavity lined by epithelium and filled with fluid or semifluid content and may either locate in soft tissue or within the jaw bone, originating in odontogenic or nonodontogenic tissues. Jaw bones show predilection for odontogenic cysts, whereas nonodontogenic cysts are uncommon. Both odontogenic and nonodontogenic cysts produce radiolucent defects causing destruction of osseous structure. Hence it is essential to understand clinical behavior and management strategies, and failure to treat at the right time may increase patient morbidity. This article focuses on the clinical presentation, investigation findings, and treatment options of nonodontogenic cysts of the jaw. The conditions discussed in this article are listed in **Box 1**.

Nasopalatine Duct Canal Cyst

Nasopalatine duct canal cyst is also known as an incisive canal cyst or median palatine cyst when it is located more posterior in the palate (**Fig. 1**). These cysts are

Disclosure: The authors have nothing to disclose.
Oral & Maxillofacial Surgery, Lincoln Medical & Mental Health Center, 234 East 149th Street, Bronx, NY 10451, USA
* Corresponding author.
E-mail address: rawle.Philbert@nychhc.org

Dent Clin N Am 64 (2020) 63–85
https://doi.org/10.1016/j.cden.2019.08.006
0011-8532/20/© 2019 Elsevier Inc. All rights reserved.

dental.theclinics.com

Box 1
Types of nonodontogenic cysts discussed in this article

- Nasopalatine duct canal cyst
- Nasolabial cyst
- Traumatic bone cyst
- Stafne cyst
- Aneurysmal bone cyst
- Focal osteoporotic bone marrow defect
- Epidermoid cyst
- Dermoid cyst
- Pilar cyst
- Sebaceous cyst

typically located in the nasopalatine canal or in the palatal soft tissues where the canal opens. This cyst is the most common nonodontogenic cyst in the oral cavity. Prevalence of this cyst is 2.2% to 11.6% of the population, or 1 out of every 100 individuals.[1] A nasopalatine duct canal cyst forms from the proliferation of the right and left palatine processes to the premaxilla. Anatomically, the exit of the canal is slightly posterior to the incisive papilla. Typically, the nasopalatine duct degenerates in humans; however, the epithelial remnants remain and have the potential for cystic enlargement. The most likely cause of the nasopalatine duct canal cyst is persistence of the epithelial remnants following duct degeneration.[2] The exact stimulus to cystic formation at this time is unknown.

PATIENT HISTORY

Nasopalatine duct canal cyst has a male predilection of 3:1.[1,3,4] Median palatine cyst has a male predilection of 4:1.[5] They are most common in the fourth to sixth decades,

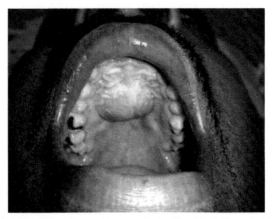

Fig. 1. Midline palatal swelling. (*From* Manzon S, Graffeo M, Philbert R. Median palatal cyst: case report and review of literature. J Oral Maxillofac Surg. 2009;67:926–30; with permission.)

although they can be seen at any age. Median age is 42.5 years.[2] Usually they are identified as an asymptomatic palatal midline swelling by the patient or the dentist on clinical examination. The patient may complain of symptoms if the cyst is secondarily inflamed or infected.

INTRAORAL EXAMINATION

Cysts present as symmetric swelling in the anterior region of the midline palate or as midline radiolucency on radiographs (**Fig. 2**). They are usually asymptomatic, with midline swelling that is suspicious for a lesion on clinical examination. Symptoms can arise from secondary infection. Sinus formation and drainage at the palatine papilla may be seen if infected. The rates of symptomatic lesions are variable in the literature and do not follow any predictable patterns, such as age or size.[6]

IMAGING AND ADDITIONAL TESTING

Radiographically, the lesion is a well-circumscribed, round, ovoid, or heart-shaped radiolucency near the maxillary incisors (**Figs. 3** and **4**).The nasopalatine duct cysts range in size from several millimeters to centimeters; the average size is 1.5 cm.[7] Lamina dura of adjacent teeth is intact, but lesions can cause divergence of the roots of the maxillary incisor teeth and less commonly are known to cause external root resorption. The lesion can appear heart-shaped because of the superimposition of the anterior nasal spine. Histopathologically, the epithelial lining of this cyst ranges from stratified squamous to pseudostratified columnar in areas close to the nasal cavity. The connective tissue contains a nasopalatine neurovascular bundle composed of arteries and nerves (**Fig. 5**).

TREATMENT

Treatment via surgical enucleation is curative without recurrence.[5] Marsupialization of larger lesions before enucleation can be considered. The recurrence rate of this lesion is low.

Nasolabial Cyst

Nasolabial cysts are soft tissue cysts of the upper lip. These cysts are very rare, comprising 0.7% of all jaw cysts.[8,9] The cyst is found in the upper lip, lateral to the midline or in the region of the lateral and canine teeth. The pathogenesis of the cyst

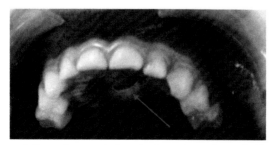

Fig. 2. Clinical presentation of nasopalatine duct canal cyst (*arrow*). (*From* Abramowicz S, Padwa BL. Pediatric head and neck tumors: benign lesions. In Bagheri SC, Bell RB, Khan HA, editors. Current therapy in oral and maxillofacial surgery. St. Louis: Saunders; 2012. p. 813–20; with permission).

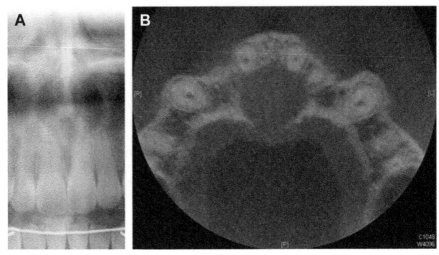

Fig. 3. (*A*) Nasopalatine duct canal cyst on panorex. Note the heart-shaped radiolucency. (*B*) Nasopalatine duct canal cyst on computed tomography axial view, bony window. (*From* Jones RS, Dillon J. Nonodontogenic cysts of the jaws and treatment in the pediatric population. Oral Maxillofacial Surg Clin N Am 2016;28:31–44; with permission)

is unclear; although a few theories do exist. One theory suggests that this cyst arises from nasolacrimal duct ectopic epithelium.[4] Another theory suggests that this cyst arises from epithelial remnants at the fusion line of the medial and lateral nasal processes during embryogenesis.[10]

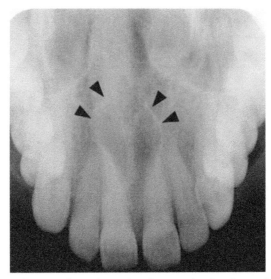

Fig. 4. Nasopalatine duct canal cyst (arrowhead) on occlusal radiograph. (*From* Kaneda T, Weber AL, Scrivani SJ, et al. Cysts, tumors, and nontumorous lesions of the jaw. In Som, PM, Curtin, HD, editors. Head and neck imaging. 5th ed. St. Louis: Mosby; 2011. p. 1469–1546; with permission.)

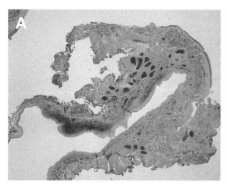
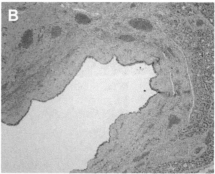

Fig. 5. (A) Histopathology of nasopalatine duct canal cyst; low power (hematoxylin-eosin [H&E], original magnification ×20). (B) Histopathology of nasopalatine duct canal cyst; high power. Note nasopalatine neurovascular bundle in connective tissue (H&E, original magnification ×100). (Courtesy of Elizabeth Philipone, DMD, Oral Pathology Residency Program Director, Columbia University Medical Center, New York, NY.)

PATIENT HISTORY

This lesion is generally noted in the fourth and fifth decades. There is a female predilection of nearly 4:1. It is usually asymptomatic, unless it becomes secondarily infected.

INTRAORAL EXAMINATION

This lesion presents as upper lip swelling, elevated ala of the nose, obliteration of the vestibule, and elevation of the mucosa of the nasal vestibule[7] (**Fig. 6**). Patients commonly complain of facial deformity.[11] Nasolabial cysts are bilateral in 10% of cases[12] (**Fig. 7**).

IMAGING AND ADDITIONAL TESTING

Because nasolabial cysts are soft tissue lesions, they are not seen on traditional plain film radiographs. Cone beam computed tomography (CT), traditional CT, and MRI

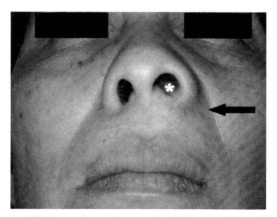

Fig. 6. Unilateral nasolabial cyst shows characteristic blunting of nasolabial fold (asterisk), elevation of nasal ala, and protrusion of upper lip (arrow). (From Yuen H, Julian C, Samuel C. Nasolabial cysts: clinical features, diagnosis, and treatment. Br J Oral Maxillofac Surg. 2007;45(4):293–7; with permission).

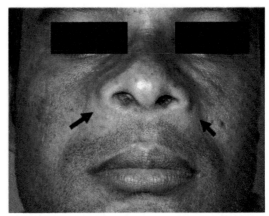

Fig. 7. Rare case of bilateral nasolabial cysts (*arrows*). (*From* Yuen H, Julian C, Samuel C. Nasolabial cysts: clinical features, diagnosis, and treatment. Br J Oral Maxillofac Surg. 2007;45(4):293–7; with permission).

show a well-circumscribed soft tissue mass of varying size[7] (**Fig. 8**). Histopathologically, the epithelial lining of the cyst is pseudostratified columnar epithelium with abundant goblet cells. Some cysts have stratified squamous epithelium as well as cuboidal epithelium[4] (**Fig. 9**).

TREATMENT

The traditional approach to treatment is surgical excision via an intraoral or sublabial approach.[7] Because of proximity to nasal mucosa and floor, nasal mucosa may need to be excised in order to completely remove the cyst. This treatment can lead to an oronasal fistula, which requires surgical repair. Endoscopic marsupialization via a transnasal approach is another treatment modality.[7]

PSEUDOCYSTS
Traumatic Bone Cyst

This lesion is also known as a simple bone cyst, hemorrhagic cyst, intraosseous hematoma, idiopathic bone cyst, extravasation bone cyst, solitary bone cyst, or solitary bone cavity.[7] The term cyst is a misnomer because this lesion lacks an epithelial lining. The pathogenesis of traumatic bone cyst formation is not known. Some cases can be attributed to prior trauma, which results in hematoma formation within the intramedullary region of bone. Rather than going through the organization process, the clot breaks down, leaving an empty cavity. Other causes include cystic degeneration of primary tumors of bone, such as central giant cell granuloma; ischemic necrosis of bone; and calcium metabolism disorders.[13]

Patient history
Teenagers are most commonly affected, but traumatic bone cysts have been reported in many age ranges.[7] There is an equal gender predilection,[7] and it can be associated with swelling. Patients are usually asymptomatic. It can be seen in association with florid osseous dysplasia.

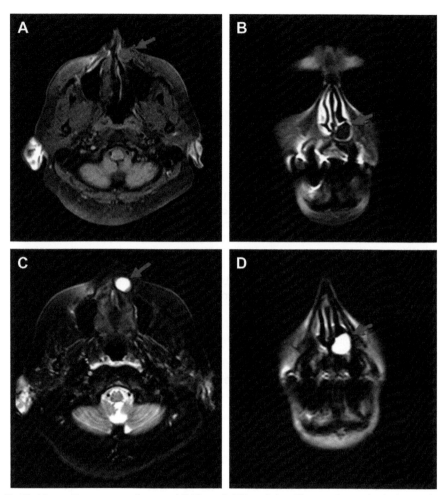

Fig. 8. Magnetic resonance images. (*A*) The axial T1-weighted image shows the lesion with a homogeneous hypointensity (*arrow*). (*B*) The coronal T1-weighted image shows the lesion with hypointense area in the lower left nasal fossa (arrow). (*C*) The axial T2-weighted image shows the well-circumscribed lesion with a homogeneous hyperintensity (*arrow*). (*D*) The coronal T2-weighted image shows the lesion with hyperintense area in the lower left nasal fossa (*arrow*). (*From* Sumer AP, Celenk P, Sumer M, et al. Nasolabial cyst: case report with CT and MRI findings. Oral Surg Oral Med Oral Pathol Oral Radiol Endod. 2010;109(2):e92–4; with permission).

Intraoral examination

Traumatic bone cyst usually presents as an asymptomatic lesion. Traumatic bone cavity is an empty dead space in medullary bone. It is most frequently reported in the mandible, with a predilection for the anterior region.[7] There are a few reports of bilateral cases. Surrounding teeth are usually vital.

Imaging and additional testing

Traumatic bone cyst is most often found as an incidental finding on dental radiographs.[7] On dental radiographs, the lesion is a well-circumscribed irregularly shaped

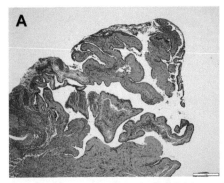
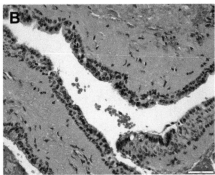

Fig. 9. (*A*) Histopathology of nasolabial cyst; low power (H&E, original magnification ×40). (*B*) Histopathology of nasolabial cyst; high power. Note pseudostratified columnar epithelium with goblet cells (H&E, original magnification ×400). (*Courtesy of* Elizabeth Philipone, DMD, Oral Pathology Residency Program Director, Columbia University Medical Center, New York, NY.)

area of radiolucency with poorly defined borders (**Fig. 10**). Inter-radicular scalloping and mild root resorption may be seen. Histopathologically, minimal amounts of fibrous tissue from the bony wall may be seen (**Fig. 11**). Lesions can be empty or include blood or sanguinous fluid.[14] This cyst lacks epithelial lining, and hence is called a pseudocyst. Giant cells adjacent to the bone surface are seen in some cases.[15]

Treatment
The lesion is managed by a surgical procedure, and surgical entry into the lesion initiates bleeding to assist in normal healing. Blood clot formation results in bony repair without recurrence.

Stafne Bone Cyst

Stafne cyst is a pseudocyst.[16] It is also known as a static bone cyst. It is a developmental defect that is an anatomic indentation of the posterior lingual cortex of the mandible into the medullary space and resembles a cyst on radiographs. This bone pseudocyst usually contains submandibular salivary gland tissue or fat. The cause of the lesion is unknown. Some investigators suggest that the lesion is caused by entrapment of salivary gland or other soft tissue during mandible development. Other

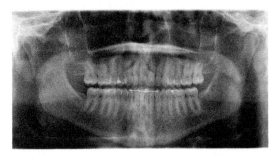

Fig. 10. Panorex of a traumatic bone cavity of the left mandibular ramus. (*From* Jones RS, Dillon J. Nonodontogenic cysts of the jaws and treatment in the pediatric population. Oral Maxillofacial Surg Clin N Am 2016;28:31–44; with permission.)

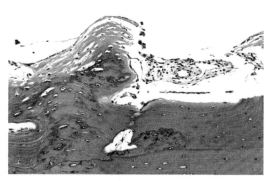

Fig. 11. Traumatic bone cyst consisting of connective tissue fragments lining surrounding bone (*bottom*). (*From* Regezi JA, Sciubba JJ, Jordan RCK. Cysts of the jaws and neck. In: Oral pathology: clinical pathologic correlations. 7th edition. St. Louis: Elsevier; 2017. p. 245–68; with permission.)

possible explanations include lingual mandibular cortical erosion from hyperplastic salivary gland tissue.

Patient history and intraoral examination
Almost all cases involve adults, most often men. The lesion is always asymptomatic and is often discovered as an incidental finding on dental panoramic radiographs. The patients are usually asymptomatic, and no specific clinical changes are observed.

Imaging and additional testing
On a dental panoramic radiograph, it appears as a well-circumscribed oval radiolucency located between the inferior alveolar canal and inferior border of the posterior mandible (**Fig. 12**). Occasionally it is bilateral and, rarely, anterior to the mandibular first molar. CT and MRI show tissue with the same appearance as fat in the defect, or salivary gland tissue from adjacent salivary gland into defect[17] (**Fig. 13**).

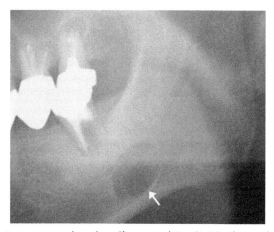

Fig. 12. Stafne cyst on panorex imaging. Shows oval "cavity" in the angle of mandible (*arrow*) below mandibular canal. (*From* Kaneda T, Weber AL, Scrivani SJ, et al. Cysts, tumors, and nontumorous lesions of the jaw. In Som, PM, Curtin, HD, editors. Head and neck imaging. 5th ed. St. Louis: Mosby; 2011. p. 1469–1546; with permission.)

A **B**

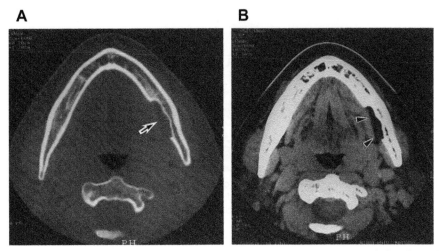

Fig. 13. Stafne bone cyst. (*A*) Axial CT (bone tissue window setting) shows a defect (*arrow*) with adjacent thinning of the lingual cortex. Note that the cortex is complete along the lateral aspect of the abnormality. (*B*) Axial CT (soft tissue window setting) shows the static bone cavity containing adjacent fat (*arrowheads*). (*From* Kaneda T, Weber AL, Scrivani SJ, et al. Cysts, tumors, and nontumorous lesions of the jaw. In Som, PM, Curtin, HD, editors. Head and neck imaging. 5th ed. St. Louis: Mosby; 2011. p. 1469–1546; with permission.)

Treatment
The appearance of Stafne bone cyst is usually pathognomonic. No treatment is required.

Aneurysmal Bone Cyst

Aneurysmal bone cyst is an uncommon lesion of the jaws, most often present in long bones. Within the craniofacial complex, approximately 40% of lesions are located in the mandible and 25% are located in the maxilla.[18] It lacks epithelial lining, and therefore is called a pseudocyst. The World Health Organization describes this lesion as an expansile, multilocular, osteolytic lesion, with blood-filled spaced separated by fibrous septa-containing osteoclast-type giant cells and reactive bone.[15] The prevalence of this lesion is 0.4%.[19] The cause is unknown, but many theories have been proposed, including vascular abnormalities leading to high-pressure hemorrhage, reactive cause, and possible genetic predisposition.[19,20] Trauma is another possible cause.

Patient history
Aneurysmal bone cyst typically occurs in patients less than 30 years old, with a peak incidence in second decade of life. Most studies find no gender predilection.[3,6,21] It commonly presents as a painless swelling. Pain is usually associated when aneurysmal bone cyst grows quickly.

Intraoral examination
Aneurysmal bone cyst is found more often in mandible than maxilla, particularly in the posterior mandible; specifically, the ramus and posterior body account for 51.7% of lesions[7] (**Fig. 14**). Aneurysmal bone cyst can also be found in the zygoma, sphenoid, ethmoid, and temporal and occipital bones.[7] Firm, nonpulsatile swelling is a common clinical sign. No associated thrill or bruit is heard on auscultation, but crepitus may be

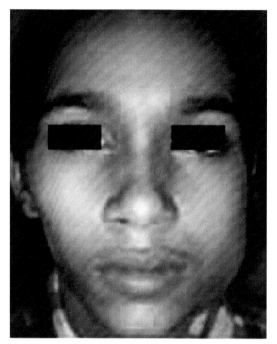

Fig. 14. Aneurysmal bone cyst of left angle of mandible. Note facial asymmetry. (*From* Kumar VV, Malik NA, Kumar DB. Treatment of large recurrent aneurysmal bone cysts of mandible: transosseous intralesional embolization as an adjunct to resection. Int J Oral Maxillofac Surg. 2009;38:671–6; with permission).

noted on firm palpation. Aspiration yields blood in some cases. Teeth remain vital; however, they can be displaced, become loose, and resorption may be seen.[22]

Imaging and additional testing
Radiographically, it is a destructive or osteolytic process with slight irregular margins (**Fig. 15**). It may be unilocular or multilocular, with or without well-defined borders. Multilocular lesions, like central giant cell granuloma, have a soap-bubble appearance. If present in the maxillary or mandibular alveolus, teeth may be displaced with or without external root resorption. Histopathologically, fibrous connective tissue stroma includes variable numbers of multinucleated giant cells (**Fig. 16**). Fibroblasts and macrophages line sinusoidal blood spaces. Aneurysmal bone cyst is similar to central giant cell granuloma. Reactive new bone formation is common.

Treatment
Excision or curettage with supplemental cryotherapy is the preferred treatment. Simple curettage has a high recurrence rate.[21]

Focal Osteoporotic Bone Marrow Defect

Focal osteoporotic bone marrow defects are also known as hematopoietic bone marrow defects. These lesions appear as radiolucencies in areas where hematopoiesis occurs. These areas include the mandibular angle and maxillary tuberosity in the jaws. The pathogenesis of this lesion is unknown, but 3 theories have been proposed. The first theory states that abnormal healing following tooth extraction may cause this

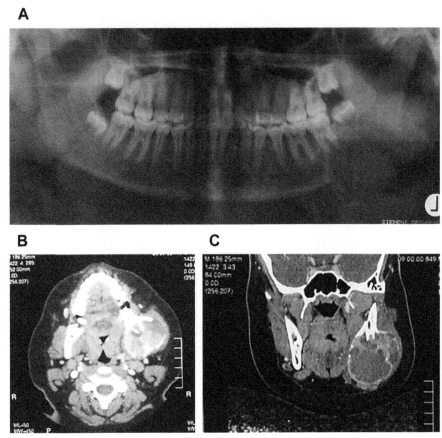

Fig. 15. (A) Panorex of an aneurysmal bone cyst of the left mandible. (B) Aneurysmal bone cyst of the left mandible. Axial-view CT with soft tissue window. (C) Aneurysmal bone cyst of the left mandible. Coronal-view CT with bone window. (*From* Jones RS, Dillon J. Nonodontogenic cysts of the jaws and treatment in the pediatric population. Oral Maxillofacial Surg Clin N Am. 2016;28:31–44; with permission.)

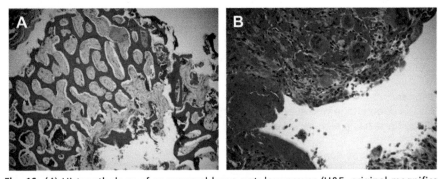

Fig. 16. (A) Histopathology of aneurysmal bone cyst; low power (H&E, original magnification ×10). (B) Histopathology of aneurysmal bone cyst; high power. Note multinucleated giant cells (H&E, original magnification ×40). (*From* Jones RS, Dillon J. Nonodontogenic cysts of the jaws and treatment in the pediatric population. Oral Maxillofacial Surg Clin N Am. 2016;28:31–44; with permission.)

lesion. The second theory states that residual remnants of fetal marrow may persist into adulthood. The third theory states that this lesion may represent a site of extramedullary hematopoiesis that becomes hyperplastic in adulthood.

Patient history and intraoral examination
This defect is asymptomatic, and is commonly found as an incidental finding on radiographs. These lesions do not commonly present with clinical symptoms or signs.

Imaging and additional testing
Radiographically, it appears as a poorly defined radiolucency (**Fig. 17**). Incisional biopsy is usually required to establish a definitive diagnosis. Histopathologically, there is an abundance of hematopoietic cells with few fat cells (**Fig. 18**). Within the cellular marrow, small lymphoid aggregates may be seen, alongside megakaryocytes.

Treatment
No treatment is required.

NONMUCOSAL CYSTS
Dermoid Cyst

Dermoid cysts are developmental lesions.[18] They occur throughout the body. In the oral cavity, they are usually located in the anterior floor of the mouth in the midline. The cause of lesions in the floor of the mouth is thought to be developmental entrapment of multipotent cells or implantation of epithelium.[18]

Patient history and intraoral examination
No gender predilection is reported. Dermoid cysts are asymptomatic and grow slowly.[18] The most common location in the oral and maxillofacial region is the periorbital lateral eyebrow area. It appears as an elevated, well-defined lesion on the skin. The clinical presentation intraorally depends on where the dermoid cyst is located. If located above the mylohyoid muscle, displacement of the tongue can occur superiorly and posteriorly[18] (**Fig. 19**). If located below the mylohyoid muscle, midline

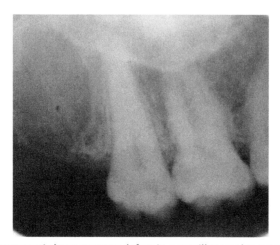

Fig. 17. Focal osteoporotic bone marrow defect in a maxillary molar extraction site. (*From* Regezi JA, Sciubba JJ, Jordan RCK. Cysts of the jaws and neck. In: Oral pathology: clinical pathologic correlations, 7th edition. St. Louis: Elsevier; 2017. p. 245–68; with permission.)

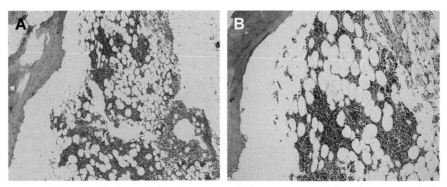

Fig. 18. (A) Histopathology of focal osteoporotic bone marrow defect; low power (H&E, original magnification ×100). (B) Histopathology of focal osteoporotic bone marrow defect; high power. Note maturing blood cells and megakaryocytes (H&E, original magnification ×200). (*Courtesy of* Elizabeth Philipone, DMD, Oral Pathology Residency Program Director, Columbia University Medical Center, New York, NY.)

swelling of the neck occurs[18] (**Fig. 20**). They are commonly small lesions, less than 2 cm in diameter, but there are reported cases of dermoid cysts as large as 12 cm. On palpation, the cyst is soft and doughy.[18]

Imaging and additional testing

Radiographically, on CT, lesions are usually hypointense and avascular and do not show contrast enhancement (**Fig. 21**). Histopathologically, dermoid cyst is lined by stratified squamous epithelium with a fibrous connective tissue wall[18] (**Fig. 22**). The cyst contains keratin and sebum within the lumen. Secondary structures, such as sebaceous glands, hair follicles, and sweat glands, may be found within the cyst, which differentiates this cyst from epidermoid cysts.[18]

Treatment

Dermoid cyst requires surgical excision. Most lesions are removed through the oral cavity, with low risk of recurrence.

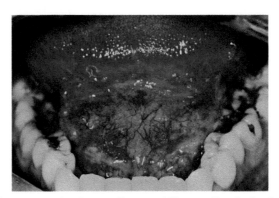

Fig. 19. Dermoid cyst presenting intraorally as a midline swelling in the floor of the mouth. (*From* Regezi JA, Sciubba JJ, Jordan RCK. Cysts of the jaws and neck. In: Oral pathology: clinical pathologic correlations, 7th edition. St. Louis: Elsevier; 2017. p. 245–68; with permission.)

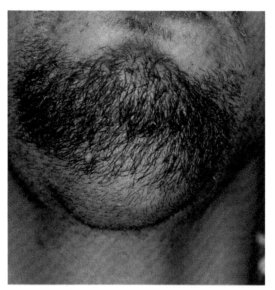

Fig. 20. Dermoid cyst presenting as a midline swelling in the neck. (*From* Regezi JA, Sciubba JJ, Jordan RCK. Cysts of the jaws and neck. In: Oral pathology: clinical pathologic correlations, 7th edition. St. Louis: Elsevier; 2017. p. 245–68; with permission.)

Epidermoid Cyst

Epidermoid cyst is a very common skin lesion and often occurs intraorally. This cyst arises from traumatic entrapment of surface epithelium or from abnormal healing of infundibular epithelium during a follicular inflammation or folliculitis.[23,24] Syndromes such as Gardner syndrome, Gorlin syndrome, and pachyonychia congenita can present with multiple cutaneous facial epidermoid cysts.[23,25]

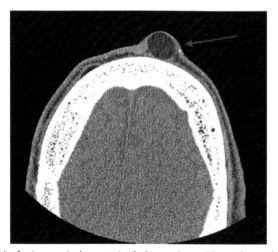

Fig. 21. Axial CT (soft tissue window setting) shows dermoid cyst (*arrow*) on the left forehead. Note dermoid cyst is well circumscribed, hypointense, and avascular.

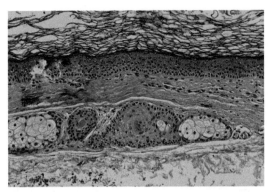

Fig. 22. Dermoid cyst lined by keratinized epithelium with sebaceous glands and rudimentary hair in the supporting connective tissue. (*From* Regezi JA, Sciubba JJ, Jordan RCK. Cysts of the jaws and neck. In: Oral pathology: clinical pathologic correlations, 7th edition. St. Louis: Elsevier; 2017. p. 245–68; with permission.)

Patient history and intraoral examination

These cysts are most common in children and young adults. They frequently present at birth and can be identified when they are large enough.[26,27] In the oral cavity, epidermoid cyst is localized to attached gingiva and is often called gingival cyst of the adult[28–31] (**Fig. 23**). Other common intraoral locations are the floor of the mouth, lateral tongue, lateral pharyngeal wall, and soft palate. Intraorally, epidermoid cyst is usually less than 1 cm in diameter and can be movable under the surface, except in bone-bound mucosa.[32] The most common extraoral presentation in the oral and maxillofacial region is the neck as a midline suprahyoid growing mass.[33] Less commonly it is also found on other regions of the face (**Fig. 24**).

Imaging and additional testing

Radiographically, epidermoid cysts have fluid attenuation on CT scan, are hypointense on T1-weighted images, and hyperintense on T2-weighted images. They are well-circumscribed lesions (**Fig. 25**). Histopathologically, epidermoid cysts lined

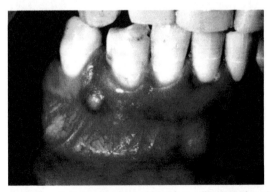

Fig. 23. Gingival cyst of the adult. Dome-shaped bluish swelling on the gingival mucosa between the right mandibular canine and first premolar. (*From* Neville BW, Damm DD, Allen CM. Odontogenic cysts and tumors. In: Gnepp DR, editor. Diagnostic surgical pathology of the head and neck, 2nd edition. Philadelphia: Saunders; 2011. p. 785–838; with permission.)

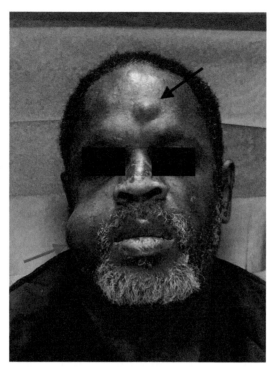

Fig. 24. Facial clinical presentation of epidermoid and dermoid cysts. Epidermoid cyst is indicated by red arrow. Dermoid cyst is indicated by black arrow. Note well-defined and elevated nature of both cysts. Histopathologic diagnosis is required for differentiating the lesions.

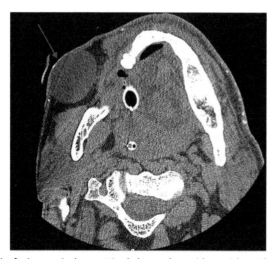

Fig. 25. Axial CT (soft tissue window setting) shows the epidermoid cyst (*arrow*) on the right cheek. Note epidermoid cyst is well circumscribed and has fluid attenuation.

with thin, stratified squamous epithelium with keratin and/or sebaceous material in the cavity occasionally contain respiratory epithelium[34] (**Fig. 26**).

Treatment
Epidermoid cyst is managed by surgical excision.

Pilar Cyst

Pilar cyst is also known as a trichilemmal cyst and wen.[35] It is a common dermal cyst and occurs in less than 10% of the population.[36] It is clinically similar to an epidermoid cyst, except that 90% of cysts occur on the scalp.[35] They arise from the epithelium located between the sebaceous gland and the arrector pili muscle.[36]

Patient history
These cysts have no racial predilection, but have a predilection for female gender and young age. Pilar cysts are slow-growing cysts.[36] A family history may be present because pilar cysts can follow an autosomal dominant inheritance pattern.[36]

Intraoral examination
Ninety percent of pilar cysts occur in the scalp (**Fig. 27**); manifestations include the face, trunk, and extremities.[35] These cysts lack an overlying punctum and they tend to be more mobile and firmer than epidermoid cysts.[35] These cysts are usually asymptomatic unless they calcify or rupture with secondary inflammatory processes.[36]

Imaging and additional testing
Diagnosis of pilar cysts is most often clinical. MRI and CT may be used to assess soft tissue and bone invasion.[36] Histopathologically, cysts are lined by stratified squamous epithelium (**Fig. 28**). Lining cells increase in size as they approach the cavity of the cyst and abruptly keratinize without forming a granular cell layer.[35] The cyst cavity contains

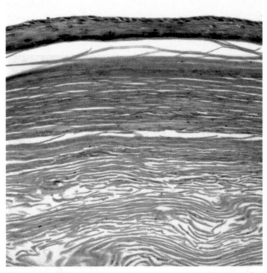

Fig. 26. Histopathology of epidermal cyst. There is a thin lining of stratified squamous epithelium with a granular cell layer and loosely woven keratin contents (H&E). (*From* Patterson, JW. Cysts, sinuses and pits. In: Weedon's skin pathology. 4th ed. Oxford: Elsevier; 2016. p. 509–29; with permission.)

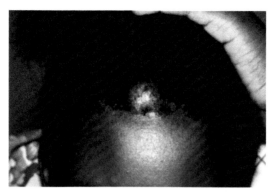

Fig. 27. Pilar cyst of the anterior scalp. (*From* Hirner JP, Martin KL. Tumors of the skin. In: Kliegman RM, St Geme JW, Blum NJ, et al, editors. Nelson textbook of pediatrics. 21st ed. Elsevier; 2019. p. 3582–7; with permission.)

homogeneous eosinophilic keratinous material; foci of calcifications can be seen in 25% of cases.[37]

Treatment
The treatment of choice is surgical enucleation.[35]

Summary

- Common dermal cyst
- Most commonly found on the scalp
- Pilar cysts have a female predilection
- Slow growing
- May show an autosomal dominant inheritance pattern
- Histopathologically lined by stratified squamous epithelium
- Treatment is surgical enucleation

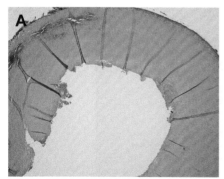
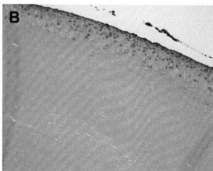

Fig. 28. (*A*) Histopathology of pilar cyst; low power (H&E, original magnification ×40). (*B*) Histopathology of pilar cyst; high power. Note lining cells increasing in size as they approach cavity of cyst (H&E, original magnification ×200). (*Courtesy of* Elizabeth Philipone, DMD, Oral Pathology Residency Program Director, Columbia University Medical Center, New York, NY.)

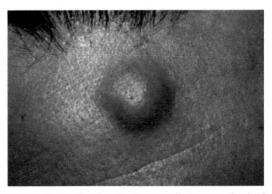

Fig. 29. Sebaceous cyst of the forehead. Note well-circumscribed, dome-shaped, skin-colored cyst. (*From* Hirner JP, Martin KL. Tumors of the skin. In: Kliegman RM, St Geme JW, Blum NJ, et al, editors. Nelson textbook of pediatrics. 21st ed. Elsevier; 2019. p. 3582–7; with permission.)

Sebaceous Cyst

Sebaceous cyst is also known as steatocystoma.[38] This lesion is a benign dermal cyst that is associated with sebaceous glands.[38] Sebaceous glands produce sebum, which coats the skin and hair. Sebaceous cysts usually arise from damage or blockage of sebaceous glands. This damage or blockage can be caused by local trauma. These cysts may arise as solitary lesions, known as steatocystoma simplex,[39] or as multiple lesions, known as steatocystoma multiplex.[40]

Patient history and intraoral examination

This lesion usually presents in the second and third decades of life.[38] There is no gender predilection.[38] There is no racial tendency noted with these cysts.[29] Family history may be present in some patients because sebaceous cysts can follow an autosomal dominant inheritance pattern. Sebaceous cysts often appear as skin-colored to translucent, smooth, 1-mm to 5-mm papules on the skin[38] (**Fig. 29**). They are usually movable and soft to the touch. These cysts are typically asymptomatic, unless they are very large or secondarily infected. The most common sites

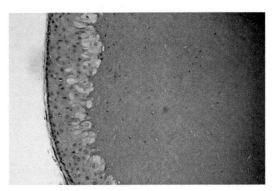

Fig. 30. Histopathology of sebaceous cyst. Lined by stratified squamous epithelium exhibiting trichilemmal keratinization. (H&E). (*From* Patterson, JW. Cysts, sinuses and pits. In: Weedon's skin pathology. 4th ed. Oxford: Elsevier; 2016. p. 509–29; with permission.)

of occurrence, in decreasing order, are the face, scalp, neck, upper limb, back, and lower limb.[39]

Imaging and additional testing
Fluid attenuation can be observed on CT scan. On MRI, the lesion appears as a well-defined subcutaneous mass of intermediate signal intensity on T1-weighted images and heterogeneously high signal intensity on T2-weighted images.[41,42] If aspirated, contents reveal sebum. On histopathology they are lined by thin squamous epithelium, with mature sebaceous glands attached to the wall of the lesion[38] (**Fig. 30**). The cyst lumen contains sebaceous material, keratin, and rare vellus hair fragments.[38]

Treatment
Surgical enucleation is the treatment of choice.

SUMMARY

Although nonodontogenic cysts are uncommon, radiolucent defects of jawbone can be seen in larger lesions. Nasopalatine duct is the most commonly encountered type of nonodontogenic cyst in dental practice. Early identification of the condition and timely referral to oral surgical services reduce morbidity.

REFERENCES

1. Suter V, Sendi P, Reichart P, et al. Expansive nasopalatine duct cysts with nasal involvement mimicking apical lesions of endodontic origin: a report of two cases. J Endod 2011;37(9):1320–6.
2. Swanson K, Kaugars G, Gunsolley J. Nasopalatine duct cyst: an analysis of 334 cases. J Oral Maxillofac Surg 1991;49(3):268–71.
3. Kaffe I, Naor H, Calderon S, et al. Radiological and clinical features of aneurysmal bone cyst of the jaws. Dentomaxillofac Radiol 1999;28:167.
4. Allard R, Van Der Kwast W, Van der Waal I. Nasopalatine duct cyst: review of the literature and report of 22 cases. Int J Oral Surg 1981;10(6):447–61.
5. Manzon S, Graffeo M, Philbert R. Median palatal cyst: case report and review of literature. J Oral Maxillofac Surg 2009;67:926–30.
6. Ariffin S, Yunus N. Aneurysmal bone cyst of the mandible: a case report. Pediatr Dent J 2014;24(3):178–83.
7. Jones RS, Dillon J. Nonodontogenic cysts of the jaws and treatment in the pediatric population. Oral Maxillofacial Surg Clin N Am 2016;28:31–44.
8. Chao W, Huang C, Chang P, et al. Management of nasolabial cysts by transnasal endoscopic marsupialization. Arch Otolaryngol Head Neck Surg 2009;135: 932–5.
9. el-Din K, el-Hamd AA. Nasolabial cyst: a report of eight cases and a review of the literature. J Laryngol Otol 1999;113:747–9.
10. Allard RHB. Nasolabial cyst. Review of the literature and report of 7 cases. Int J Oral Surg 1982;11:351–9.
11. Yuen H, Julian C, Samuel C. Nasolabial cysts: clinical features, diagnosis, and treatment. Br J Oral Maxillofac Surg 2007;45(4):293–7.
12. Neville BW. Developmental defects of the oral and maxillofacial region. Oral and maxillofacial pathology. St Louis (MO): Saunders/Elsevier; 2009. p. 27–8.
13. Hatakeyama D, Tamaoki N, Iida K, et al. Simple bone cyst of the mandibular condyle in a child: report of a case. J Oral Maxillofac Surg 2012;70(9):2118–23.

14. Sciubba J, Fantasia J, Kahn L. Tumors and cysts of the jaws. Am Registry Pathol 2001.
15. Vered M, Buchner A, Dayan D. Central giant cell granuloma of the jawbones – new insights into molecular biology with clinical implications on treatment approaches. Histol Histopathol 2008;23:1151–60.
16. Stafne E. Bone cavities situated near the angle of the mandible. J Am Dent Assoc 1942;29:1969–72.
17. Wood NK, Goaz PW. Differential diagnosis of oral and maxillofacial lesions. St Louis (MO): Mosby; 1997.
18. Regezi JA, Sciubba JJ, Jordan RCK. Oral pathology: clinical pathologic correlations. 7th edition. St Louis (MO): Elsevier; 2017. p. 245–68.
19. Biesecker J, Marcove R, Huvos A, et al. Aneurysmal bone cysts: a clinicopathologic study of 66 cases. Cancer 1970;26:615.
20. Panoutsakopoulos G, Pandis N, Kyriazoglou I, et al. Recurrent (16;17)(q22;p13) in aneurysmal bone cysts. Genes Chromosomes Cancer 1999;26:265.
21. Wakasa T, Kawai N, Aiga H, et al. Management of florid cemento-osseous dysplasia of the mandible producing solitary bone cyst: report of a case. J Oral Maxillofac Surg 2002;60(7):832–5.
22. Motamedi M, Behroozian A, Aziz T, et al. Assessment of 120 maxillofacial aneurysmal bone cysts: a nationwide quest to understand this enigma. J Oral Maxillofac Surg 2014;72:1523–30.
23. Elder DE, Elenitsas R, Johnson BL, et al. Lever's histopathology of the skin. Philadelphia: Lippincott Williams & Wilkins; 2004.
24. Golden BA, Zide MF. Cutaneous cysts of the head and neck. J Oral Maxillofac Surg 2005;63:1613–9.
25. Gorlin RJ, Cohen MM, Raoul CM, et al. Syndromes of the head and neck. Oxford (United Kingdom): Oxford University Press; 2001.
26. Eppley BL, Bell MJ, Sclaroff A. Simultaneous occurrence of dermoid and heterotopic intestinal cysts in the floor of the mouth of a newborn. J Oral Maxillofac Surg 1985;43:880–3.
27. Gibson WS, Fenton NA. Congenital sublingual dermoid cyst. Arch Otolaryngol 1982;108:745–8.
28. Neville BW, Damm DD, Allen CM, et al. Oral and maxillofacial pathology. Philadelphia: WB Saunders; 2008.
29. Buchner A, Hansen LS. The histomorphologic spectrum of the gingival cyst in the adult. Oral Surg Oral Med Oral Pathol 1979;48:532–9.
30. Nxumalo TN, Shear M. Gingival cyst in adults. J Oral Pathol Med 1992;21:309–13.
31. Breault LG, Billman MA, Lewis DM. Report of a gingival surgical cyst developing secondarily to a subepithelial connective-tissue graft. J Periodontol 1997;68:392–5.
32. Shaari CM, Ho BT, Shah K, et al. Lingual dermoid cyst. Otolaryngol Head Neck Surg 1995;112:476–8.
33. Som P. Cystic lesion of the neck. Postgrad Radiol 1987;7:211–31.
34. Seward GR. Dermoid cysts of the floor of the mouth. Br J Oral Surg 1965;3:36–47.
35. James W, Dirk EM, Treat JR, et al. Andrews diseases of the skin. 13th edition. Elsevier; 2020. p. 679.
36. Aboud D, Patel B. Pilar cyst. [online] Ncbi.nlm.nih.gov. 2019. Available at: https://www.ncbi.nlm.nih.gov/books/NBK534209/. Accessed April 21, 2019.
37. Kliegman RM, St Geme JW, Blum NJ, et al. Nelson textbook of pediatrics. 21st edition. Elsevier; 2020. p. 3582–7.

38. Brinster NK, Liu V, Diwan AH, et al. Dermatopathology: high-yield pathology. 1st edition. Saunders; 2011. p. 313.
39. Brownstein MH. Steatocystoma simplex. A solitary steatocystoma. Arch Dermatol 1982;118:409–11.
40. Requena L, Martin L, Renedo G, et al. A facial variant of steatocystoma multiplex. Cutis 1993;51:449–52.
41. Iglesias A, Arias M, Santiago P, et al. Benign breast lesions that simulate malignancy: magnetic resonance imaging with radiologic-pathologic correlation. Curr Probl Diagn Radiol 2007;36:66–82.
42. Regezi JA, Sciubba JJ, Pogrel MA. Atlas of oral and maxillofacial pathology. Philadelphia: WB Saunders; 2000.

Salivary Gland Diseases

Orrett E. Ogle, DDS[a],*

KEYWORDS

- Sialolithiasis • Sialadenitis • Sialadenosis • Sjögren syndrome • Xerostomia
- Xerogenic medications • Pleomorphic adenoma

KEY POINTS

- Sialolithiasis is the most common problem in the salivary gland.
- Dry mouth is associated with xerogenic medications, dehydration, exposure to radiation, and smoking.
- Infections are either bacterial or viral.
- Most salivary tumors are benign.
- Several systemic diseases can cause enlargement of salivary glands.

There are 3 pairs of major salivary glands: parotid, submandibular, and sublingual glands and thousands of minor salivary glands dispersed throughout the oral cavity. The parotid is the largest of the major salivary gland and is situated lateral to the ramus of the mandible and anterior to the sternocleidomastoid muscle. This gland is encapsulated and secretes serous saliva. The submandibular glands are the second largest and are located below the angle of the mandible in the submandibular triangle of the neck and makes up part of the floor of the mouth. This gland secretes a mixed serous and mucous saliva. The sublingual glands are the smallest of the major salivary glands and lies below the mucosa of the floor of the mouth above the mylohyoid muscle. Unlike the parotid and the submandibular glands, the sublingual gland is not encapsulated and it is dispersed throughout the sublingual space. The sublingual gland secretes mucous saliva. The minor salivary glands are composed of 800 to 1000 small salivary glands concentrated along the buccal mucosa, labial mucosa, lingual mucosa, soft/hard palate, and floor of mouth.[1] These clusters of glands secrete primarily mucous saliva (**Box 1**).

SALIVARY GLAND DISEASES

A variety of disease processes, ranging from painful obstructions, infections, to benign and malignant tumors, can occur within the salivary glands. Despite the rarity in which

Disclosure: The author has nothing to disclose.
[a] University of The West Indies, Kigston, Jamaica
* 4974 Golf Valley Court, Douglasville, GA 30135.
E-mail address: oeogle@aol.com

Dent Clin N Am 64 (2020) 87–104
https://doi.org/10.1016/j.cden.2019.08.007
0011-8532/20/© 2019 Elsevier Inc. All rights reserved.

Box 1
Functions of saliva

Aids in digestion and taste perception

Moistens food bolus to assist swallowing

Lubricate the oral soft tissues to assist the movement against each other and against the teeth.

Neutralizes bacterial acids by its buffering action.

Promotes enamel remineralization

Protects the teeth and the oral mucosa by the presence of immunoglobulin's tissue repair factors and antibacterial system[2]

---

salivary gland diseases are encountered in the practice of general dentistry, it is essential that general dentists be knowledgeable about salivary gland function, abnormalities, and the diseases that can affect these glands. They should be able to recognize and diagnose problems involving the major and minor salivary glands as well as in the management of certain problems such as oral dryness associated with salivary problems and stones and other problems related to the ducts of the glands. This article reviews several important diseases affecting the glands, their clinical presentations, trends in diagnosis, and their general management (**Table 1**).

CLINICAL EXAMINATION, LABORATORY STUDIES, AND IMAGING

A careful history is the first step in the diagnosis of salivary gland conditions (**Table 2**). Nearly all diseases that affect the salivary glands present as painful or painless swelling of the gland. In addition, there may be dryness of the mouth (xerostomia), as well as local and systemic symptoms of an infection.

In a lot of cases the clinical examination by itself can provide a diagnosis. A ranula or mucocele is easily identified on clinical examination. Salivary stones and tumors can also usually be visualized and/or palpated and a good educated conditional diagnosis established (**Box 2**).

Laboratory Studies

For most of the salivary gland diseases, laboratory testing is not indicated. If Sjögren syndrome or sarcoidosis is suspected, however, then antinuclear antibodies, SS-A or SS-B (Sjögren syndrome antibodies to duct epithelium), and angiotensin-converting enzyme levels would be the indicated laboratory tests.[3] The workup of a suspected infection would consist of complete blood count with differential blood count and C-reactive protein. Salivary secretion rate is indicated in the assessment of xerostomia. Fine-needle aspiration biopsy is used to obtain tissue for the histologic diagnosis of neoplasms.

Imaging

Conventional radiography has a very limited role in the diagnosis of salivary gland pathology and is useful only for identifying salivary stones. Intraoral occlusal radiograph is useful in diagnosis and localization of stones in the submandibular duct.

Sialography is used to evaluate the ductal system of salivary glands using a contrast medium injected into the duct. It is useful in the assessment of salivary gland dysfunction secondary to obstructive disorders. Because of the risks in the use of contrast medium, this technique is no longer favored and is contraindicated in acute conditions

Table 1 Classification of salivary gland diseases	
Inflammatory Disorders	
Acute sialadenitis	Chronic sialadenitis
Viral:	• Granulomatous:
Mumps	TB
Coxsackie	Cat scratch disease
Cytomegalovirus	• Actinomycosis
Paramyxovirus	• Sarcoidosis
• Bacterial: *Staphylococcus aureus* (acute	• HIV
suppurative parotitis)	• Abscess (parotid and submandibular)
	• Recurrent subacute parotitis
	• Radiation sialadenitis
Noninflammatory Enlargement	
• Parotitis	
○ Associated with alcohol cirrhosis	
○ Diabetes mellitus	
○ Bulimia	
○ Malnutrition	
Obstructive Disorders	
Traumatic	• Mucocele
	• Ranula
	• Traumatic strictures of major ducts
Stones	Mostly submandibular
Impaction of foreign body into a duct	
Secretory Disorders	
Dry mouth (xerostomia)	Excess saliva (sialorrhea)
• Inflammation	• Neuromuscular disorders
• Fibrosis of major glands	• Psychosomatic problems
• Dehydration states	• Insertion of new dentures
• Drug therapy	• Decreased vertical dimension
• Autoimmune diseases	
• Chemotherapy	
• Postradiation changes	
• Alcoholism	
• Malnutrition	
Systemic Diseases	
Autoimmune	Sjörgen
	Mikulicz
	Sarcoidosis
Benign lymphoepithelial lesions	Amyloidosis
Fibrocystic disease (mucoviscidosis)	HIV-associated benign lymphoepithelial cysts
	of the parotid glands
	Rare
Drug and Hypersensitivity Reactions	
Clonidine (Catapres)	Causes a reduction of saliva production or
Methyldopa (Aldomet)	secretion
Tranquilizers	
Antihistamines	
Anticholinergics	

(*continued on next page*)

Table 1 (continued)	
Neoplasms	
Benign	Malignant
• Pleomorphic adenoma	• Mucoepidermoid
• Monomorphic adenoma	• Acinic cell
• Warthin tumor	• Adenocarcinoma
• Oncocytoma	• Adenoid cystic
	• Malignant pleomorphic
	• Squamous cell
	• Malignant oncocytoma
	• Lymphoma
	• Metastatic

Abbreviation: HIV, human immunodeficiency virus.

of salivary glands.[4] Instead of sialography, sialoendoscopy and magnetic resonance Sialography can be used for evaluation of the ductal system of the salivary glands (**Table 3**).

INFLAMMATORY DISORDERS

Sialadenitis can be due to either infectious or noninfectious factors. Viruses and bacteria are the most common cause of acute sialadenitis. The parotid glands are most commonly involved and to a lesser extent the submandibular glands. Children, adolescents, and debilitated adults are the groups most commonly affected.

Viral infections are less common than bacterial infections. Viruses causing sialadenitis include paramyxoviruses (mumps—the most common), cytomegalovirus, Coxsackie virus, human immunodeficiency virus (HIV), parainfluenza types I and II, influenza A, and herpes.[6] The most important viral pathogens are the mumps virus and cytomegalovirus (**Fig. 1**). (Mumps is a rare problem today because of the MMR vaccine).Dental treatment is not indicated during an acute viral infection.

Staphylococcus aureus is the most common cause for acute bacterial parotitis. The infection is caused by a retrograde spread of infection up the duct secondary to

Table 2 Patient evaluation	
History	• Painful diffuse swelling suggests sialadenitis
• Onset, duration, and course	
• Is it painful?	• Painful swelling that fluctuates with meals suggests sialolithiasis
• Other concurrent symptoms	
• History of systemic diseases	• Nonpainful swelling suggests tumor
• Medication history	Dry mouth
	Diabetes, HIV, HCV, alcoholism
	Drug-induced disorders
Physical Examination	Bilateral swelling indicates systemic disease
• Is the mass unilateral/bilateral	Diffused swelling is usually inflammatory
• Is swelling diffuse or well circumscribed	Tenderness suggests inflammation
• Is swelling tender	• Enlarged lymph nodes
• Are there associated head and neck findings	• Palpable calculi
	• Other signs of diseases

Abbreviation: HCV, hepatitis C virus.

Box 2
Quick summary: generalizations

- Diseases of the salivary glands can be diagnosed by lumps in the submandibular area, lumps on the side of the face in front of the ear. *OR:* lumps, ulcers, or fluid-filled sacks inside the mouth.

- With the submandibular gland the most common reason for lumps is stone formation. Tumors are less common.

- Benign salivary gland tumors grow slowly over months or even years.

- Salivary gland tumors occur with a higher incidence in the upper lip than in the lower lip.

- Lower lip masses are most frequently cystic masses.
  - Upper lip: tumor
  - Lower lip: cyst

- Palate—most common site of intraoral tumor. Pleomorphic adenoma—most common tumor.

- Malignancy should be suspected if the growth has been short or if there is any pain.

- Ulcerations should be considered malignancy until proved otherwise.

---

decreased salivary flow or ductal obstruction. Bacterial sialadenitis is most commonly seen in the elderly and chronically ill especially those with xerostomia or who are dehydrated. Sialadenitis presents as pain, tenderness, redness, and gradual localized swelling of the affected gland. Pus may drain through the duct into the mouth[6] (**Fig. 2**). Dental treatment unrelated to the infection should not be done.

Treatment

Most viral infections are benign, usually self-limiting, and will generally go away on their own. Treatment will be supportive care and the management of symptoms. Bacterial infections will require antibiotic, increasing fluid intake, and good oral hygiene.

Table 3
Imaging techniques

Ultrasonography	Displays high-definition images. Useful in evaluating the superficial structures of the affected salivary gland
Sonoelastography	Measures the elasticity of the glandular parenchyma and is useful in evaluating the hypofunction of saliva especially in postradiation hypofunction of salivary glands
Computed tomography (CT)	Useful in delineating the extent and location of a lesion. CT scans are helpful in differentiating benign and malignant tumors of salivary glands by delineating the characteristic irregular tumor margin and surrounding tissue infiltration of malignancy
MRI	The wide variety of soft tissue signals differences and multiplanar image acquisition have made MRI the most effective imaging modality for assessment of salivary gland tumors. MRI scans delineate the intraparotid course of facial nerve, which is an important landmark for surgeons operating on parotid glands[5]
Scintigraphy	Salivary gland scintigraphy uses Tc-99m pertechnetate to assess salivary gland dysfunction
PET	A PET scan focuses on areas of high cellular activity suggesting a sign of tumor growth. It aids in the diagnosed cancer.

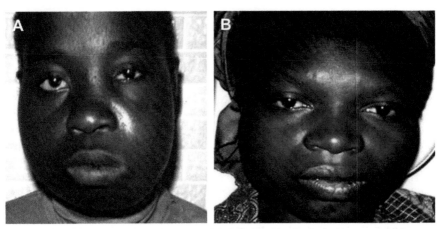

Fig. 1. Unilateral (*A*) and bilateral mumps (*B*) ("chipmunk cheeks"). (*Courtesy of* Orrett E. Ogle, DDS, Atlanta, GA.)

HIV infections can involve the salivary glands, most commonly the parotid (**Fig. 3**). The condition is chronic and generally presents as a progressive unilateral or bilateral parotid enlargement with associated xerostomia. The swelling is most often localized, painless, and sometimes fluctuant. The enlargement of the salivary glands is due to the formation of benign lymphoepithelial cysts within the gland.[7] These patients can receive routine dental care with adherence to Standard Precautions.

Radiation sialadenitis occurs as a result of exposure to radiation treatment of head and neck cancer. The symptoms will be xerostomia and mucositis. The serous parotid gland is considerably more radiation sensitive than the submandibular gland with its seromucous structure or the purely mucous sublingual gland.[8] The dental treatment will be management of the mucositis and xerostomia.

NONINFLAMMATORY ENLARGEMENT

Sialadenosis is a noninfectious, noninflammatory gland enlargement usually affecting the parotid bilaterally. This swelling is generally painless but in some instances it can

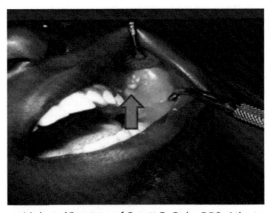

Fig. 2. Pus from parotid duct. (*Courtesy of* Orrett E. Ogle, DDS, Atlanta, GA.)

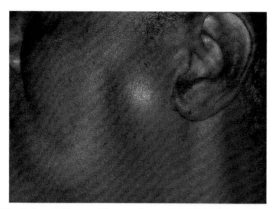

Fig. 3. Lymphoepithelial cyst of parotid secondary to HIV. (*Courtesy of* Orrett Ogle, DDS, Atlanta, GA and Earl I. Clarkson, DDS, Woodhull Hospital, Brooklyn, NY.)

be tender. Dental practitioners need to be able to differentiate sialadenosis from an inflammatory or neoplastic process to prevent unnecessary referrals.

Sialadenosis may be idiopathic or may be associated with the following:

1. Chronic malnutrition
2. Obesity
3. Diabetes mellitus
4. Alcoholism
5. Liver disease (usually advanced liver disease and hepatitis C virus infection)
6. Eating disorders (bulimia)
7. Drugs (ie, antihypertensives)[9]

The disease is most frequent in 3 distinct groups of patients: alcoholics, diabetics, and the malnourished. Diabetes mellitus and alcoholism are the most common causes. To establish a diagnosis the dentist should first question the patient regarding any endocrine or nutritional disorders, the chronic use of alcohol, or any other factors that are known to be associated with sialadenosis such as hepatic diseases. If the dentist is unable to explain bilateral parotid enlargement from the history, the patient should then be referred to an oral and maxillofacial surgeon or an otorhinolaryngologist. A medical consult may also be necessary.

Patients with sialadenosis may sometimes complain of reduced salivary flow. The treatment is the management of the underlying systemic condition. Dental treatment is not contraindicated. But the dentist should be aware of the possibility of coagulation issues in alcoholism.

OBSTRUCTIVE DISORDERS

Obstructive sialadenitis is the most frequently encountered salivary gland disease in dental practice. Stones in the excretory ducts are most frequently the cause of the obstruction. Other less frequent causes are impaction of the duct orifice, trauma to the orifice, idiopathic inflammatory stenosis, and radioiodine-induced stenosis.[10] The symptoms are usually very characteristic, consisting of recurrent swelling of the affected gland, particularly with meals, which may be associated with postprandial salivary pain. Bacterial infection of the gland may at times be the first presenting symptom.

Sialoliths are more frequently located in the submandibular gland (84%), than in the parotid gland (13%). Most of the submandibular stones are located in Wharton duct (90%) (**Figs. 4** and **5**), whereas parotid stones are more often located within the gland itself[11] (**Fig. 6**). Salivary stones consist of an amorphous mineralized nucleus, surrounded by concentric laminated layers of organic and inorganic substances. The organic components of salivary stones include collagen, glycoproteins, amino acids, and carbohydrates. The major inorganic components are hydroxyapatite, carbonate apatite, whitlockite, and brushite.[11]

Diagnosis in the dental office will be based on history of pain and swelling associated with eating. The swelling will be present in the region of the duct behind the stone and will slowly dissipate after meal time. Stones in the region of the Wharton duct may be visualized through the thin mucosa of the floor of the mouth or/and palpated at examination. Occlusal radiograph and, sometimes, panoramic imaging will visualize the stone. Other more sophisticated diagnostic methods are ultrasonography, non–contrast-enhanced computed tomography, magnetic resonance sialography, and sialendoscopy. Digital subtraction sialography, combined with ultrasonography, is the method of choice in visualization of salivary gland calculi[12] when the stone cannot be detected by occlusal radiographs or by palpation. Sialography is a very old and controversial diagnostic method, but it still seems to be the best diagnostic tool in the imaging of salivary gland duct system in dental practice. It is inexpensive and capable of demonstrating subtle anatomy within the salivary gland ductal system.

Treatment

Treatment consists of first treating any acute infection if present, followed by surgical removal of the stone. Stones that are located from near the orifice up to the hilum in the submandibular gland can be removed transorally, but stones near the hilum of the gland will require gland excision. Sialendoscopy (a 0.8–1.6 mm semirigid endoscope is introduced into the salivary duct and is used to remove the stone) is an alternative to open surgery. Some studies have demonstrated its superiority over open surgery in stone clearance, symptom resolution, gland preservation, and safety.[13,14] Stones in the parotid duct is best treated with Extracorporeal shockwave lithotripsy.

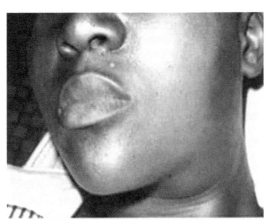

Fig. 4. Stone in Wharton duct. Swelling of submandibular gland at meal time. (*Courtesy of* Orrett E. Ogle, DDS, Atlanta, GA.)

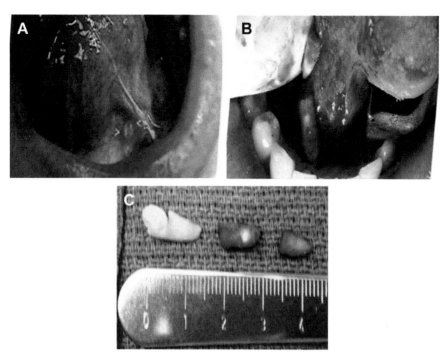

Fig. 5. (*A*) Stone at orifice of Wharton duct. (*B*) Stones removed from duct. (*C*) Stones. (*Courtesy of* Orrett E. Ogle, DDS, Atlanta, GA.)

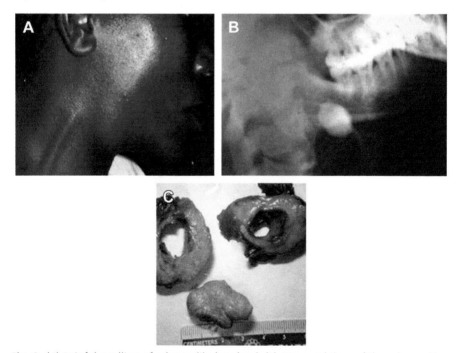

Fig. 6. (*A*) Painful swelling of submandibular gland. (*B*) Stone at hilum of the submandibular gland. (*C*) Specimen of dilated duct and stone. Gland was removed extraorally. ([*C*] *Courtesy of* Orrett E. Ogle, DDS, Atlanta, GA.)

Mucocele

The mucocele is caused by rupture of a duct of a minor salivary gland, most commonly on the lower lip, typically due to trauma resulting in spillage of mucin into the adjacent tissues. Typically, it appears as a bluish thin walled lesion that is fluctuant (**Figs. 7** and **8**).

Ranula

A ranula is a type of mucocele found in the floor of the mouth. It is an extravasation cyst consisting of collected mucin from a traumatic rupture of a duct of a sublingual salivary gland. The occurrence is unilateral and the swelling is away from the midline. Ranulas are classified as oral, plunging, or mixed based on their site of presentation. Oral ranulas are confined to the floor of the mouth, whereas plunging ranulas descend below the mylohyoid muscle to be seen below the inferior border of the mandible or as a lateral neck swelling termed a cervical ranula (**Figs. 9** and **10**).

SECRETORY DISORDERS

The normal daily production of saliva is between 0.5 and 1.5 L (**Table 4**). The submandibular glands are the major contributors to resting (unstimulated) saliva, and the parotid glands are the major contributors to stimulated saliva. The contribution of sublingual glands to unstimulated and stimulated whole saliva is low.[15]

Secretory disorders can be caused by a wide range of factors. The most frequent causes of dry mouth among dental patients are the use of xerogenic medications, head and neck radiotherapy, and Sjögren syndrome.[16]

Xerostomia is a combination of signs and symptoms in which the patient complains of a sensation of dry mouth. Women have a significantly higher rate than men, and the condition usually results in a lower quality of life. Xerostomia is associated with dental caries, oral candidiasis, and bacterial infection, along with the functional problems of dysgeusia (distortion of the sense of taste) and dysphagia (difficulty swallowing) (**Tables 5** and **6**).

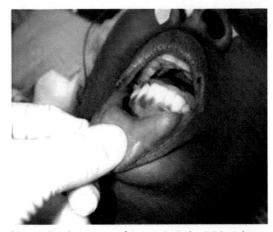

Fig. 7. Mucocele of lower lip. (*Courtesy of* Orrett E. Ogle, DDS, Atlanta, GA.)

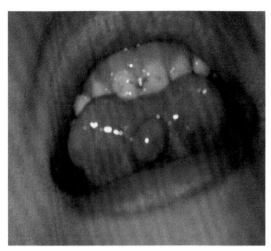

Fig. 8. Mucocele on the midline ventral surface of the tongue involving the glands of Blandin and Nuhn. (*Courtesy of* Orrett E. Ogle, DDS, Atlanta, GA and Earl I. Clarkson, DDS, Woodhull Hospital, Brooklyn, NY.)

Treatment of Xerostomia-Associated Problems

Dental caries: use of fluorinated dentifrice (0.05% NaF)/fluoride gel in the concentration of 1% NaF; 0.4% stannous fluoride application; 0.5% sodium fluoride varnish to teeth; and regular use of remineralizing tooth paste. Dental examination every 6 months and bitewing radiograph once a year for early diagnosis of dental caries.[17]

The dry mouth should be hydrated regularly using water, sucking ice cubes, or lozenges with citric acid to stimulate salivation, artificial salivary substitutes (Biotene and Roxane), lubricants such as lanolin-based product Vaseline or lip balm, and oral gels such as oral balance. Mouthwashes and sprays, sugar-free gums, mint water, or ice chips are also recommended. Sialogogues such as pilocarpine, 5 mg, 3 times a day

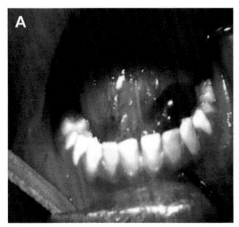
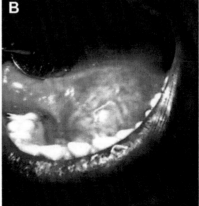

Fig. 9. (*A*, *B*) Ranula in the floor of mouth. (*Courtesy of* Orrett E. Ogle, DDS, Atlanta, GA.)

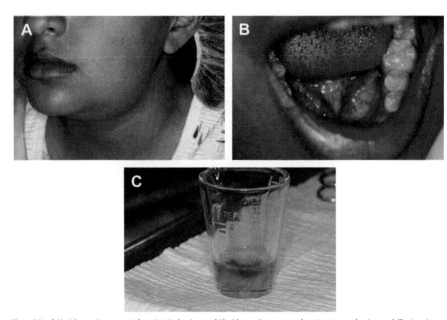

Fig. 10. (*A*) Plunging ranula. Facial view. (*B*) Plunging ranula. Intraoral view. (*C*) Aspirant from submandibular swelling. (*Courtesy of* Orrett E. Ogle, DDS, Atlanta, GA.)

and cevimeline, 30 mg, 3 times a day may be used in conditions where there is some functional gland remaining. Use of saliva substitute solutions mainly containing electrolytes stimulates natural saliva (eg, Salivart, OraLube, Xero Lube), Plax may also be recommended.[17]

Sialorrhea is salivary hypersecretion. The diagnosis is difficult to make and the condition is rare. The most common cause is neuromuscular dysfunction. Mental retardation and cerebral palsy are conditions in which sialorrhea may be seen in children, whereas in adults, Parkinson disease is the most common cause. In most cases of drooling there is not an increase of salivary flow but the oral handling of the saliva is disturbed. Dental-related causes could be due to insertion of new dentures or decreased vertical dimension in complete dentures.

Anticholinergic medications, such as glycopyrrolate and scopolamine, can be used to reduce drooling, but their side effects may limit their use. The injection of botulinum

Table 4 Salivary gland flow rates	
Unstimulated whole saliva flow rate in a normal person	0.3–0.4 mL/min
Abnormal unstimulated flow rate	<0.1 mL/min
Flow rate during eating, chewing, and other stimulating activities	4–5 mL/min
Abnormal stimulated saliva flow rate	<0.5 mL per gland in 5 min

Data from Coulthard P, Horner K, Sloan P, et al. Salivary gland disease. In: Oral and maxillofacial surgery, radiology, pathology and oral medicine. 3rd ed. Edinburgh: Churchill Livingstone/Elsevier; 2013. p. 296.

Table 5 Causes of xerostomia	
Reversible Causes	**Irreversible Causes**
Anxiety and depression	Sjogrens syndrome:
Drugs	Radiotherapy
Ductal obstruction—stones	Nerve damage
Infections	Parkinson disease
Dehydration	
Nutritional deficiencies	
Snoring and mouth breathing	
Smoking	

toxin type A into the parotid and submandibular glands is safe and effective in controlling drooling, but the effects fade in several months, and repeat injections are necessary.[18]

SYSTEMIC DISEASES

The salivary glands are affected by systemic diseases because they are secretory glands that are part of the gastrointestinal system. The diseases most frequently described are Sjögren syndrome and Mikulicz disease. Xerostomia will be the major presenting symptom.

Sjögren Syndrome

Sjögren syndrome is an autoimmune disorder. The primary presenting symptoms are dry eyes and dry mouth. Depending on the studies, female to male ratio varies from as high as 20:1 to 9:1. The disease is more prevalent in Caucasian women, and, although it may present at any age, the mean age of onset is usually in the fourth to fifth decade.[19]

The prevalence of primary Sjögren syndrome in a US population was estimated to be between 2 and 10 per 10,000 inhabitants.[20]

Table 6 Some of the most commonly prescribed drugs that causes xerostomia	
Anticholinergic	Atropine, scopolamine
Antidepressant	Tricyclic antidepressants (amitriptyline, doxepin, nortriptyline, amoxapine), selective serotonin reuptake inhibitors (Lexapro, Prozac, Paxil, Zoloft), and lithium (Lithobid)
Antihistamine	Alavert, Allegra, Atarax Benadryl, Chlor-Trimeton, Claritin, Dimetane, Vistaril, Xyzal, and Zyrtec
Antihypertensive	Atenolol (Tenormin), clonidine (Catapres, Kapvay, Nexiclon XR), methyldopa (Aldomet), prazosin (Minipress), and propranolol (Inderal, InnoPran, Propranolol HCl Intensol).
Antiparkinsonian drugs	Procyclidine, Sinemet (carbidopa-levodopa)
Benzodiazepines (commonly used to treat epilepsy, panic disorders [anxiety])	Diazepam (Valium), alprazolam (Xanax), clonazepam (Klonopin), lorazepam (Ativan), clorazepate (Tranxene)

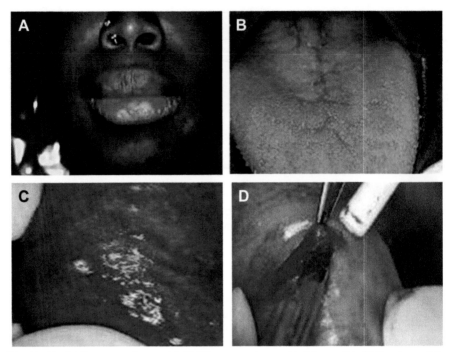

Fig. 11. (*A, B*) Sjögren syndrome. (*C, D*) Sjögren syndrome. Lip biopsy. ([*A, B*] *Courtesy of* Orrett E. Ogle, DDS, Atlanta, GA.)

The diagnosis is often based on a lip biopsy showing lymphocytes around salivary glands (**Fig. 11**). The other tests are Schirmer test, Rose Bengal dye test, sialography, and sialochemistry.[17]

The dental treatment should be aimed at relief of symptoms by the administration of saliva substitutes, fluoride applications, and good oral hygiene.

Mikulicz Disease

Mikulicz disease is of unknown cause, but is believed to be autoimmune by some authorities. The disease resembles Sjögren syndrome except that the salivary and lacrimal depletion in secretion is far less than that seen in Sjögren syndrome. Patients

Table 7	
Neoplasms of salivary glands	
Benign Neoplasms	**Malignant Neoplasms**
Pleomorphic adenoma	Mucoepidermoid carcinoma
Monomorphic adenoma	Adenoid cystic carcinoma
Papillary cystadenoma lymphomatosum (Warthin tumor)	Malignant pleomorphic adenoma
Oncocytoma	Acinic cell carcinoma
Canalicular adenoma	Adenocarcinoma
Myoepithelioma	
Sebaceous adenoma	
Ductal papilloma	

Box 3 Generalization of salivary gland neoplasms		
	Benign	**Malignant**
Parotid	80%	20%
Submandibular	60%	40%
Sublingual	10%	90%
Minor glands[a]	20%	80%
Benign labial salivary gland neoplasms are more common in the upper lip, and malignant labial tumors are more common in the lower lip.		
[a] Number varies widely in published reports.		

with Mikulicz disease will have asymptomatic, bilateral swelling of the parotid, submandibular salivary glands, and lacrimal glands.

The diagnosis of Mikulicz disease is based on the following criteria: (1) symmetric and persistent swelling of the lacrimal glands and either or both of the major salivary glands (parotid and submandibular) and (2) the exclusion of other diseases that may mimic this presentation, such as Sjögren syndrome, sarcoidosis, viral infection, or lymphoproliferative disorders.[21] Laboratory test will distinguish between the two.

The dental treatment would be the same as for Sjögren syndrome.

NEOPLASMS

Salivary gland tumors most often present as painless, slow-growing masses (**Table 7**). Most of the salivary neoplasms are benign with only 20% being malignant (**Box 3**). Eighty percent of major salivary gland tumors occur in the parotid glands, and most minor salivary gland tumors are located in the palate.[22] The most common benign tumor is the pleomorphic adenoma, also called benign mixed tumor (**Fig. 12**). It occurs in both major and minor salivary glands. The commonest malignant salivary tumor in the parotid gland is mucoepidermoid carcinoma (**Fig. 13**). Adenoid cystic carcinoma is the commonest cancer in the submandibular and minor salivary glands, although mucoepidermoid carcinoma is not uncommon (**Fig. 14**).

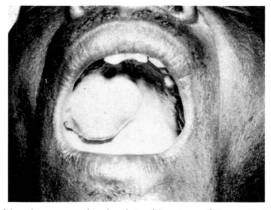

Fig. 12. Pleomorphic adenoma on hard palate. (*Courtesy of* Orrett E. Ogle, DDS, Atlanta, GA.)

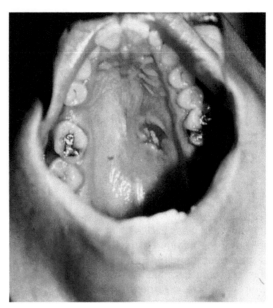

Fig. 13. Mucoepidermoid carcinoma of palate. (*Courtesy of* Orrett E. Ogle, DDS and Earl I. Clarkson, DDS, Woodhull Hospital, Brooklyn, NY.)

Diagnosis is made from biopsy specimen. Clinically, the overlying mucosa is normal in appearance unless it has been traumatized. Fine-needle aspiration biopsy is the preferred biopsy technique but requires equipment that most likely will not be available in dental offices. An incisional biopsy is an alternative if fine-needle aspiration does not provide a large enough tissue sample for a definitive diagnosis. Treatment of salivary gland tumors is surgical excision.

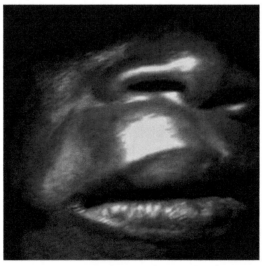

Fig. 14. Adenoid cystic carcinoma (cylindroma) of upper lip. (*Courtesy of* Orrett E. Ogle, Atlanta, GA.)

REFERENCES

1. Som PM, Brandwin-Gensler MS. Anatomy and pathology of the salivary glands. In: Som PM, Curtin HD, editors. Head and neck imaging. 5th edition. St Louis (MO): Mosby; 2011. p. 2449.
2. Schenkels LC, Veerman EC, Nieuw Amerongen AV. Biochemical composition of human saliva in relation to other mucosal fluids. Crit Rev Oral Biol Med 1995; 6(2):161–75.
3. Iro H, Zenk J. Salivary gland diseases in children. GMS Curr Top Otorhinolaryngol Head Neck Surg 2014;13:Doc06. Available at: https://www.ncbi.nlm.nih.gov/pmc/articles/PMC4273167/. Accessed April 2019.
4. Rastogi R, Bhargava S, Mallarajapatna GJ, et al. Pictorial essay: salivary gland imaging. Indian J Radiol Imaging 2012;22(4):325–33.
5. Chu J, Zhou Z, Hong G, et al. High-resolution MRI of the intraparotid facial nerve based on a microsurface coil and a 3D reversed fast imaging with steady-state precession DWI sequence at 3T. AJNR Am J Neuroradiol 2013; 34(8):1643–8.
6. Jothi S. Salivary gland infection. MedlinePlus; 2015. Available at: http://www.nlm.nih.gov/medlineplus/ency/article/001041.htm. Accessed March 2019.
7. Shanti RM, Aziz SR. HIV-associated salivary gland disease. Oral Maxillofac Surg Clin North Am 2009;21(3):339–43.
8. Dreyer JO, Sakuma Y, Seifert G. Radiation-induced sialadenitis stage classification and immunohistology. Pathologe 1989;10:165–70. Springer Verlag [Article in German]. Available at: kfkronenberg.com/Sialadenitis-Eng.pdf. Accessed March 2019.
9. Chen S, Benjamin C, Myssiorek D. An algorithm approahc to diagnosing bilateral parotid enlargement. Otolaryngol Head Neck Surg 2013;148(5): 732–9.
10. Koch M, Iro H, Zenk J. Sialendoscopy-based diagnosis and classification of parotid duct stenoses. Laryngoscope 2009;119(9):1696–703.
11. Kraaij S, Karagozoglu KH, Forouzanfar T, et al. Salivary stones: symptoms, aetiology, biochemical composition and treatment. Br Dent J 2014;217(11):1038–54.
12. Rzymska-Grala I, Stopa Z, Grala B, et al. Salivary gland calculi – contemporary methods of imaging. Pol J Radiol 2010;75(3):25–37.
13. Wilson KF, Meier JD, Ward PD. Salivary gland disorders. Am Fam Physician 2014; 89(11):882–8.
14. Luers JC, Grosheva M, Reifferscheid V, et al. Sialendoscopy for sialolithiasis: early treatment, better outcome. Head Neck 2012;34(4):499–504.
15. Navazesh M. Salivary gland hypofunction in elderly patients. J Calif Dent Assoc 1994;22(3):62–8.
16. Miranda-Rius J, Brunet-Llobet L, Eduard Lahor-Soler E, et al. Salivary secretory disorders, inducing drugs, and clinical management. Int J Med Sci 2015; 12(10):811–24.
17. Krishnamurth S, Vasudeva SB, Vijayasarathy S. Salivary gland disorders: a comprehensive review. World J Stomatol 2015;4(2):56–71.
18. Hockstein NG, Samadi DS, Gendron K, et al. Sialorrhea: a management challenge. Am Fam Physician 2004;69(11):2628–35.
19. Patel R, Shahane A. The epidemiology of Sjögren's syndrome. Clin Epidemiol 2014;6:247–55.

20. Maciel G, Crowson CS, Matteson EL, Cornec D. Prevalence of primary Sjögren's syndrome in a US population-based cohort. Arthritis Care Res 2017;69(10): 1612–6.
21. Lee S, Tsirbas A, McCann JD, et al. Mikulicz's disease: a new perspective and literature review. Eur J Ophthalmol 2006;16(2):199–203.
22. Speight PM, Barrett AW. Salivary gland tumours. Oral Dis 2002;8(5):229–40.

Odontogenic Cysts

Arvind Babu Rajendra Santosh, BDS, MDS

KEYWORDS

- Odontogenic cysts • Periapical cyst • Dentigerous cyst • Odontogenic keratocyst
- Lateral periodontal cyst • Calcifying odontogenic cyst

KEY POINTS

- Odontogenic cysts occur exclusively in tooth-bearing regions of maxilla and mandible.
- Odontogenic cysts are usually asymptomatic, slow-growing, painless swellings of jaw bone.
- Larger lesions may cause pain or discomfort. Pain is usually caused by secondary infection.
- Palpation of affected area of the jaw swelling may show bony, hard consistency with normal-appearing overlying mucosa.
- Early recognition and diagnosis of the jaw cyst may minimize the resorption and destruction of jaw bone.

INTRODUCTION

Odontogenic cysts are unique disorder that affects oral and maxillofacial tissues. They arise as a result of inflammatory or developmental pathogenic causes associated with epithelium of tooth-forming apparatus. The 4 most frequently occurring odontogenic cysts are periapical cysts (PCs), dentigerous cysts, residual cysts, and odontogenic keratocysts (OKCs). However, other conditions, such as lateral periodontal cyst (LPC) and buccal bifurcation cyst, are included because they may be commonly seen in general practice. Glandular odontogenic cysts and calcifying odontogenic cysts are included in this article because they have a propensity to behave aggressively and recur frequently.

A United States study on oral biopsies from a dental school pathology service stated that the prevalence of cystic lesions was 10.7%.[1] A demographic study from Canada stated that PCs were the most common odontogenic cysts (65.15%), followed by dentigerous cyst (24.08%) and OKC (4.88%).[2] A study from the United Kingdom reported that a diagnosis of odontogenic cysts was made on 12.8% of the samples received by an oral pathology service.[3] A Brazilian study reported a frequency of odontogenic cysts of 13.9%, with the most common being PCs.[4]

School of Dentistry, Faculty of Medical Sciences, The University of the West Indies, Mona campus, Kingston 7, Jamaica, West Indies
E-mail address: arvindbabu2001@gmail.com

Dent Clin N Am 64 (2020) 105–119
https://doi.org/10.1016/j.cden.2019.08.002
0011-8532/20/© 2019 Elsevier Inc. All rights reserved.

Jaw cysts are more common among men than among women, with a ratio of 1.6:1. Most cases are reported in the fourth to sixth decade of life. Most odontogenic cysts are encountered in the maxillary anterior region, followed by the mandibular molar region. Periapical/radicular cysts, dentigerous cysts, residual cysts, and OKCs are the most frequently reported odontogenic cysts.[5] Clinical misdiagnoses are possible because of the similar clinical and radiological presentations of theses cysts. However, a careful understanding and interpretation of clinical and radiological presentations helps in the recognition of jaw cysts and accurate diagnoses can be obtained through oral and maxillofacial pathology services.

For convenience, the types of odontogenic cysts are listed in **Box 1**. No classifications are listed in this article, although there are many classifications that have been published. The intention is to provide specific information on the conditions that are discussed to aid the memory and understanding of commonly encountered jaw cysts.

Periapical Cyst (Radicular Cyst)

PCs are the most common cyst of the jaw and are caused by inflammatory processes. All PCs are associated with nonvital teeth and identified at the apices of teeth (ie, the PC). Either carious process or trauma triggers the residual epithelial remnants at the periapical region and stimulates and proliferates the remnants, leading to cyst formation. These cysts are well identified through radiological investigations. Most cases are managed either by root canal treatment and periapical surgery or by extractions.[6]

Clinical features

The carious or traumatic condition leads to the death of dental pulp tissue. However, carious or discolored teeth are often associated with PCs. The inflammatory stimulus from a pulpal region reaches a periapical region to cause stimulation of epithelial cell rests of Malassez, eventually forming a PC. The symptoms of the PC depend on the status of inflammation. Careful palpation over the mucosa at the periapical zone of the offending tooth may provide a clue to swelling, which may guide cortical plate expansion. PC are most often associated with unicortical plate expansion; that is, either buccal/labial or palatal/lingual cortical bones. Bilateral occurrence of PCs has also been documented (**Fig. 1**).[7] A tooth with acute inflammatory exacerbation is symptomatic and presents with pain or discomfort. Displacement of the tooth may be seen clinically when the cyst is large. Pulp testing and radiography are compulsory for diagnosing PC. Teeth associated with PCs must be nonvital and do not respond to thermal or electric pulp testing methods. Lymph nodes must be palpated during

---

Box 1
Odontogenic cysts

1. Periapical cyst/residual cyst

2. Eruption cyst

3. Dentigerous cyst

4. OKC/orthokeratinized odontogenic cyst/nevoid basal cell carcinoma

5. Buccal bifurcation cyst/paradental cyst

6. Lateral periodontal cyst

7. Glandular odontogenic cyst

8. Calcifying odontogenic cyst

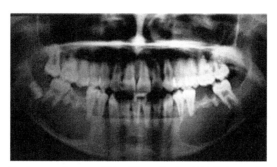

Fig. 1. Bilateral radicular cyst in mandible. (*From* Parkar MI, Belgaumi UI, Suresh KV, et al. Bilaterally symmetrical infected radicular cysts: Case report and review of literature. J Oral Maxillofac Surg Med Pathol. 2017;29(5):458–62; with permission.)

clinical examination. Regional lymph nodes may be enlarged in cases of PC. PCs are rare in deciduous tooth because deciduous teeth are usually resorbed. However, a radiolucent zone may be seen at the bifurcation or inter-radicular space of the deciduous tooth when infected.

Diagnostic modalities

Pulp testing, radiographs, and histopathologic evaluation are helpful in achieving an accurate diagnosis. PCs are radiologically recognized by well-defined, well-circumscribed, unilocular radiolucency that is closely associated with the apex of the affected tooth. Loss of lamina dura and a faint or thin radiopaque line (sclerotic border) that encircles the cystic region are also important radiographic markers for securing a diagnosis. Root resorption can be seen in cases with cytokine-related inflammatory action of the cyst. Cases with large radiolucent areas can be observed when the lesion is aggressive or left untreated for a long period. PCs with large radiolucency often flatten out as they reach the adjacent tooth; PCs rarely displace the adjacent tooth. Very few PC cases have reported radiopaque foci within the radiolucent area.[8]

Misdiagnosis of PC may happen with periapical cemento-osseous dysplasia (PCOD). This condition has a similar radiological presentation: unilocular radiolucency at the periapical region of a tooth. Misdiagnosis can be easily prevented by the dentist subjecting the offending tooth to the pulp testing method. The tooth in PCOD usually responds to the thermal or electric pulp testing method. Misdiagnosis of PC may lead to unnecessary root canal treatment. Several cases have been reported of the misdiagnosis of PC in cases of PCOD.[9–11]

Microscopically radicular cyst is observed with stratified squamous nonkeratinized epithelium often surrounded by an inflamed connective tissue stroma. Inflammatory hyperplasia of epithelium shows a characteristic loop-and-arcade pattern. The connective tissue stroma may show cholesterol clefts or Rhuston bodies.

Differential diagnosis

The differential diagnosis may include periapical granuloma, because both periapical granulomas and PCs occur at the apex of nonvital teeth and radiologically appear as unilocular radiolucent areas. Although PCs usually appear larger than periapical granulomas, size should be considered as a definitive diagnostic criterion. In other words, periapical granulomas are usually tiny or small. Periapical granuloma lacks the radiopaque border; that is, the sclerotic area around the radiolucent zone. The periapical type of cemento-osseous dysplasia must be considered in the anterior mandibular region. Lateral radicular cysts appear as discrete radiolucent areas along the lateral side of the affected tooth because of lateral accessory canals. LPC should be considered when a lateral radicular cyst is observed.[12] The exclusion can be made with pulp testing. PC does not respond to thermal testing, but LPCs do respond.

Management

PCs are usually managed with conventional root canal treatment with periapical surgery; that is, apicoectomy (removal of tooth apex). Extraction with curettage is another mode of treatment. Inadequate curettage may lead to persistent radiolucent cavity (residual cyst).[13,14]

Residual Cyst

Cyst that remains in the jaw bone on completion of exodontia is termed residual cyst. In addition, extraction with inadequate curettage may also lead to persistent cyst in jaw, leading to formation of residual cyst. The cyst may remain asymptomatic unless the cyst enlarges and causes pressure effects. Radiologically residual cyst shows well-defined, unilocular radiolucency at the site of previous extraction. A thin radiopaque border may surround radiolucent area. Cysts may degenerate with time and may lead to radiopaque masses (dystrophic calcification) within the cystic cavity (ie, radiolucent area). Symptomatic cases and larger residual cysts need to be managed through the surgical approach.[15]

Paradental Cyst

Paradental cyst is another type of cyst that originates from inflammation. This cyst is commonly associated with erupted teeth with periodontal pockets. The inflammation from the gingival sulcus of the pocket may trigger the cystic process. A radiologically radiolucent area is observed in the lateral aspect of the erupted tooth and in most cases the periodontal ligament space is not widened.[16–18] Teeth associated with a paradental cyst are vital and react to thermal/pulp testing normally. Paradental cysts are commonly encountered in wisdom molars. Paradental cysts seldom recur. Paradental cysts associated with wisdom molars can be extracted; however, benign-appearing paradental cysts can be treated with cystic enucleation without removing the tooth (**Fig. 2**).

Eruption Cyst

Eruption cysts are commonly seen in the deciduous incisor or permanent mandibular first molar region. Eruption cysts occur because of fluid collection in the follicular

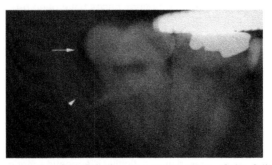

Fig. 2. Intraoral periapical radiograph showing preservation of the follicle space (*arrow*) with distobuccal location of the cyst around the lower right third molar tooth (*arrowhead*). (*From* Colgan CM, Henry J, Napier SS, et al. Paradental cysts: a role for food impaction in the pathogenesis? A review of cases from Northern Ireland. Br J Oral Maxillofac Surg. 2002;40(2):163–8; with permission.)

space of an erupting tooth and appear blue to purplish brown.[19,20] This cyst is normally considered as a soft tissue cystic variant of dentigerous cyst. No treatment is required because these cysts rupture and spontaneously degenerate. Watchful waiting is an option. Simple surgical excision of the cystic roof should be done when cysts do not rupture.

Dentigerous Cyst

Dentigerous cyst is the second most common cyst of the jaw and has a developmental origin. Almost all of the dentigerous cyst encloses the crown of an unerupted tooth and the radiolucent area is attached to the tooth at the cementoenamel junction (CEJ).[21] The cyst occurs because of fluid accumulation between the crown of the unerupted tooth and follicular epithelium (reduced enamel epithelium). These cysts are well-defined unilocular radiolucent areas associated with the crowns of unerupted teeth. Management of dentigerous cyst is done by enucleation of the cyst along with the removal of associated unerupted tooth. If the eruption path of an associated tooth is feasible, then the tooth may be left in the jaw.

Clinical presentation

The cyst occurs because of accumulation of fluid between the crown of an unerupted tooth and follicular epithelium. Dentigerous cysts are predominantly asymptomatic unless the condition is secondarily infected (**Fig. 3**). Mandibular third molars and maxillary canines are the most frequently affected.[22] Because of their asymptomatic nature, most cases are detected during routine radiographic examinations or accidental discovered during radiological investigation. Symptomatic cases are identified in larger cysts because of enlargement of the cyst. Symptoms such as pain and swelling may present. The enlargement of the cysts may show either unicortical or bicortical expansion. Larger cysts usually hollow out the affected jaw bone, which may lead to eggshell cracking on palpation. Pathologic fractures may be seen in larger

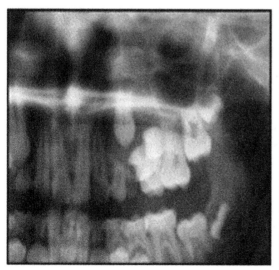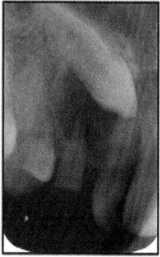

Fig. 3. Periapical (*right*) and panoramic (*left*) radiographs showing dentigerous cyst of maxillary canine. (*From* Narang RS, Manchanda AS, Arora P, et al. Dentigerous cyst of inflammatory origin—a diagnostic dilemma. Ann Diagn Pathol. 2012;16(2):119–23; with permission.)

cysts. Lymph nodes are palpable when the cyst is secondarily infected. Bilateral or multiple dentigerous cysts are observed in cleidocranial dysplasias and Maroteaux-Lamy syndrome. Cases have been reported of aggressive dentigerous cysts with transformation of squamous cell carcinomas or mucoepidermoid carcinomas.[6,23] Few cases have been reported of dentigerous cyst being associated with adenomatoid odontogenic tumor.[24,25] Supernumerary teeth are considered to be one of the common developmental disturbances, hence impacted supernumerary teeth have a risk for dentigerous cyst.[26,27]

Diagnostic modalities
Radiological and histopathologic examinations are helpful in achieving accurate diagnosis. Dentigerous cysts are classically characterized by the unilocular radiolucent areas associated with the crowns of unerupted teeth at the level of CEJ. The radiolucent cavity is well defined and well circumscribed with a sclerotic border (radiopaque). The dentigerous cyst with secondary infection may show ragged margins or ill-defined borders. Roots of adjacent teeth may show resorption or displacement caused by the pressure from dentigerous cysts. Larger cysts may have a multiloculated appearance and should be considered in the differential diagnosis of ameloblastoma. Three types of radiographic appearance can be observed in dentigerous cysts: (1) central, (2) lateral, and (3) circumferential. Central radiographic appearance is the most commonly encountered. This appearance is characterized by the radiolucent cavity that surrounds the crown of an unerupted tooth. Lateral variant is characterized by radiolucent cavity observed laterally along the root surface and partially covers the crown of the unerupted tooth. Circumferential variant is challenging for diagnosing dentigerous cysts because the radiolucent cavity surrounds the entire tooth. Most clinicians are familiar with the radiolucent cavity being associated with the crown of an unerupted tooth and extending up to the level of the CEJ.[28]

Microscopically, dentigerous cyst is observed with thin (2–3 layers) nonkeratinizing cystic epithelium. Scattered mucous cells may be observed. The fibrous capsule is loosely arranged and may show small inactive-appearing odontogenic epithelial islands. Inflamed dentigerous cysts may show multilayered cystic epithelium with hyperplastic rete peg formation. Complications associated with dentigerous cysts are ameloblastoma from potential transformation of odontogenic epithelial cell nests, mucoepidermoid carcinoma (a malignant salivary gland tumor that may arise as potential complication from mucous cells observed in the lining epithelium of cyst), and squamous cell carcinoma from the lining epithelium.[29]

Differential diagnosis
Differential diagnosis of radiolucency covering the crown of an unerupted tooth should include OKC and unicystic ameloblastoma. Ameloblastic fibroma should be considered in younger individuals. However, adenomatoid odontogenic tumor must be considered in the differential diagnosis of dentigerous cyst for pericoronal radiolucency observed on maxillary or mandibular canines.

Management
Management involves careful enucleation of cyst along with extraction of associated unerupted tooth. Large cysts with extensive jaw destruction are managed with a marsupialization procedure.[30]

Odontogenic Keratocyst

OKC arises from the remnants of dental lamina either in mandible or maxilla. Posterior mandible is the most frequent site of involvement. Although OKCs are characterized by cavity filled with fluid, because of the higher recurrence rate, aggressive clinical behavior, and other biochemical protein content, OKCs are considered to be cystic neoplasm and termed as keratocystic odontogenic tumors. Association of multiple OKCs with multiple basal cell carcinomas is termed Nevoid Basal Cell Carcinoma (NBCC). OKCs have less tendency to expand buccolingually, but have a tendency to spread anteroposteriorly and have a tendency to cross the midline of the jaw bone.[31] OKCs are usually recognized as multilocular radiolucencies; however, unilocular radiolucencies can be observed. OKCs are managed by surgical excision with peripheral osseous curettage or ostectomy.

Clinical presentation

OKCs can be observed in any adult age group but are most commonly observed in the second, third, or fourth decades of life. Children are rarely affected. OKCs more frequently affect mandible than maxilla. Posterior ramus is the most common region in the mandible, whereas in maxillae it is the third molar and cuspid region. Multiple OKCs are observed in association with NBCC syndrome. Most cases are asymptomatic. However, patients may present with pain or soft tissue swelling in infected OKCs. Bony expansion (buccal or lingual) and paresthesia of the lips are reported in fewer cases.

Diagnostic modalities

Radiological and histopathologic examinations are helpful in achieving accurate diagnosis. OKCs are characterized by well-defined unilocular or multilocular radiolucent areas with a clear peripheral radiopaque rim (**Fig. 4**). The borders are usually scalloped. Displacement of roots may be seen, and root resorption of adjacent tooth is uncommon. Radiologically, OKCs can be differentiated as 4 types: replacement, envelopmental, extraneous, and collateral. OKC that forms in the location of a tooth are termed the replacement type. OKCs that embrace an adjacent unerupted tooth are the envelopmental type. The envelopmental type usually mimics the radiographic appearance of dentigerous cyst. OKCs occurring in ascending ramus (ie, away from the teeth) are extraneous type. OKCs occurring adjacent to the root surfaces are the collateral type. The collateral type radiographically mimics the LPC.[32,33]

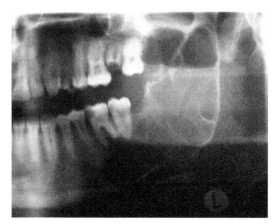

Fig. 4. Panoramic radiograph showing multilocular radiolucent lesion. No evidence of root resorption. (*From* Giuliani M, Grossi GB, Lajolo C, et al. Conservative management of a large odontogenic keratocyst: report of a case and review of the literature. J Oral and Maxillofac Surg. 2006;64(2):308–16; with permission.)

Microscopically, OKCs show a characteristic lining of parakeratinized stratified epithelium 6 to 11 cells thick. The surface of the lining epithelium is usually corrugated. The basal layer is lined by tall columnar cells with a nuclear palisading arrangement. The epithelium-fibrous wall interface is flat and detachment of portions of epithelium from the fibrous wall is also observed. Chronic inflammatory cell infiltrate can be seen in the fibrous wall.

Differential diagnosis

Differential diagnosis may include dentigerous cyst and ameloblastoma because of the posterior ramus molar region. However, resorption is more common in dentigerous cysts and ameloblastomas than in OKCs. The envelopmental type of OKCs usually mimic dentigerous cyst because of their pericoronal radiolucency. Radiographic differentiation of the collateral type of OKCs with LPCs is challenging, especially when observed in the mandibular canine-premolar region.

Management

OKCs are managed via surgical care with careful complete excision of cyst because of the higher recurrence rate. Surgical challenges of OKCs are caused by the thin and friable cyst lining. Osseous curettage is done to prevent recurrences.[34] Recurrence of OKCs is caused by incomplete removal of cystic lesion, epithelial remnants, and the basal cell layer of the oral epithelium, and the association of nevoid basal cell syndrome.[35] Because of the high recurrence potential of OKC, chemical fixation with Carnoy solution has been used.[36]

Lateral Periodontal Cyst

LPC is a developmental odontogenic cyst derived from rests of dental lamina. The name LPC implies that the cyst occurs in a lateral periodontal location. This cyst is development and hence an inflammatory origin must be excluded. It is an uncommon but well-recognized type of developmental cyst. Discussion of this cyst is important to rule out lateral PC and the collateral type of OKC. This cyst tends to occur in the mandibular premolar region. The cyst is usually identified as well-defined unilocular radiolucency between roots of vital mandibular premolars with or without root divergence. Vitality of the pulp must be tested to rule out lateral PC. LPCs are treated by the conservative surgical approach through cyst enucleation.[37]

Clinical presentation

LPCs are predominantly observed in adult patients (fifth to seventh decades) with higher predilection for mandibular premolars.[38] A few cases show labial mass because of the labial position of LPCs. The surface or overlying mucosa of the mass appears normal. The lesion is usually asymptomatic and detected during routine radiographic investigation. LPCs can show signs of draining abscess when secondarily infected.[12]

Diagnostic modalities

LPCs are well-defined radiolucent cyst cavities with thin radiopaque sclerotic borders. The radiographic size of LPCs do not exceed 1 cm in diameter. Multilocular radiolucency area may be observed in polycystic LPCs. The polycystic type of LPC is termed botryoid odontogenic cyst. Radiolucency in LPCs is in the periodontal tissues lateral to roots of affected teeth, and pulp chambers appear normal (**Fig. 5**).

Microscopically, LPCs are recognized by thin nonkeratinized epithelium with a thickness of 1 to 5 layers. Focal thickening of epithelial cells (ie, plaque) is easily recognized. The fibrous capsule is thick and shows minimal or no inflammatory cells.

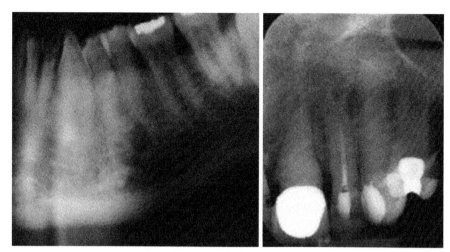

Fig. 5. LPC on mandibular and maxillary arch from 2 patients. (*From* Nikitakis NG, Brooks JK, Melakopoulos I, et al. Lateral periodontal cysts arising in periapical sites: a report of two cases. J Endod. 2010;36(10):1707–11; with permission.)

Differential diagnosis

Differential diagnosis may include lateral PC, OKC, gingival cyst in adults, and unicystic ameloblastoma. Lateral PC reacts negatively to the pulp vitality test, whereas LPCs show a normal response. Collateral OKCs radiographically mimic LPCs and it is challenging to differentiate them; however, LPC may be more likely based on the location (ie, mandibular premolar region).[39] Gingival cysts in adults show clinically recognizable swelling over the labial gingiva of affected teeth. The swelling usually consists of clear fluid material, whereas LPCs are intraosseous and do not show clinical swelling. However, labial mass is reported in a few cases of LPC, and in such cases it can be differentiated with the absence of clear fluid content in the mass. Few cases have been reported mimicking the appearance of LPCs with unicystic ameloblastoma because of smaller size and well-defined unilocular radiolucency in lateral surfaces of roots of mandibular premolars.[40]

Management

LPCs are managed by surgical enucleation. LPCs are associated with minimal or low recurrence rates.[41]

Glandular Odontogenic Cyst

Glandular odontogenic cyst (GOC) is an unusual type of odontogenic cyst of developmental origin. These cysts can show aggressive behavior. GOC predominantly occurs in the mandibular anterior region with a tendency to cross the midline. It is frequently seen in middle-aged adults, and uncommon among younger individuals. GOC is well recognized in radiographic investigation. Because of the aggressive behavior of this cyst, surgical therapy such as enucleation or curettage is used in managing this condition. The lesion can be identified in the periapical zone of mandibular anterior teeth and can be mistaken for PC. Hence it is important for general dentists to learn this condition to avoid misdiagnosis.[42]

Clinical presentation

GOCs are frequently reported in the mandibular anterior region; however, they can occur in any part of the teeth-bearing region of the jaw. Mandibular lesions tend to cross the midline, which is one of the important diagnostic features. GOC clinically presents as an asymptomatic swelling with slow growth rate. Jaw expansions are reported, especially in mandibular lesions. The lesion is aggressive and has recurrence potential.

Diagnostic modalities

GOCs are characterized by multilocular radiolucency with sclerotic radiopaque rim and scalloped border. However, unilocular radiolucent GOCs are also reported (**Fig. 6**).[43] The radiolucent area may be as small as PCs or extend more widely to involve bilateral spread.

Microscopically, GOCs are recognized by nonkeratinized epithelium with focal thickening of epithelium. Epithelium consists of cuboidal and mucosal cells. Because of the presence of mucosal cells, the cyst is considered to have a glandular origin. The cyst usually shows a mucinous pool.[44]

Differential diagnosis

GOCs are to be considered in diagnosis when an individual reports a slow-growing swelling in the anterior teeth-bearing region of the jaw, especially crossing the midline. The mucosa covering the swelling appearing mucus filled or bluish is another significant finding. Differential diagnosis of GOC includes OKC, unicystic ameloblastoma, periapical cyst, or residual cyst. OKC is considered in the differential diagnosis of GOC because both lesions tend to cross the midline. Unicystic ameloblastoma can be considered in the differential diagnosis of unilocular radiolucent-appearing GOC.[45] Periapical or residual cyst is also considered in the differential diagnosis in

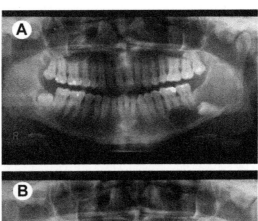
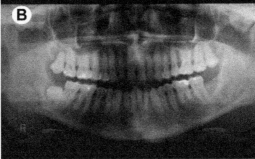

Fig. 6. (*A*) Panoramic radiograph showing well-defined, unilocular radiolucency in left mandibular body and ramus with an impacted third molar. Resorption of roots of first molar is observed. (*B*) Postoperative follow-up radiograph. (*From* Kaplan I, Gal G, Anavi Y, et al. Glandular odontogenic cyst: Treatment and recurrence. J Oral Maxillofac Surg. 2005;63(4):435-41; with permission.)

patients in whom the lesion is noticed at the periapical region of anterior or missing teeth.[46]

Management
GOCs are managed through surgical enucleation or the curettage approach because of their recurrence rate. Periodic postsurgical follow-up is important in evaluating prognosis.[47]

Calcifying Odontogenic Cyst

Calcifying odontogenic cyst (COC) is another uncommon odontogenic tumor with a developmental origin. COC shows variable clinical behavior and shows recurrence. COC reflects dual behavior (ie, cyst and tumor), and hence reports have called this lesion a cystic neoplasm: calcifying cystic odontogenic tumor. COC presents with unpredictable clinical behavior; therefore, this condition is managed with a more extensive surgical approach than simple curettage. The lesion can be identified in routine radiographic investigation (ie, periapical radiograph), hence it is important for general dentists to be aware of this condition.[48]

Clinical presentation
COCs are frequently reported in the maxillary anterior region with a male predilection. COC may present either as intraosseous or extraosseous. The intraosseous form is more common and may be identified with or without presentation of a swelling, whereas the extraosseous form usually presents with a clinical swelling.[49] COC therefore has variable clinical presentation and behavior. COC is more commonly identified in individuals less than 40 to 50 years of age. COCs can be associated with other odontogenic tumors, such as ameloblastoma and OKC.[50,51]

Diagnostic modalities
COCs may present as unilocular or multilocular radiolucencies with radiopaque structures within the lesion (**Fig. 7**). The radiopaque structures either appear irregular or as toothlike structures. Unerupted maxillary canines may be seen in the radiolucent area. Root resorption and divergence are also noted in a few cases.

Microscopically, COCs are recognized by cystic proliferation with a fibrous capsule. The thickness of lining epithelium may vary between 4 and 10 layers. Areas of calcification and ghost cells can be observed.[52]

Differential diagnosis
Differential diagnosis of COCs varies based on the stages. In early stage, radiolucent changes are observed. In such instances, differential diagnosis of OKC and ameloblastoma can be considered, whereas, in late stage a mixed appearance (radiolucent-radiopaque) is observed. During late stage, differential diagnosis of dentigerous cyst and adenomatoid odontogenic tumor can be considered because of association of the unerupted tooth. When radiopaque structures in the lesion have irregular radio density, then differential diagnosis of odontoma, calcifying epithelial odontogenic tumor, or ameloblastic fibro-odotoma may be considered.

Management
Thorough surgical management is required for the COC because of its aggressive clinical behavior and high recurrence rate. Postsurgical follow-up should monitor further recurrences.[53] However, peripheral or extraosseous forms are managed through conservative surgical approach because recurrences are not a routine feature.[54]

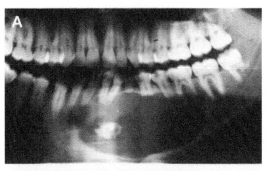

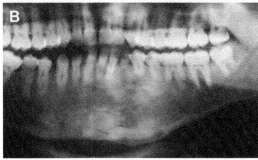

Fig. 7. (*A*) Panoramic radiograph showing well-defined, unilocular, radiolucent condition extending from lower left first molar to right lateral incisor region. Note the lesion crossing midline of the mandible. (*B*) Postoperative follow-up (41 months) of the patient following to marsupialization. (*From* Souza LN, Souza ACRA, Gomes CC, et al. Conservative treatment of calcifying odontogenic cyst: report of 3 cases. J Oral Maxillofac Surg. 2007;65(11):2353–6; with permission.)

SUMMARY

General dentists are the first point of contact for patients with dental complaints. However, individuals also visit for routine dental checks with no dental complaints. Odontogenic cysts are commonly reported in the adult age group, and they can be detected early through routine oral examination at general dental offices. Odontogenic cysts may be either symptomatic or asymptomatic and are identified during routine radiographic investigation. Although odontogenic cysts are difficult to diagnose because this requires a certain level of clinical exposure and experience in examining or managing, these conditions can be identified in routine clinical and radiological investigations. Hence, it is essential for general dentistry practitioners to have updated knowledge on odontogenic cysts for both management of these conditions and providing referral to oral surgery and oral pathology clinics at appropriate times.

REFERENCES

1. Das S, Das AK. A review of pediatric oral biopsies from a surgical pathology service in a dental school. Pediatr Dent 1993;15(3):208–11.
2. Daley TD, Wysocki GP, Pringle GA. Relative incidence of odontogenic tumors and oral and jaw cysts in a Canadian population. Oral Surg Oral Med Oral Pathol 1994;77(3):276–80.
3. Jones AV, Craig GT, Franklin CD. Range and demographics of odontogenic cysts diagnosed in a UK population over a 30-year period. J Oral Pathol Med 2006; 35(8):500–7.

4. da Silva LP, Gonzaga AK, Severo ML, et al. Epidemiologic study of odontogenic and non-odontogenic cysts in children and adolescents of a Brazilian population. Med Oral Patol Oral Cir Bucal 2018;23(1):e49–53.
5. Tamiolakis P, Thermos G. Demographic and clinical characteristics of 5294 jaw cysts: a retrospective study of 38 years. Head Neck Pathol 2019. [Epub ahead of print].
6. Bilodeau EA, Collins BM. Odontogenic cysts and neoplasms. Surg Pathol Clin 2017;10(1):177–222.
7. Parkar MI, Belgaumi UI, Suresh KV, et al. Bilaterally symmetrical infected radicular cysts: Case report and review of literature. J Oral Maxillofac Surg Med Pathol 2017;29(5):458–62.
8. Sridevi K, Nandan SRK, Ratnakar P, et al. Residual cyst associated with calcifications in an elderly patient. J Clin Diagn Res 2014;8(2):246–9.
9. Huh J-K, Shin S-J. Misdiagnosis of florid cemento-osseous dysplasia leading to unnecessary root canal treatment: a case report. Restor Dent Endod 2013;38(3):160–6.
10. Smith S, Patel K, Hoskinson AE. Periapical cemental dysplasia: a case of misdiagnosis. Br Dent J 1998;185(3):122–3.
11. Delai D, Bernardi A, Felippe GS, et al. Florid cemento-osseous dysplasia: a case of misdiagnosis. J Endod 2015;41(11):1923–6.
12. de Carvalho LF, Lima CF, Cabral LAG, et al. Lateral periodontal cyst: a case report and literature review. J Oral Maxillofac Res 2011;1(4):e5.
13. Dandotikar D, Peddi R, Lakhani B, et al. Nonsurgical management of a periapical cyst: a case report. J Int Oral Health 2013;5(3):79–84.
14. Dwivedi S, Dwivedi C, Chaturvedi T, et al. Management of a large radicular cyst: a non-surgical endodontic approach. Saudi Endod J 2014;4(3):145–8.
15. Karam N, Karam F, Nasseh I, et al. Residual cyst with a misleading clinical and radiological appearance. J Oral Maxillofac Radiol 2013;1(1):17–20.
16. Kanno CM, Gulinelli JL, Nagata MJ, et al. Paradental cyst: report of two cases. J Periodontol 2006;77(9):1602–6.
17. da Graca Naclerio-Homem M, Deboni MC, Simoes AW, et al. Paradental cyst: case report and review of the literature. J Clin Pediatr Dent 2004;29(1):83–6.
18. Colgan CM, Henry J, Napier SS, et al. Paradental cysts: a role for food impaction in the pathogenesis? A review of cases from Northern Ireland. Br J Oral Maxillofac Surg 2002;40(2):163–8.
19. Shamim T, Shabeer KPO. Eruption cyst associated with right maxillary deciduous first molar. Pan Afr Med J 2018;30:285.
20. Sen-Tunc E, Acikel H, Sonmez IS, et al. Eruption cysts: a series of 66 cases with clinical features. Med Oral Patol Oral Cir Bucal 2017;22(2):e228–32.
21. Vasiapphan H, Christopher PJ, Kengasubbiah S, et al. Bilateral dentigerous cyst in impacted mandibular third molars: a case report. Cureus 2018;10(12):e3691.
22. Narang RS, Manchanda AS, Arora P, et al. Dentigerous cyst of inflammatory origin—a diagnostic dilemma. Ann Diagn Pathol 2012;16(2):119–23.
23. Panneerselvam K, Parameswaran A, Kavitha B, et al. Primary intraosseous squamous cell carcinoma in a dentigerous cyst. South Asian J Cancer 2017;6(3):105.
24. Rajendra Santosh AB, Coard KCM, Williams EB, et al. Adenomatoid odontogenic tumor: clinical and radiological diagnostic challenges. J Pierre Fauchard Acad 2017;31(2):115–20.
25. Majumdar S, Uppala D, Rao AK, et al. Dentigerous cyst associated with adenomatoid odontogenic tumour. J Clin Diagn Res 2015;9(5):ZD01–4.

26. Navarro BG, Jane Salas E, Olmo IT, et al. Maxillary dentigerous cyst and supernumerary tooth. Is it a frequent association? Oral Health Dent Manag 2014;13(1): 127–31.
27. Bandaru B, Thankappan P, Kumar Nandan S, et al. The prevalence of developmental anomalies among school children in Southern district of Andhra Pradesh, India. J Oral Maxillofac Pathol 2019;23(1):160.
28. Thompson LD. Dentigerous cyst. Ear Nose Throat J 2018;97(3):57.
29. Meleti M, van der Waal I. Clinicopathological evaluation of 164 dental follicles and dentigerous cysts with emphasis on the presence of odontogenic epithelium in the connective tissue. The hypothesis of "focal ameloblastoma". Med Oral Patol Oral Cir Bucal 2012;18(1):e60–4.
30. Gendviliene I, Legrand P, Nicolielo LFP, et al. Conservative management of large mandibular dentigerous cysts with a novel approach for follow up: two case reports. Stomatologija 2017;19(1):24–32.
31. Wright JM, Odell EW, Speight PM, et al. Odontogenic tumors, WHO 2005: where do we go from here? Head Neck Pathol 2014;8(4):373–82.
32. Borghesi A, Nardi C, Giannitto C, et al. Odontogenic keratocyst: imaging features of a benign lesion with an aggressive behaviour. Insights Imaging 2018;9(5): 883–97.
33. Veena KM, Rao R, Jagadishchandra H, et al. Odontogenic keratocyst looks can be deceptive, causing endodontic misdiagnosis. Case Rep Pathol 2011;2011:3.
34. Abdullah WA. Surgical treatment of keratocystic odontogenic tumour: a review article. Saudi Dent J 2011;23(2):61–5.
35. Giuliani M, Grossi GB, Lajolo C, et al. Conservative management of a large odontogenic keratocyst: report of a case and review of the literature. J Oral Maxillofac Surg 2006;64(2):308–16.
36. Ogle OE, Santosh AB. Medication management of jaw lesions for dental patients. Dent Clin North Am 2016;60(2):483–95.
37. Govil S, Gupta V, Misra N, et al. Bilateral lateral periodontal cyst. BMJ Case Rep 2013;2013 [pii:bcr2013009383].
38. Nikitakis NG, Brooks JK, Melakopoulos I, et al. Lateral periodontal cysts arising in periapical sites: a report of two cases. J Endod 2010;36(10):1707–11.
39. Esen A, Kilinc A, Guler Y, et al. Keratocystic odontogenic tumor mimicking lateral periodontal cyst: a case report. Clin Surg 2016;1:1045.
40. Majid OW. Unicystic ameloblastoma mimicking a lateral periodontal cyst. Oral Surg 2013;6(2):83–7.
41. Kumuda Arvind Rao HT, Shetty SR, Babu S. Unusual clinicoradiographic presentation of a lateral periodontal cyst. J Dent (Tehran) 2012;9(4):265–9.
42. Anchlia S, Bahl S, Shah V, et al. Glandular odontogenic cyst: a rare entity revealed and a review of the literature. BMJ Case Rep 2015;2015 [pii:bcr2015211502].
43. Kaplan I, Gal G, Anavi Y, et al. Glandular odontogenic cyst: treatment and recurrence. J Oral Maxillofac Surg 2005;63(4):435–41.
44. Fowler CB, Brannon RB, Kessler HP, et al. Glandular odontogenic cyst: analysis of 46 cases with special emphasis on microscopic criteria for diagnosis. Head Neck Pathol 2011;5(4):364–75.
45. Cousin T, Bobek S, Oda D. Glandular odontogenic cyst associated with ameloblastoma: Case report and review of the literature. J Clin Exp Dent 2017;9(6): e832–6.
46. Shah M, Kale H, Ranginwala A, et al. Glandular odontogenic cyst: a rare entity. J Oral Maxillofac Pathol 2014;18(1):89–92.

47. Krishnamurthy A, Sherlin HJ, Ramalingam K, et al. Glandular odontogenic cyst: report of two cases and review of literature. Head Neck Pathol 2009;3(2):153–8.
48. Zornosa X, Müller S. Calcifying cystic odontogenic tumor. Head Neck Pathol 2010;4(4):292–4.
49. Resende RG, Brito JAR, Souza LN, et al. Peripheral calcifying odontogenic cyst: a case report and review of the literature. Head Neck Pathol 2010;5(1):76–80.
50. Basile JR, Klene C, Lin YL. Calcifying odontogenic cyst with odontogenic keratocyst: a case report and review of the literature. Oral Surg Oral Med Oral Pathol Oral Radiol Endod 2010;109(4):e40–5.
51. Muddana K, Maloth AK, Dorankula SP, et al. Calcifying cystic odontogenic tumor associated with ameloblastoma – a rare histological variant. Indian J Dent Res 2019;30(1):144–8.
52. Arruda J-A, Silva L-V, Silva L, et al. Calcifying odontogenic cyst: a 26-year retrospective clinicopathological analysis and immunohistochemical study. J Clin Exp Dent 2018;10(6):e542–7.
53. Souza LN, Souza ACRA, Gomes CC, et al. Conservative treatment of calcifying odontogenic cyst: report of 3 cases. J Oral Maxillofac Surg 2007;65(11):2353–6.
54. Balaji SM, Rooban T. Calcifying odontogenic cyst with atypical features. Ann Maxillofac Surg 2012;2(1):82–5.

Odontogenic Tumors

Arvind Babu Rajendra Santosh, BDS, MDS[a],*, Orrett E. Ogle, DDS[b]

KEYWORDS

- Odontogenic tumors • Odontoma • Ameloblastoma • Impacted tooth
- Posterior mandible

KEY POINTS

- Early stages of odontogenic tumors are usually asymptomatic and slow-growing swelling.
- Late stages of odontogenic tumors can cause facial asymmetry, symptomatic progressive swelling, pain, or bicortical plate expansion.
- Odontomas and ameloblastomas are the most frequently reported odontogenic tumors across the globe.
- Most odontogenic tumors are associated with unerupted/impacted tooth. Thus, exploring the cause of impaction through radiographic investigation may unravel odontogenic pathologies when detected.
- Surgical approach is recommended in the management of odontogenic tumors.

INTRODUCTION

Odontogenic tumors are pathologic outcomes from tissue elements that are part of the tooth-forming apparatus, that is, odontogenic tissues. These tumors occur exclusively in the bones of the jaw particularly around the teeth-bearing segments. Patients with odontogenic tumors usually present with symptomatic or asymptomatic swelling in the oral and maxillofacial region. Most of these swellings have either tooth-associated symptoms or tooth-associated radiological changes.[1] The general dentist possesses a unique opportunity to be the first health care professional to see anatomic or radiographic changes in the maxillofacial region due to proximity of the neighboring structures that they routinely treat. Because general dentists serve as the preliminary point of patient contact and see patients on a regular basis, it is imperative that they become familiar with the recognition and diagnosis of odontogenic tumors. Although dentists have the examination skills and the knowledge regarding swelling and ulcerative conditions, the art of examination skills and the knowledge of differential diagnosis may have faded due to the relatively low prevalence of such

Disclosure Statement: The authors have nothing to disclose.
[a] School of Dentistry, Faculty of Medical Sciences, The University of the West Indies, Mona campus, Kingston 7, Jamaica, West Indies; [b] 474 Golf Valley Court, Douglasville, GA 30135, USA
* Corresponding author.
E-mail address: arvindbabu2001@gmail.com

Dent Clin N Am 64 (2020) 121–138
https://doi.org/10.1016/j.cden.2019.08.008
0011-8532/20/© 2019 Elsevier Inc. All rights reserved.

conditions in general dental practice. Peter Morgan stated that "one reason that the field of odontogenic tumors appear so esoteric to the non-expert clinician or pathologist is that new entities appear and apparently standard well understood names are jettisoned, as if on a whim.[2]" This adds another layer of complexity while diagnosing such conditions in dental practice.

Odontogenic tumors comprise neoplastic growths of benign, malignant, or tumor-like malformations originating from odontogenic tissues. The interactions between ectodermal and mesenchymal elements from odontogenic tissues can initiate tumor formation due to disturbance in signaling mechanism for their growth and proliferation.[1,3] This article presents relevant knowledge on clinical presentation, diagnostic criteria, and management details on commonly encountered odontogenic tumors. The correlation of the history, clinical presentation, radiographic presentation, and histological details are important factors in achieving an accurate diagnosis. The list of the odontogenic tumors is shown in **Box 1**. Although there are many published classifications of odontogenic tumors, the have purposefully omitted them because their intention is to provide the general dentist with useful information on the conditions that will be discussed as aid to memory and understanding commonly encountered odontogenic tumors.

Odontoma

Odontoma is a benign tumor of mixed odontogenic origins consisting of both odontogenic hard and soft tissue. It is thought to be the most frequently encountered odontogenic tumor. Odontomas are composed of both epithelial and ectomesenchymal components that contribute to enamel- and dentinlike structures within the lesion.[4] Although odontomas may consist of normal-appearing enamel/dentin structures, they have defects in their structural arrangement and hence they are considered as hamartomas, or tumorlike malformations, rather than true neoplasms.

The odontoma is seen predominantly in the second and third decade of life and has a slight female predilection. There are 2 main types: compound and complex. The

---

Box 1
Odontogenic tumors

1. Odontoma
2. Keratocystic odontogenic tumor
3. Ameloblastoma
4. Malignant ameloblastoma, ameloblastic carcinoma
5. Adenomatoid odontogenic tumor
6. Calcifying epithelial odontogenic tumor (Pindborg tumor)
7. Ameloblastic fibroma
8. Ameloblastic fibroodontoma
9. Central odontogenic fibroma
10. Peripheral odontogenic fibroma
11. Odontogenic myxoma
12. Cementoblastoma
13. Calcifying cystic odontogenic tumor (calcifying odontogenic cyst, Gorlin cyst)

lesion is easily recognized in radiographic examinations and appears as a radiopaque mass with thin radiolucent rim. Odontomas are usually managed by conservative enucleation but more extensive surgical procedures may be necessary for larger, more extensive lesions.[5]

Clinical features

Odontomas are slow-growing, expanding, and painless intrabony lesions. Pain and inflammation may, however, result from secondary infection. The 2 types of odontomas are complex and compound odontoma. The distinction between these 2 types is based on either the appearance of toothlike structures or disorganized mass of dental tissue. The complex type is unrecognizable as dental structures, appearing as a radiopaque mass with varying densities. The compound odontoma has recognizable enamel, dentin, and cementum and consists of individual recognizable small teeth. The complex odontomas are located in the posterior mandible and identified based on disorganized mass of dental tissues, that is, enamel and/or dentine (**Fig. 1**A). Compound odontomas are located in the anterior maxillae and identified based on well-organized, multiple toothlike structures (**Fig. 1**B, C). Odontomas can also be associated with other odontogenic tumors such as calcifying odontogenic cyst, ameloblastic fibroodontoma (AFO), and odontogenic fibromas.[6,7] The association of odontoma with Gardner syndrome and coronoid hypoplasia has also been reported.[8,9]

Diagnostic modalities

In most cases odontomas can be diagnosed based on their radiographic appearance alone. The radiologic appearance depends on the stage of the lesion. The first stage is characterized by a radiolucent appearance due to lack of calcification. Partial calcification or radiopacity are seen in second or intermediate stage. The third stage is characterized by predominance of radiopaque masses of dental hard tissues with a thin radiolucent zone.[10] Resorption or adjacent tooth or roots are uncommon. Association with unerupted teeth may be seen. Radiographically compound odontomas seem as collection of multiple toothlike structures of varying size and shape with periphery of narrow radiolucent zone,[11] whereas complex odontomas seem as calcified mass with radiodensity of tooth structures with periphery of narrow radiolucent zone (**Fig. 2**).[8]

Microscopically odontomas are observed with multiple mineralized structures resembling small, single-rooted teeth with loose fibrous matrix. Pulp tissue may be seen in coronal and radicular zone of toothlike structures.[12]

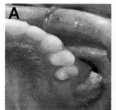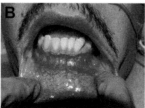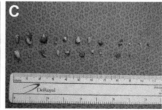

Fig. 1. (*A*) A growth observed in left posterior maxillae that is hard and rough mass. (*B*) Asymptomatic presentation of compound odontoma in anterior mandible with crowding of dentition. (*C*) Multiple toothlike structures excised from compound odontoma in anterior mandible. ([*A*] *From* Zhuoying C, Fengguo Y. Huge erupted complex odontoma in maxilla. Oral Maxillofac Surg Cases 2019;5(1):100096; with permission; and [*B, C*] *Courtesy of* Orrett E. Ogle, DDS, Woodhull Hospital, Brooklyn, NY.)

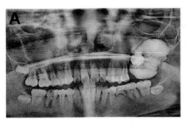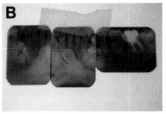

Fig. 2. (*A*) Panoramic radiograph showing a large irregular radiopaque mass in left posterior maxillae. (*B*) Intraoral periapical radiograph showing a multiple toothlike structures in anterior mandible. ([*A*] *From* Zhuoying C, Fengguo Y. Huge erupted complex odontoma in maxilla. Oral Maxillofac Surg Cases 2019;5(1):100096; with permission; and [*B*] *Courtesy of* Orrett E. Ogle, DDS, Woodhull Hospital, Brooklyn, NY.)

Differential diagnosis

Differential diagnosis may include supernumerary tooth, AFO, and osteomas. Based on formation and the number of toothlike structures present, a supernumerary tooth can be easily differentiated from odontomas. Distinguishing AFO from odontoma can be challenging. Radiographically, the radiopacity seen in AFO is usually scattered, whereas the odontomas will have a central area of radiopacity. Radiographic appearance of complex odontoma may be confused with osteoma due to mineralized mass of tissue. However, the radiolucent zone at the periphery of the odontoma, which represents the dental follicle along with the radiodensity of the mass having a density similar to teeth, will differentiate odontomas from osteomas.[13]

Management

Odontomas are managed with conservative surgical excision and special surgical considerations are given for large odontomas. The prognosis of the condition is usually excellent with minimal to no recurrence.[14]

Keratocystic Odontogenic Tumor (Formally Known as the Odontogenic Keratocyst)

Keratocystic odontogenic tumor (KCOT) is a controversial benign intraosseous cystic neoplasm of the jaw, which was formerly called odontogenic keratocyst but was reclassified under a new designation in order to better convey its neoplastic nature due to its aggressive and recurrence nature. KCOT is radiographically recognized as a unilocular radiolucent area with scalloped borders or multilocular radiolucent lesion in the posterior jaw. KCOT tend to grow more in anteroposterior direction rather than in buccal-lingual expansion (**Fig. 3**).[15] Because of its aggressive clinical behavior and high recurrence rate, the odontogenic keratocyst was considered to be a neoplasm.[16] However, in 2018 both a World Health Organization and International Agency for Research on Cancer consensus concluded that further research is needed to explore the genetic changes in the KCOT/OKC for it to be classified as a neoplasm. Because of insufficient evidence to support neoplastic origins of keratocystic odontogenic tumor, the condition was again reclassified as a cyst, and in 2019 the appropriate name is again odontogenic keratocyst and it has been removed from the classification of odontogenic tumors.[17] The clinical and diagnostic details of keratocystic odontogenic tumor are discussed in Arvind Babu Rajendra Santosh's article, "Odontogenic Cysts," in this issue.

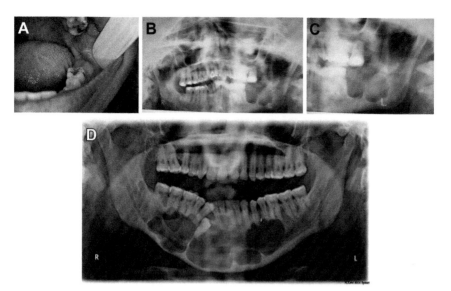

Fig. 3. (*A*) Asymptomatic bony expansion in left mandibular angle region (odontogenic keratocyst). (*B*) Large multilocular radiolucent defect with scalloped borders in left mandibular angle region. (*C*) Large multilocular radiolucent defect with scalloped borders in left mandibular angle region. (*D*) Large multilocular radiolucent defect crossing midline, that is, extending anteroposterior direction. ([*A–C*] *Courtesy of* Orrett E. Ogle, DDS, Woodhull Hospital, Brooklyn, NY; and [*D*] *From* Pogrel MA. The keratocystic odontogenic tumour (KCOT)–an odyssey. Int J Oral Maxillofac Surg. 2015;44(12):1566; with permission.)

Ameloblastoma

Ameloblastomas are the second most common benign odontogenic tumor. They are potentially aggressive, locally invasive, slow-growing benign tumors that may originate from cell rests of dental lamina, epithelium from the enamel organ, epithelial lining of odontogenic cyst (ie, dentigerous cyst), and basal cell layer of oral mucosa. Based on clinical, radiologic, histologic, and prognosis aspects, ameloblastomas are classified as (1) classic/solid/multicystic ameloblastomas, (2) unicystic type, (3) peripheral, and (4) desmoplastic ameloblastoma. Histopathologic examination is mandatory for confirmation of diagnosis. Ameloblastomas are managed by wide surgical resection, and recurrences have been reported.

Clinical features

Ameloblastomas are uncommon among children and is predominantly seen in third and fourth decades of life with a male predilection. The posterior mandible is the most commonly affected site, although one of the authors (OEO) have noted that the parasymphysis/symphysial area is the most common sites in patients seen in Central and East Africa. Ameloblastoma is a slow-growing, painless swelling of the jaw. The clinical signs such as pain and disfigurement may be seen as the lesion advances in the size. The pain occurs due to pressure effects from the mass size on peripheral nerves and secondary infection. Ameloblastomas that present with large expansile mass of the jaw can cause thinning of cortical plate, and crepitation or egg shell crackling may be elicited while palpating jaw.[18] Rarely the lesion can perforate jaw bone leading to ulcerated growth in oral cavity and sometimes the skin. Peripheral ameloblastomas present as painless, slow-growing gingival swelling that may produce shallow depression in the underlying bone rather than infiltration.[19]

Diagnostic modalities

Radiographic examination can greatly assist in the diagnosis of ameloblastomas. The frequent presentation type of ameloblastoma is solid/multicystic type, which appears as multilocular radiolucent destruction of bone. A well-defined, small or large radiolucent area in the bone gives the appearance of honeycomb or soap bubble appearance. The destructive changes of the jaw bone may be either confined to alveolar bone or half the mandible. Buccal and lingual cortical plate expansions are observed. Cortical plate expansions can be well recognized in occlusal radiographs. Resorption of adjacent roots of teeth is frequently observed. Association of unerupted tooth is common and adds a layer of complexity in differentiating ameloblastoma with circumferential type of dentigerous cyst. Although ameloblastoma frequently shows irregular scalloping border, this is not a consistent finding in all the cases. Mixed radiographic appearance is due to osseous septa in the lesion but not a true mineralized content in the lesion. Unicystic ameloblastoma shows a large unilocular radiolucent destruction of the involved jaw bone (**Fig. 4**).[20,21]

Microscopic examination shows ameloblast-like cells and stellate reticulum–like cells with fibrous stroma. Histologic variants of ameloblastomas include follicular, plexiform, acanthomatous, granular cell, desmoplastic, clear cell, basal cell,

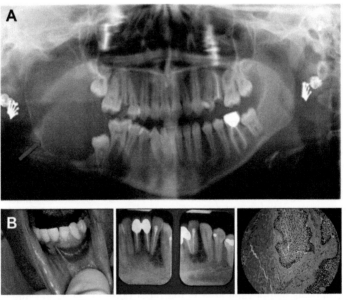

Fig. 4. (*A*) Panoramic radiograph showing a large radiolucent defect involving right mandibular body. (*B*) Asymptomatic swelling and labial cortical plate expansion of lower anterior region. The intraoral periapical radiograph showing small multilocular radiolucent defect (honeycomb appearance) in lower left central incisor to canine region. The histopathology specimen showing follicular ameloblastoma with peripheral ameloblast-like cells and central stellate reticulum–like cells. ([A] *From* Almajid EA, Alfadhel AK. Management of large pediatric ameloblastoma: conservative approach with 4-years follow up. Oral Maxillofac Surg Cases 2019;5(1):100093; with permission; and [B] Courtesy of Earl I. Clarkson, DDS, and Orrett E. Ogle, DDS, Woodhull Hospital, Brooklyn, NY.)

keratoameloblastoma, papilliferous type, mucous cell, hemangiomatous, and extra-gnathic types.

Differential diagnosis

Differential diagnosis of ameloblastoma can be categorized into radiolucency with and without mineralization changes.[22] Differential diagnosis of uni-/multilocular radiolucency without mineralization includes odontogenic keratocyst, central giant cell granuloma, and dentigerous cyst, whereas differential diagnosis panel of uni-/multilocular radiolucency with mineralization includes odontogenic myxoma, calcifying odontogenic cyst, and calcifying epithelial odontogenic tumor. One must look for size, location, and presence/absence of mineralization while formulating differential diagnosis. Central giant cell granulomas are commonly reported in anterior mandible, whereas ameloblastomas are seen in posterior region. Odontogenic keratocyst has a tendency to expand in anteroposterior region, whereas ameloblastomas tend to expand in a buccal-lingual direction. Dentigerous cyst tends to show pericoronal radiolucency, whereas ameloblastomas show impacted tooth in the lesion, not necessarily pericoronal radiolucency. Mineralization density is greatly appreciated in calcifying epithelial odontogenic tumor and calcifying odontogenic cyst.[20]

Management

Multicystic ameloblastomas are treated by wide range of surgical options ranging from simple enucleation to en-bloc resection.[23] Peripheral ameloblastomas are managed by surgical excision and curettage of the bone at the base.[2] Ameloblastomas have a tendency to recur, hence careful postsurgical follow-up visits are necessary.

Malignant Ameloblastoma and Ameloblastic Carcinoma

Ameloblastoma sometimes exhibit behavior of metastases that are most often found in the lungs. The diagnosis of malignant ameloblastoma should be made when a tumor in both primary and metastatic locations demonstrate histopathologic features of ameloblastoma.[24]

The diagnosis of ameloblastic carcinoma should be made when microscopic examination of ameloblastoma cases shows cytologic features of malignancy in the primary tumor. Ameloblastic carcinomas show local aggressive behavior but do not demonstrate the character of metastasis.[25]

Adenomatoid Odontogenic Tumor

Adenomatoid odontogenic tumor (AOT) is a benign odontogenic tumor arising from odontogenic apparatus showing odontogenic epithelium with mature fibrous stroma and without ectomesenchyme. AOT was formerly considered to be a variant of ameloblastoma. However, because of clinical and biological behavior, AOT is considered as a separate entity from ameloblastoma. Based on radiological features, 3 variants of AOT are recognized: (1) follicular/pericoronal, (2) extrafollicular/extracoronal, and (3) peripheral types.[26] Microscopic examination is mandatory for confirmation of diagnosis. AOT usually responds well to surgical excision due to encapsulation of the lesion that can be enucleated from the adjacent bone. Aggressive behavior and recurrences are rarely reported.

Clinical features

AOTs are uncommon, benign, slow-growing, painless swelling of the jaw bone. Adenomatoid odontogenic tumors are sometimes referred as "two-thirds tumors," because two-thirds of AOTS occur before second decade of life, two-thirds of cases are in anterior maxillae, two-thirds of cases are reported in women, two-thirds of AOTs surround an impacted tooth, and two-thirds of the time that impacted tooth is canine.[26] Peripheral variant of AOT appears as small, sessile, exophytic mass over the labial gingiva of the maxillae.

Diagnostic modalities

AOTs are frequently recognized during radiographic examination of unerupted maxillary canine tooth. Radiolucent defect with mandible canine impaction is also observed (**Fig. 5**).[27] The lesion is predominantly intraosseous and shows variation in radiographic location. Based on the location of the lesion, it can be extrafollicular type (no relation to tooth structures); interradicular; adjacent to roots; superimposed on the root apex (periapical type); superimposed at midroot level; or peripheral type (extraosseous/gingival) with slight erosion of alveolar crest of bone. The follicular type is the most common type of AOT presentation. Radiographically, follicular type presents as well-defined, unilocular (oval or round) radiolucency associated with the crown of an unerupted tooth mimicking dentigerous cyst. Radiographic examination can greatly assist in the diagnosis of AOT.[28] The intraoral periapical radiograph is the best radiograph to show radiopacities in AOT. Cone beam computed tomography seems to possess the best potential for diagnosing AOT.

Microscopic examination of AOT shows encapsulation, and multiple ducts such as structures and spindle-shaped tumor cells form sheets, strands, or rosette pattern. Calcifications and amyloid deposits may be seen.

Differential diagnosis

Radiographic differential diagnosis of AOT includes dentigerous cyst, unicystic ameloblastoma, calcifying epithelial odontogenic tumor, calcifying odontogenic cyst, and AFO. Dentigerous cyst should be considered in differential diagnosis when radiolucency envelopes crown of unerupted tooth. AOTs can be distinguished from dentigerous cyst when radiolucency is extending beyond the crown-root junction. Although unilocular radiolucent area may mimic unicystic ameloblastoma, both location and calcifications in the lesion may be helpful in distinguishing between AOT and unicystic ameloblastoma. AOTs sometimes present as multilocular radiolucent areas. In such instances calcifying odontogenic tumor, calcifying odontogenic cyst, AFO, and odontogenic keratocyst should be considered in the differential and will require further evaluation of the multilocular radiolucency with or without mineralization.[26]

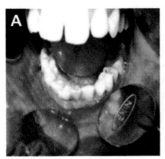 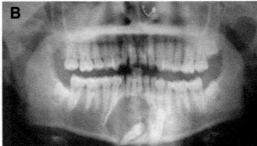

Fig. 5. (*A*) Swelling in right anterior region crossing midline. (*B*) Panoramic radiograph showing radiolucent defect with cortical borders with impacted mandibular canines and resorption of lower border of anterior mandible. (*From* Neha S, Santosh M, Sachin MG, et al. Adenomatoid odontogenic tumour: an enigma. Saudi Dent J. 2018;30(1):96; with permission.)

Management

AOTs are managed by surgical enucleation or curettage. Because of the presence of encapsulation the lesion can be easily shelled out from the adjacent bone. Aggressive behavior and recurrence of the lesion are uncommon features.[29]

Calcifying Epithelial Odontogenic Tumor

Calcifying epithelial odontogenic tumor (CEOT) is an uncommon odontogenic tumor arising from odontogenic epithelium. CEOT presents as a mixed radiographic appearance and frequently occurs in posterior mandible in association with an unerupted tooth. The clinical behavior of CEOT is less aggressive than ameloblastoma, hence careful conservative surgical approach is followed in the management of this condition.[30]

Clinical features

CEOT is an uncommon aggressive, benign, slow-growing, painless tumor of the jaw bone **(Fig. 6)**,[31] frequently reported in the third to fifth decade of life with equal sex predilection. Predominant number of cases is observed in posterior mandible. Peripheral lesions observed on gingiva shows sessile, painless, slow-growing mass usually seen on anterior maxillae **(Fig. 7)**.[32]

Diagnostic modalities

CEOT is well recognized on radiographic examination. Occlusal and panoramic radiographs typically show a well-defined mixed radiopaque-radiolucent lesion with bicortical expansion. The radiolucent defect also shows calcified structures of varying density and size giving mixed radiographic pattern. The calcification or opacity observed in this condition shows a streaking pattern termed as "driven-snow" appearance.[33]

The lesion is predominantly intraosseous with unilocular or multilocular radiolucent appearance. The unilocular pattern is predominant among maxillary posteriors. Mandibular lesions generally have a well-defined multilocular appearance with scalloped margins due to lytic changes.

Microscopic examination of CEOT shows tumor lesion cells in the form of sheets or strands appearing polyhedral-shaped with prominent intercellular bridges. Amyloid and calcification deposits are frequently observed.

Differential diagnosis

The differential diagnosis of CEOT includes calcifying odontogenic cyst and AFO due to the mixed radiographic appearance. Root resorption and divergence of adjacent

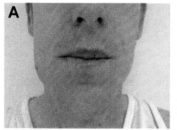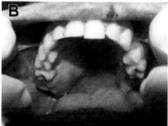

Fig. 6. (*A*) Extraoral swelling of the right side of posterior maxillae. (*B*) Intraoral appearance of swelling in posterior region of maxillae. (*From* Gruber K, de Freitas Filho SAJ, Dogenski LC, et al. Surgical management of a large calcifying epithelial odontogenic tumor in the maxilla: a case report. Int J Surg Case Rep. 2019;57:198. Creative Commons Attribution License (CC BY): http://creativecommons.org/licenses/by/4.0/)

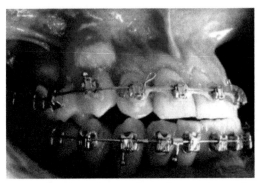

Fig. 7. Solitary swelling in the gingival area of maxillary canine region. (*From* Rahman N, Cole E, Webb R. Calcifying epithelial odontogenic tumour presenting at a surgical site: case report. Br J Oral Maxillofac Surg. 2013;51(8):e278; with permission.)

roots may be seen in calcifying odontogenic cyst but not in CEOT cases. AFO is more common among children age group and predominantly presents as unilocular radiolucent defect of posterior mandible, whereas CEOT presents as multilocular radiolucent defect of posterior mandible. There are a few cases in which calcifications are not present, and this feature may lead to misdiagnosis as squamous cell carcinoma.

Management
The clinical behavior of CEOT is aggressive but less so than ameloblastoma because CEOT does not infiltrate into the intertrabecular bony spaces as ameloblastoma. Small tumors can be managed by enucleation and curettage, whereas larger ones require local resection. However, posterior maxillary lesions are treated more aggressively because maxillary tumors tend to be more aggressive, spread rapidly, and may involve the surrounding vital structures. Adequate resection of the lesion with disease-free surgical margins and long-term follow-up is recommended. Recurrence of the lesions has been reported,[34] but CEOT has a much lower recurrence rate than ameloblastoma.

Ameloblastic Fibroma

Ameloblastic fibroma (AF) is a rare benign odontogenic tumor that originates from both epithelial and mesenchymal elements of odontogenic tissues. This lesion is discussed in this article because early developing stages of odontoma often appear as AF. The differentiation between early odontoma and AF is important so as to avoid unnecessary potentially destructive surgery. The AF has the potential for recurrence and malignant transformation to ameloblastic fibrosarcoma, which would require more aggressive surgery.

Microscopic examination of biopsied tissue is required for confirmation of clinical and/or radiographic diagnosis. Because of reported higher recurrence rate and the potential for malignant transformation the lesion is managed surgically through aggressive approaches.

Clinical features
AF presents as an asymptomatic, slow-growing, painless swelling of jaw. The posterior mandible is frequently affected. Cases are reported commonly in first and second decades of life. Gingival lesions are uncommon.[35]

Diagnostic modalities
AF is radiographically characterized as well-defined unilocular or multilocular radiolucent defect in posterior mandible extending into the ascending ramus. The radiolucent lesion is associated with a sclerotic border. An association with an unerupted tooth is not uncommon.[36]

Microscopic examination shows mesenchyme appearance of dental papilla of developing tooth bud. The odontogenic epithelium appears as long and narrow cords.

Differential diagnosis
Early developmental stage of odontoma should be considered in the AF. This is because early stages of odontoma appear as radiolucent defect.[11]

Management
AF is managed by a more conservative surgical excision when compared with amelo-blastoma. Initially AF was treated by simple surgical excision however due to the consideration of its recurrence rate; aggressive surgical approach is now the recommendation.

Ameloblastic Fibroodontoma

AFO is a relatively rare mixed odontogenic tumor arising from both odontogenic epithelial and mesenchyme elements (**Fig. 8**). The lesion is similar to AF with an addition of mineralized mass. The mineralized mass observed in AFO is enamel and dentin. This lesion usually occurs in people younger than 20 years with no gender predilection. AFO is commonly reported in posterior mandible followed by posterior maxillae.

Radiographically, AFO is recognized as a well-defined unilocular radiolucent defect with multiple mineralized opacities of tooth densities. Multiple small radiopacities may aggregate to form a large solid mass in radiolucent defect.[37]

Microscopic examination of biopsied tissue shows a presentation identical to AF with an addition of calcifying element of enamel and dentin matrix structures. The lesion is managed by conservative curettage. The lesion has minimal tendency for recurrence.[11,38]

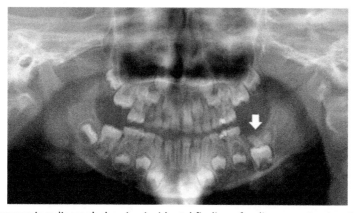

Fig. 8. Panoramic radiograph showing incidental finding of radiopaque structure in the left first mandibular molar in a 6-year-old patient. (*From* Otsugu M, Okawa R, Nomura R, et al. Ameloblastic fibro-odontoma in mandibular molar region: a case report. Pediatr Dent J. 2019;29(1):38; with permission.)

Central Odontogenic Fibroma

Central odontogenic fibroma (COF) is a rare odontogenic tumor arising from mature odontogenic ectomesenchyme. The 2 variants of odontogenic fibroma are central or intraosseous and peripheral or extraosseous forms. Radiographically, COF presents as a multilocular or a unilocular radiolucency covering the crown of unerupted tooth. Few cases show a sclerotic border. Distinguishing COF with dentigerous cyst is sometimes challenging and radiographic features are not diagnostic. Because of similarity of appearance with dentigerous cyst, COF is discussed in this article.

Clinical features

COF is a painless, slow but progressive swelling of the jaw. Small lesions are asymptomatic, and larger lesions may present symptoms due to cortical plate expansion. Tooth mobility is reported in few cases. Female predilection is observed in COF. Predominant number of cases are reported in maxillary anterior region (**Fig. 9**) followed by posterior mandible.[39,40]

Diagnostic modalities

COF is radiologically characterized by well-defined unilocular radiolucency pericoronal area of unerputed teeth or periradicular area of erupted teeth. Few cases also show sclerotic border. In cases with periradicular radiolucency, root resorption or root divergence may be seen. In larger lesions with buccal lingual expansion the radiograph may show a multilocular radiolucency similar to that of the ameloblastoma. Few cases reported calcifications within radiolucent areas. Smaller COF also mimics the features of hyperplastic dental follicle.[41]

Microscopic examination of tumor stroma either shows stellate-shaped fibroblasts or cellular with collagen fibers in interlacing fashion. Long strands of odontogenic epithelium are also seen.

Differential diagnosis

Radiographic appearance of COF mimics dentigerous cyst due to pericoronal radiolucency with radiopaque sclerotic border, whereas larger long-standing lesions mimic ameloblastoma. Differential diagnosis of dentigerous cyst must be considered in

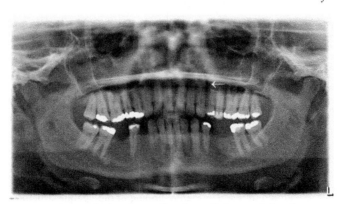

Fig. 9. Panoramic radiograph showing unilocular radiolucent defect between maxillary left canine and first premolar. (*From* De Matos FR, De Moraes M, Neto AC, et al. Central odontogenic fibroma. Ann Diagn Pathol. 2011;15(6):482; with permission.)

cases with suspicion of COF. Because of similarity in radiographic appearance it is very difficult to distinguish from dentigerous cyst. Hence radiographic examination is not diagnostic, and microscopic examination of biopsied specimen is the only way to achieve a definitive diagnosis.

Management
COF is managed by surgical enucleation and curettage. Prognosis is usually good. Few cases were reported with recurrence.

Peripheral Odontogenic Fibroma

Peripheral odontogenic fibroma (POF) is an extraosseous variant of central odontogenic fibroma that arises within the gingival mucoperiosteum. The lesions predominantly appear on gingiva and some lesions have mineralization within the mass. Cases have been documented with recurrence after surgical removal.

Clinical features
POF appears clinically as asymptomatic, painless, small, slow-growing, exophytic, firm, and sessile gingival swelling with normal color of mucosa.[42] The lesion shows slight predilection and is observed on facial aspect of gingiva than lingual or palatal side.

Diagnostic modalities
Radiographic appearance is generally not diagnostic, but horizontal bone loss may be seen. Where mineralized has occurred, a soft tissue shadow may be seen. Few POF cases show mineralized material.

Microscopic examination of POF is characterized by gingival epithelium cellular fibrous connective tissue with interlacing collagen fibers and long strands of odontogenic. The features are similar to COF except for the presence of gingival epithelium.[43]

Differential diagnosis
Differential diagnostic list includes gingival lesions such as healing stage of pyogenic granuloma, peripheral giant cell granuloma, and peripheral ossifying fibroma. History and clinical details are helpful in distinguishing POF with above-stated conditions but will not be diagnostic. Peripheral ossifying fibroma should be considered when mineralized spicules in the lesion are observed in palpation of gingival lesions. Peripheral giant cell granuloma can be excluded when foci of bluish changes are not observed in the gingival swelling. Cases of healing stage of pyogenic granuloma may give a history of bleeding to touch in the early stages of the lesion. Microscopic diagnosis is required for confirmatory diagnosis.

Management
POF is managed by surgical excision with underlying mucoperiosteum. Prognosis is excellent. Few cases have reported about recurrence of lesion.

Odontogenic Myxoma

Odontogenic myxoma (OM) is a rare odontogenic tumor that arises from odontogenic ectomesenchyme. Although this is a rare neoplasm, it is discussed in this article because the lesion can be seen in periradicular regions of premolar-molar teeth of maxillae or mandible. In addition, the lesion tends to be accidently discovered in routine radiographic examination.

Clinical features

Smaller OM presents as asymptomatic and is usually discovered in routine dental radiographic examination. Larger lesions may cause cortical plate expansion, facial asymmetry with or without painless ulcerative changes. OM occurs in individuals over a wide age range with predominance to posterior region of mandible or maxillae.[44]

Diagnostic modalities

Radiologically smaller OM lesions are characterized by unilocular radiolucent area with scalloped margin. Larger myxomas show striking multilocular appearance due to numerous opaque mineralized septa resulting in honeycomb or soap bubble appearance.[45] The mineralization in OM occur perpendicular to each other mimicking a step-ladder appearance.

Microscopic examination is characterized by loose myxomatous stroma with intersecting mineralized tissue. The myxomatous tissue is gelatinous, hence the specimen tends to stick to metal instruments while surgical operation or sectioning in laboratory.

Differential diagnosis

The unilocular radiolucent appearance of the lesion in between tooth and periradicular region may possess challenge to differentiate with lateral periodontal cyst or periapical cyst. Histopathology will be required for definitive diagnosis.

Management

OM is managed by enucleation and wide curettage of the normal surrounding bone. The lesion is not encapsulated, hence it requires more attention during surgical procedure to assure complete removal of the tumor. One-fourth of lesions tend to recur; however, the overall prognosis is good.

Cementoblastoma

Cementoblastoma is a benign odontogenic neoplasm originating from cementoblasts. Hence the name cementoma is also preferable. The features of cementoblastoma are similar to osteoblastoma; the difference is that cementoblastoma occurs in association with teeth, whereas the former does not. Although this condition is rare, general dentist should be aware of this lesion because it occurs at the periapical region of tooth. In addition, the cementoblastoma is hard tissue that attaches to the apex of tooth and possesses challenges when such tooth is indicated for extraction.

Clinical features

Cementoblastoma is closely associated with the apex of one or more tooth roots. The growth is usually painless with or without cortical plate expansion. Although the lesion cam presents as asymptomatic, approximately about two-thirds of cases present with pain and cortical plate expansion. Displacement of adjacent teeth can occur. When maxillary premolar or molars are affected, the tumor can displace the floor of the maxillary sinus. The permanent dentition is predominantly affected and deciduous dentition is rarely affected.[46]

Diagnostic modalities

Radiographic appearance is diagnostic because the mass seems as periapical radiopaque structure at one or more tooth roots, and usually the mass is fused with the tooth. The lesion is surrounded by a thin radiolucent rim. Root resorption of the affected tooth is common; however, the feature is hidden because the mineralized mass tends to fuse with associated root of affected teeth (**Fig. 10**).[47]

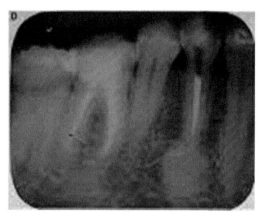

Fig. 10. Intraoral radiograph showing radiopaque mass attached to root of affected tooth. (*From* Borges DC, Rogerio de Faria P, Junior HM, Pereira LB. Conservative treatment of a periapical cementoblastoma: a case report. J Oral Maxillofac Surg. 2019;77(2):272.e2; with permission.)

Microscopic examination of the tissue resembles osteoblastoma with difference of teeth involvement. The lesion is characterized by multiple mineralized areas with the background of connective tissue stroma.

Differential diagnosis

Differential diagnosis of cementoblastoma should be made on the grounds of periapical or periradicular radiopaque appearance. Hypercementosis, condensing osteitis, osteoid osteoma, periapical cemento-osseous dysplasia (PCOD) can be considered in differential diagnosis depending on case situation. Condensing osteitis cases usually show thermal response of nonvital tooth. PPCOD should be considered in differential diagnosis in cases occurring in anterior region. PCOD usually shows mixed radiographic appearance with predominance of radiopaque structure in the background of radiolucent zone. Osteoid osteoma cases may be located near the apex of teeth. However, patients with osteoid osteoma may report nocturnal pain that may be relieved by taking aspirin. Hypercementosis is usually found at the apex of teeth that have no opposing tooth.

Management

Symptomatic and asymptomatic cementoblastoma are managed by surgical extraction of tooth and associated mass. It seems important that the involved tooth be removed, because if it remains, there is a risk of the growth reappearing. Root amputation, surgical excision of the mass, and endodontic treatment are also treatment options due to the low recurrence rate. However, cases that are endodontically managed with root amputation must be closely monitored for any recurrence of lesion at the apex of affected teeth.

Calcifying Cystic Odontogenic Tumor

Calcifying cystic odontogenic tumor (CCOT) is also known as calcifying odontogenic cyst because the condition reflects dual behavior, that is, cyst and neoplastic. CCOT is listed in this article because CCOT can be accidently discovered in routine radiographic examination. Two variants of CCOT are reported: peripheral and extraosseous. Extraosseous variant presents as a gingival swelling, whereas intraosseous forms may or may not present any clinically abnormal enlargement.

The radiographic examination is characterized by either unilocular or multilocular radiolucent defect depending on the size of the lesion. The radiolucent defect shows multiple mineralized opacities of tooth densities.[7]

CCOT are managed by aggressive surgical approach due to clinical behavior and recurrence rate. The clinical and diagnostic details of CCOT are discussed in Arvind Babu Rajendra Santosh's article, "Odontogenic Cysts," in this issue.

SUMMARY

Odontogenic neoplasm is a group of conditions with heterogeneous clinical behavior and radiological appearances. Although general dentist do not manage odontogenic tumors in their practice, the knowledge on these conditions are important because early stages are detectable in intraoral periapical radiographic examination when they occur near the dental tissues of jaw bone. The recognition of odontogenic tumors will seem challenging to the general dentist because of their relatively low prevalence, the reclassification or appearance of new entities, and the fact that long-standing names are subjects for renaming or changing categories such as cyst to tumor or tumor to cyst through academic discussions. However, regardless of reclassifications and name changes the fundamental concepts on diagnostics and clinical presentations remain the same. It is worth noting that odontogenic tumors possess characteristic clinical patterns and behavior along with demonstrable radiographic appearances, which makes clinicopathologic correlation possible for diagnosis. Hence a general dentist with sound knowledge on the diagnostic information with good radiographic interpretation skills will be able to detect these conditions when observed in their practice. Early identification, timely referral, and adequate treatment will greatly reduce severity of disease, extensive surgery, and patient cost.

REFERENCES

1. Wright JM, Soluk Tekkesin M. Odontogenic tumors: where are we in 2017 ? J Istanb Univ Fac Dent 2017;51(3 Suppl 1):S10–30.
2. Morgan PR. Odontogenic tumors: a review. Periodontol 2000 2011;57(1):160–76.
3. Santosh ABR, Jones TJ. The epithelial-mesenchymal interactions: insights into physiological and pathological aspects of oral tissues. Oncol Rev 2014;8(1):239.
4. Satish V, Prabhadevi MC, Sharma R. Odontome: a brief overview. Int J Clin Pediatr Dent 2011;4(3):177–85.
5. Gedik R, Müftüoğlu S. Compound odontoma: differential diagnosis and review of the literature. West Indian Med J 2014;63(7):793–5.
6. Radheshyam C, Alokenath B, Kumar H, et al. Calcifying cystic odontogenic tumor associated with an odontome - a diverse lesion encountered. Clin Cosmet Investig Dent 2015;7:91–5.
7. Muddana K, Maloth A, Dorankula S, et al. Calcifying cystic odontogenic tumor associated with ameloblastoma – A rare histological variant. Indian J Dent Res 2019;30(1):144–8.
8. Dar MA, Alaparthi R, Yalamanchili S, et al. Bilateral coronoid hypoplasia and complex odontoma: a rare concurrence of developmental pathology and odontogenic tumour of the mandible. BMJ Case Rep 2015;2015 [pii:bcr2015212022].
9. Koh K-J, Park H-N, Kim K-A. Gardner syndrome associated with multiple osteomas, intestinal polyposis, and epidermoid cysts. Imaging Sci Dent 2016;46(4):267–72.

10. Zhuoying C, Fengguo C. Huge erupted complex odontoma in maxilla. Oral Maxillofac Surg Cases 2019;5(1):100096.
11. Cohen DM, Bhattacharyya I. Ameloblastic fibroma, ameloblastic fibro-odontoma, and odontoma. Oral Maxillofsc Surg Clin North Am 2004;16(3):375–84.
12. Soluk Tekkesin M, Pehlivan S, Olgac V, et al. Clinical and histopathological investigation of odontomas: review of the literature and presentation of 160 cases. J Oral Maxillofac Surg 2012;70(6):1358–61.
13. Thulasirman SK, Thuasidoss G, Prabhu NK, et al. A rare case of ameloblastic fibro-odontoma of mandible with literature review. Ann Maxillofac Surg 2018; 8(2):324–6.
14. Pacifici A, Carbone D, Marini R, et al. Surgical management of compound odontoma associated with unerupted tooth. Case Rep Dent 2015;2015:902618.
15. Pogrel MA. The keratocystic odontogenic tumour (KCOT)–an odyssey. Int J Oral Maxillofac Surg 2015;44(12):1565–8.
16. Ogle OE, Santosh AB. Medication management of jaw lesions for dental patients. Dent Clin North Am 2016;60(2):483–95.
17. Speight PM, Takata T. New tumour entities in the 4th edition of the World Health Organization Classification of Head and Neck tumours: odontogenic and maxillofacial bone tumours. Virchows Arch 2018;472(3):331–9.
18. McClary AC, West RB, McClary AC, et al. Ameloblastoma: a clinical review and trends in management. Eur Arch Otorhinolaryngol 2016;273(7):1649–61.
19. Santosh ABR, Boyd D, Laxminarayana KK. Proposed clinico-pathological classification for oral exophytic lesions. J Clin Diagn Res 2015;9(9):ZE01–8.
20. Neyaz Z, Gadodia A, Gamanagatti S, et al. Radiographical approach to jaw lesions. Singapore Med J 2008;49(2):165–76 [quiz: 177].
21. Almajid EA, Alfadhel AK. Management of large pediatric ameloblastoma: conservative approach with 4-years follow up. Oral Maxillofac Surg Cases 2019;5(1): 100093.
22. Scholl RJ, Kellett HM, Neumann DP, et al. Cysts and cystic lesions of the mandible: clinical and radiologic-histopathologic review. Radiographics 1999; 19(5):1107–24.
23. Neagu D, Escuder-de la Torre O, Vázquez-Mahía I, et al. Surgical management of ameloblastoma. Review of literature. J Clin Exp Dent 2019;11(1):e70–5.
24. Dao TV, Bastidas JA, Kelsch R, et al. Malignant ameloblastoma: a case report of a recent onset of neck swelling in a patient with a previously treated ameloblastoma. J Oral Maxillofac Surg 2009;67(12):2685–9.
25. Smitha T, Priya NS, Hema KN, et al. Ameloblastic carcinoma: a rare case with diagnostic dilemma. J Oral Maxillofac Pathol 2019;23(Suppl 1):69–73.
26. Babu A, Coard KCM, Williams EB, et al. Adenomatoid odontogenic tumor: Clinical and radiological diagnostic challenges. J Pierre Fauchard Acad 2017;31: 115–20.
27. Neha S, Santosh M, Sachin MG, et al. Adenomatoid odontogenic tumour: an enigma. Saudi Dent J 2018;30(1):94–6.
28. Laheji A, Sakharde S, Chidambaram S, et al. Adenoameloblastoma: a dilemma in diagnosis. J Contemp Dent Pract 2012;13(6):925–9.
29. Awange DO. Adenomatoid odontogenic tumour (adenoameloblastoma)–a review. East Afr Med J 1991;68(3):155–63.
30. Bilodeau EA, Seethala RR. Update on odontogenic tumors: proceedings of the North American Head and Neck Pathology Society. Head Neck Pathol 2019; 13(3):457–65.

31. Gruber K, de Freitas Filho SAJ, Dogenski LC, et al. Surgical management of a large calcifying epithelial odontogenic tumor in the maxilla: a case report. Int J Surg Case Rep 2019;57:197–200.
32. Rahman N, Cole E, Webb R. Calcifying epithelial odontogenic tumour presenting at a surgical site: case report. Br J Oral Maxillofac Surg 2013;51(8):e277–8.
33. Narwal A, Devi A, Gupta S, et al. A radiolucent lesion presenting calcification histopathologically: a classical case of CEOT. J Exp Ther Oncol 2018;12(4):317–22.
34. Vigneswaran T, Naveena R. Treatment of calcifying epithelial odontogenic tumor/ Pindborg tumor by a conservative surgical method. J Pharm Bioallied Sci 2015; 7(Suppl 1):S291–5.
35. Rao SP, Srivastava G, Smitha B. Ameloblastic fibroma. J Oral Maxillofac Pathol 2012;16(3):444–5.
36. de Castro J-F-L, Correia A-V-L, Santos L-A-M, et al. Ameloblastic fibroma: a rare case appearing as a mixed radiographic image. J Clin Exp Dent 2014;6(5): e583–7.
37. Otsugu M, Okawa R, Nomura R. Ameloblastic fibro-odontoma in mandibular molar region: a case report. Pediatr Dent J 2019;29(1):37–41.
38. Singh AK, Kar IB, Mishra N, et al. Ameloblastic fibroodontoma or complex odontoma: two faces of the same coin. Natl J Maxillofac Surg 2016;7(1):92–5.
39. Eversole LR. Odontogenic fibroma, including amyloid and ossifying variants. Head Neck Pathol 2011;5(4):335–43.
40. de Matos FR, de Moraes M, Neto AC, et al. Central odontogenic fibroma. Ann Diagn Pathol 2011;15(6):481–4.
41. Santoro A, Pannone G, Ramaglia L, et al. Central odontogenic fibroma of the mandible: a case report with diagnostic considerations. Ann Med Surg (Lond) 2015;5:14–8.
42. Prasanth T, Chundru NS, Arvind Babu RS, et al. Peripheral ossifying fibroma: report of 2 cases. Dentaires Revista 2012;4(2):22–5.
43. Siwach P, Joy T, Tupkari J, et al. Controversies in odontogenic tumours: review. Sultan Qaboos Univ Med J 2017;17(3):e268–76.
44. Shivashankara C, Nidoni M, Patil S, et al. Odontogenic myxoma: a review with report of an uncommon case with recurrence in the mandible of a teenage male. Saudi Dent J 2017;29(3):93–101.
45. Nandan SRK, Chundru NS, Arvind Babu RS, et al. Odontogenic myxoma of the anterior maxilla : an unusual case report with review of literature. Dentaires Revista 2014;4(1):9–14.
46. Çalışkan A, Karöz TB, Sumer M, et al. Benign cementoblastoma of the anterior mandible: an unusual case report. J Korean Assoc Oral Maxillofac Surg 2016; 42(4):231–5.
47. Borges DC, Rogerio de Faria P, Junior HM, et al. Conservative treatment of a periapical cementoblastoma: a case report. J Oral Maxillofac Surg 2019;77(2): 272.e1-7.

Mucocutaneous Diseases

Michal Kuten-Shorrer, DMD, DMSc[a], Reshma S. Menon, BDS, DMSc[b],*,
Mark A. Lerman, DMD[c]

KEYWORDS

- Lichen planus • Pemphigus vulgaris • Mucous membrane pemphigoid
- Oral mucocutaneous diseases • Dermatoses • Oral cavity

KEY POINTS

- Oral manifestations of mucocutaneous diseases may be the first, only, and/or most significant sign of disease.
- Although some clinical features are pathognomonic for a specific disease, others are nonspecific. Diagnostic tests, including histopathology and immunofluorescence studies, are crucial in achieving a definitive diagnosis.
- Because of the systemic nature of mucocutaneous diseases, a multidisciplinary approach in management is necessary.

INTRODUCTION

The oral mucosa originates in large part from an invagination of the ectoderm and is therefore comparable with the skin. Both structures are composed of highly specialized stratified squamous epithelium, mainly comprising keratinocytes adhering to one another and to the underlying basement membrane and connective tissue. Mucocutaneous conditions are a group of disorders mostly confined to the epithelium, thereby involving the skin and oral mucosa. Other mucosal sites, such as genital mucosa, nasal mucosa, and conjunctiva, are also affected.

Oral mucosal manifestations vary and may be the initial feature, most prevalent and/or symptomatic feature, or only sign of disease. Although mucocutaneous disorders are mainly observed in the dermatology practice, a multidisciplinary approach is critical for effective care. Based on the clinical presentation, the dental practitioner may be the first to identify oral lesions and hence plays an important role in the early diagnosis and management of disease.

Disclosure: The authors have nothing to disclose.
[a] Division of Oral Medicine, Department of Diagnostic Sciences, Tufts University School of Dental Medicine, 1 Kneeland Street, Boston, MA 02111, USA; [b] Department of Oral Medicine, Infection and Immunity, Harvard School of Dental Medicine, 188 Longwood Avenue, Boston, MA 02115, USA; [c] Division of Oral Pathology, Department of Diagnostic Sciences, Tufts University School of Dental Medicine, 1 Kneeland Street, Boston, MA 02111, USA
* Corresponding author.
E-mail address: Reshma_menon@hsdm.harvard.edu

Dent Clin N Am 64 (2020) 139–162
https://doi.org/10.1016/j.cden.2019.08.009
0011-8532/20/© 2019 Elsevier Inc. All rights reserved.

Mucocutaneous disorders can be broadly categorized based on cause into developmental (genodermatoses), infectious, inflammatory, immune-mediated or autoimmune, and neoplastic conditions. These diseases are autoimmune/immune mediated or inflammatory, and are characterized by frequent and early involvement of the oral mucosa. This article discusses the more common and clinically significant mucocutaneous conditions and provides overview information on less common conditions (**Box 1**).

LICHEN PLANUS
Epidemiology

Lichen planus (LP) is a chronic inflammatory disorder that most frequently involves the skin and/or oral mucosa.[1,2] Compared with cutaneous disease, oral LP (OLP) tends to be more chronic, with a mean age at onset in the fifth to sixth decades and a slight female predilection.[1,3] Data on the prevalence of OLP are limited, with estimates ranging between less than 1% and up to 3% of the population, making OLP the most common mucocutaneous condition in the mouth.[4]

Pathobiology

OLP is considered a T cell–mediated reaction directed against epithelial basal cells, but the target antigen, whether endogenous or exogenous, is unknown.[5–10] Following antigen recognition, both cluster of differentiation (CD) 4+ T-helper cells and CD8+ cytotoxic T cells are activated, with a predominance of CD8+ cells within the epithelium. The exact mechanism of the ensuing basal keratinocytes apoptosis remains unknown; however, it is thought to be triggered by granzyme B release, tumor necrosis factor alpha secretion, and Fas Ligand expression. Aside from these antigen-specific processes, the development of OLP also is thought to involve mast cell degranulation and matrix metalloproteinase activation, leading to basement membrane disruption and migration of lymphocytes through the epithelium.

Several causal factors have been implicated in OLP, including (1) psychological stress; (2) local and systemic inducers of cell-mediated hypersensitivity; and (3) infectious agents. Acute exacerbations of OLP have been linked to psychological stress, and anxiety and depression are reported to be more common in patients with OLP compared with normal controls.[11,12] Lichenoid mucositis is an umbrella term for

---

Box 1
Mucocutaneous diseases

Most common

Lichen planus

Pemphigus vulgaris

Mucous membrane pemphigoid

Less common

Erythema multiforme

Systemic lupus erythematosus

Epidermolysis bullosa

Psoriasis

Chronic ulcerative stomatitis.

lichenoid hypersensitivity reactions, presenting with clinical and histologic features almost identical/very similar to OLP.[10,13–16] Oral lichenoid contact lesions (OLCLs) are typically triggered by dental restorative materials (mainly amalgam) or food flavoring (usually cinnamic aldehyde). Oral lichenoid drug reactions (OLDRs) arise in temporal association with exposure to certain medications, such as oral hypoglycemic agents, diuretics, angiotensin-converting enzyme inhibitors, or nonsteroidal antiin-flammatory drugs.[15–17] Strong evidence suggests an association between hepatitis C virus (HCV) infection and OLP in some geographic regions, such as southern Europe and Japan.[18–20] The mechanism underlying this association is not clear but may be related to a pattern of immune dysregulation and could involve a cytotoxic immune response to epithelial cells infected with HCV.[21]

Clinical Presentation

Classic cutaneous LP presents with violaceous papules, sometimes polygonal, and often covered by a network of fine white lines (Wickham striae). Lesions appear mainly on the flexural aspect of the wrists and ankles and in the lumbar region. They are char-acteristically pruritic and self-limiting, remitting within 1 to 2 years in most cases.[1,2,22]

Although up to 60% of patients with cutaneous LP may show oral disease, only 15% of patients with OLP develop cutaneous lesions.[1] In these cases, lesions develop within several months after the appearance of oral disease.[23] OLP is characterized by roughly symmetric and bilateral distribution, typically affecting the buccal mucosa, gingiva, and/or tongue. This characteristic distribution allows differentiation of OLP from OLCLs (**Table 1**). Although histopathologically similar to OLP, OLCLs are often unilateral in presentation, occurring in direct topographic relationship with the offend-ing agent (**Fig. 1**).[24,25]

OLP can be classified into 6 subtypes based on clinical appearance. These sub-types may present individually or concurrently: reticular, atrophic, erosive, papular, plaque, and bullous.[26] A more recent classification groups lesions into only 3 clinical subtypes: reticular, atrophic/erythematous, and ulcerative (**Table 2, Fig. 2**).[27] By far, the reticular subtype is the most common, presenting with Wickham striae, and is generally asymptomatic. Atrophic and ulcerative forms are usually accompanied by reticulation, facilitating the differentiation process from other mucocutaneous dis-eases, such as pemphigus vulgaris or mucous membrane pemphigoid (MMP). When affecting the gingiva, atrophic OLP often presents as desquamative gingivitis, with painful diffuse erythema, erosion, and desquamation of the attached and mar-ginal gingiva. Although OLP is the leading cause, other mucocutaneous disorders can lead to desquamative gingivitis and these cases can be clinically indistinguishable (**Box 2**).[28,29]

When more than 1 site is concurrently involved, the severity of the oral disease does not necessarily correlate either with the extent of involvement or with the severity of the disease in the other sites. Furthermore, the intensity of symptoms in the oral cavity is variable and, in some cases, symptoms are expressed only when triggered by spicy or acidic foods. A sense of mucosal roughness or reduced mucosal flexibility may also be noted.

Diagnosis and Assessment

Definitive diagnosis of OLP relies on both clinical and histopathologic features. The clinicopathologic correlation is especially important considering the various OLP mimics that may present with similar clinical and/or histopathologic characteristics (see **Table 1**).[15]

Table 1
Clinical and histologic mimics of oral lichen planus

Entity	Common Clinical Presentation	Typical Histopathology	Characteristic Immunofluorescence Findings
OLP	• Bilateral, roughly symmetric distribution • Reticular, atrophic, or erosive subtypes (see **Table 2**)	• Basal cell degeneration with presence of cytoid bodies • Bandlike lymphocytic infiltrate at interface • Sawtooth rete ridges • Subepithelial clefting	• DIF: usually negative; shaggy deposits of fibrinogen at BMZ and IgM-positive colloid bodies • IIF: negative
OLCLs	• Individual lesions similar to OLP • At site of irritation, often unilateral	• Similar to OLP • Eosinophils or perivascular/paravascular inflammation may be noted	• DIF: similar to OLP • IIF: negative
OLDRs	• Similar to OLP • Temporal relationship with medications	Similar to OLP	• DIF: similar to OLP • IIF: negative
Mucous membrane pemphigoid	• Desquamative gingivitis, ulcers, bullae formation • Positive Nikolsky sign	• Subepithelial clefting with preservation of basal cells • Variable chronic inflammation	• DIF: continuous linear deposits of IgG, IgM, C3, and/or IgA along the BMZ • IIF: often negative
LP pemphigoides	• Combined features of MMP and OLP	• Similar to OLP, MMP, or both	• DIF: similar to MMP • IIF: IgG at BMZ
Pemphigus vulgaris	• Diffuse ulcers and erosions, desquamative gingivitis • Positive Nikolsky sign	• Suprabasilar clefting and acantholysis • Variable inflammation in the lamina propria	• DIF: intercellular deposits of IgG and C3 • IIF: intercellular IgG
Chronic graft-versus-host disease	• Similar to OLP • History of allogeneic hematopoietic stem cell transplant	• Similar to OLP • Lymphocytic band is usually sparse	• DIF: similar to OLP • IIF: negative
Lupus erythematosus	• Usually asymmetric lesions • Central ulceration surrounded by radiating striae	• Similar to OLP • BMZ thickening • Perivascular inflammatory infiltrate	• DIF: granular deposits of IgG, IgM, and/or C3 at BMZ • IIF: negative in discoid LE; systemic LE commonly ANA, anti–double-stranded DNA, anti-SM, RNP, Ro/SSA, and La/SSB, anti-antiphospholipid, and cardiolipin positive

Abbreviations: ANA, antinuclear antibody; BMZ, basement membrane zone; DIF, direct immunofluorescence; IIF, indirect immunofluorescence; LE, lupus erythematosus; MMP, mucous membrane pemphigoid.
Data from Refs.[14–16]

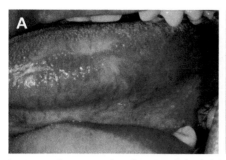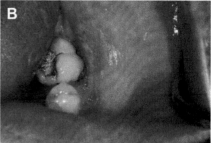

Fig. 1. Amalgam-associated OLCLs of the left lateral tongue (*A*) and posterior buccal mucosa (*B*) presenting with erythema and white striations/plaques. The amalgam is in direct contact with the affected areas. (*Courtesy of* Daliah Salem, DMD, MMSc, Boston University Goldman School of Dental Medicine, Boston, MA.)

Histopathology

The 2003 modified World Health Organization (WHO) diagnostic criteria for OLP outline 2 hallmark features (**Fig. 3**)[30]:

1. A well-defined, bandlike zone of lymphocytic infiltration confined to the superficial lamina propria
2. Liquefactive degeneration (squamatization) of the basal cell layer

Other microscopic features include hyperparakeratosis and/or orthokeratosis, acanthosis, sawtooth-rete ridges, and cytoid (colloid or Civatte) bodies. Subepithelial clefting may occur and is a common artifact caused by the weakened basal cell adhesion to the connective tissue.

Immunofluorescence

Tissue diagnosis may be challenging because the histopathologic features of OLP may be influenced by a variety of factors, including the clinical subtype and the severity of disease at the time of the biopsy. The use of direct immunofluorescence (DIF) is thus recommended as a diagnostic adjunct, and can facilitate, for example, the differentiation of OLP from vesiculobullous diseases (see **Table 1**). This differentiation is of particular importance in the case of OLP presenting solely as desquamative gingivitis,[31] or in the rare case of LP pemphigoides of the pemphigoid family,

Table 2
Oral lichen planus: clinical patterns

Type	Clinical Appearance and Common Sites	Comments
Reticular	White striations (Wickham striae), papules, or plaquelike lesions on the buccal mucosa, ventral and dorsal tongue, labial mucosa, or gingiva. Usually asymptomatic	Most common manifestation of disease
Atrophic	Areas of erythema, particularly on the gingiva (desquamative gingivitis). May be painful	Usually in conjunction with reticular lesions
Ulcerative	Ulcerations, rare bullae. May cause significant pain	In conjunction with reticular and erythematous lesions

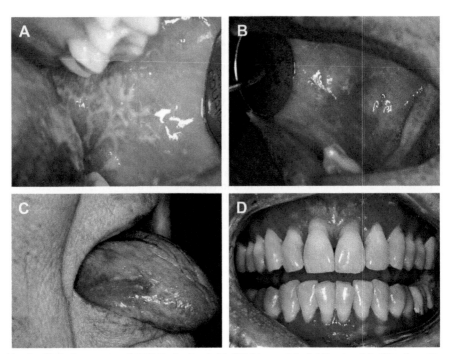

Fig. 2. Clinical patterns of OLP. Reticular (with Wickham striae) (*A*); atrophic (*B*); ulcerative (*C*); atrophic form presenting as desquamative gingivitis (*D*).

characterized by the development of vesiculobullous lesions on areas affected by LP.[32] DIF requires submission of tissue in Michel solution as opposed to the 10% formalin used to transport tissue for routine hematoxylin-eosin (H&E) staining. To this end, 2 samples should be obtained. OLP is characterized by deposition of fibrinogen in a shaggy pattern along the basement membrane zone (BMZ) with variable deposition of immunoglobulin (Ig) and complement.

Treatment

Management of OLP focuses on symptom alleviation, because no cure exists. Although not specific for OLP, patients benefit from elimination of local factors that may trigger or exacerbate symptoms. These factors may include sharp or rough restorations, ill-fitting dentures, or plaque-induced gingival disease. Oral lichenoid

---

Box 2
Differential diagnosis: desquamative gingivitis

1. OLP and lichenoid lesions

2. Vesiculobullous diseases
   a. Mucous membrane pemphigoid
   b. Pemphigus vulgaris
   c. Less common: paraneoplastic pemphigus, epidermolysis bullosa acquisita, and linear immunoglobulin A disease

3. Plasma cell gingivitis

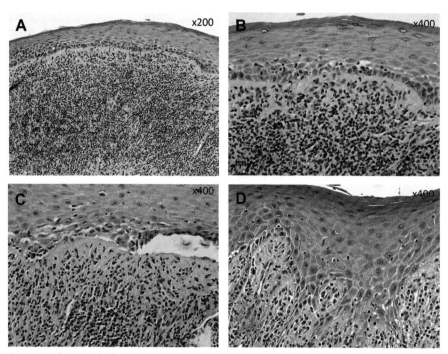

Fig. 3. OLP histopathology. (*A*) Hyperkeratosis, epithelial atrophy, and a dense bandlike lymphohistiocytic infiltrate in the superficial lamina propria (original magnification ×200). (*B*) Squamatization and degeneration of basal cells with scattered eosinophils in the inflammatory infiltrate (original magnification ×400). (*C*) Squamatization of the basal cells and a subepithelial cleft with a moderately dense lymphohistiocytic infiltrate in the lamina propria (original magnification ×400). (*D*) Acanthotic epithelium, colloid bodies, and sawtooth-shaped rete ridges with weakened cell adhesions in the basal cell layer (original magnification ×400).

reactions may resolve following identification and removal of the offending agent. Patch testing can further assist in determining alternative materials to use.

Pharmacologic therapy
Although asymptomatic OLP requires no treatment other than periodic observation, symptomatic cases are managed pharmacologically based on the extent and severity of disease. Topical corticosteroids are first-line therapy.[33–36] The potency of the agent, coupled with the delivery formulation, significantly affect the effectiveness of the treatment (**Table 3**), and maximal efficacy is ensured by providing the patient with clear instructions for use. For refractory and symptomatic localized ulcerative lesions, intralesional injections of triamcinolone acetonide (10–40 mg/mL) can be used. Alternatively, tacrolimus 0.1%, a calcineurin inhibitor, can be used topically either as an ointment or a compounded solution when topical corticosteroids alone are insufficient. Topical retinoids, tretinoin 0.1% or isotretinoin 0.1%, can also be considered as second-line treatment.[33] Because topical immunosuppressive treatment increases the risk of secondary candidiasis, prophylactic topical or systemic antifungal therapy may be required and should be considered on a case-by-case basis.[37]

The addition of systemic therapy is considered during acute severe exacerbations of localized disease, or in cases involving extraoral sites as well (eg, genitalia, skin,

Table 3
Topical corticosteroids commonly used for the management of oral manifestations of mucocutaneous diseases

Medication[a]	Instruction of Use[b]	Comments
Topical Gels, Creams, and Ointments		
Clobetasol 0.05% Fluocinonide 0.05% Betamethasone dipropionate 0.05% Triamcinolone 0.1%–0.5%	Apply to lesions 2–4 times per day. Gels can be applied with gauze and left in place 10–15 min Extensive gingival lesions can be treated with occlusive trays that hold the gel on the affected areas	Gels are preferred for intraoral use and are effective in managing limited areas of involvement
Topical Solutions		
Dexamethasone 0.1 mg/mL (5 mL) Prednisolone 3 mg/mL (5 mL)	Hold solution and swish in mouth for 4–6 min before expectoration. Repeat 2–4 times per day	For mild to moderate cases in which lesions are diffuse, numerous, or inaccessible to topical application

[a] Drugs are listed in a descending order of potency.
[b] For all cases of topical therapy, patients are instructed to wait 10 to 15 minutes after application before eating/drinking or brushing teeth.

or esophagus). Systemic prednisone (1 mg/kg/d) is generally effective and should be used for the shortest possible duration in order to mitigate potential adverse effects. If used for longer than 2 weeks, a taper is needed. Evidence to support the use of other, steroid-sparing systemic agents is sparse and generally weak.[36,38] These agents include hydroxychloroquine,[39] azathioprine,[40,41] and mycophenolate mofetil.[42]

Prognosis and Monitoring

OLP is a chronic condition, characterized by waxing and waning severity. Patients are typically followed at least annually, with the frequency of follow-up visits increasing proportionally with disease activity and symptoms. The importance of long-term monitoring and periodic repeat biopsy is further emphasized by the reported risk of malignant transformation, especially in the erosive subtype of disease. Depending on the study, the transformation rate varies between 0.4% and 5.8% over periods of observation from 0.5 to more than 20 years.[43] This variability primarily stems from the lack of concordance in the diagnostic criteria of OLP and is at the heart of the controversy surrounding its malignant potential.[38] In a recent attempt to address this problem, Aghbari and colleagues[44] conducted a meta-analysis limited to studies using the modified WHO diagnostic criteria, showing an overall 0.9% transformation rate.

PEMPHIGUS VULGARIS
Epidemiology

Pemphigus refers to a group of autoimmune acantholytic blistering disorders that affect the mucosa and skin.[45] Several variants of pemphigus have been described based on clinicopathologic correlation, including pemphigus vulgaris (PV), pemphigus foliaceus, paraneoplastic pemphigus (PNP), and other less common varieties.[46] Only PV and PNP typically have oral involvement. PV is the most common variant, preferentially affecting women in their fifth and sixth decades of life.[47,48] Showing a strong genetic component, PV is more prevalent in certain ethnic groups, particularly Ashkenazi Jews and individuals of Mediterranean and south Asian origin. The incidence of PV is extremely variable and ranges between 0.5 and 50 cases per million based on the population evaluated.[49–52]

Pathobiology

Pemphigus is understood to be predominantly familial, although sporadic cases have been reported. Many human leukocyte antigen (HLA) genetic profile studies have been performed and associations have been noted for *HLA-DRB1*0402/1401/1404*, *DQB1*0503*, and *DRB1*03/07/15* in distinct populations, among several others.[53] Although many of these phenotypes have associated risks, the correlation between the HLA status and patients' clinical outcomes is still vague.[54]

Historically, PV is thought to result from antibody-mediated acantholysis leading to suprabasal blistering. According to the compensation hypothesis, IgG serum autoantibodies are directed against desmogleins (Dsg) 1 and 3, members of the cadherin family of molecules that are present in desmosomes and are normally responsible for maintaining the structural integrity of stratified squamous epithelium.[45,55,56] In normal mucosa and skin, these are expressed throughout the thickness of the epithelium with a predominance of Dsg3 in oral mucosa. This differential expression profile of autoantibodies significantly corresponds to the patient's clinical presentation and extent of mucous membrane and cutaneous involvement. Hence, patients with oral mucosal involvement have chiefly anti-Dsg3 autoantibodies that lead to defective cell adhesion and acantholysis.[48,56,57]

Nowadays, it is thought that the pathogenesis of PV is more complex, with factors other than autoantibodies against Dsg1 and Dsg3 contributing to the development of disease.[58–60] Studies on mechanistic pathways of Dsg antibody generation have led to the identification of a synergistic model formed from a trifecta of autoantibody-guided steric hindrance of Dsg-mediated adhesion, altered desmosome assembly, and altered signaling pathways.[46,59]

Clinical Presentation

The lesions in PV typically present in a mucocutaneous fashion with extremely rare cases involving only the skin.[61] The oral mucosal lesions are usually the first to appear, followed by mucosal lesions in other sites, such as the larynx, esophagus, conjunctiva, nose, anus and genitals, or the skin. Cutaneous lesions present as flaccid bullae and erosions, commonly presenting on the head, trunk, and groin.

Exclusive oral mucosal involvement is estimated to occur in 50% of cases,[62–64] consisting of flaccid blisters, painful erosions, and superficial ulcers (**Fig. 4**). A recent study of 31 cases of PV revealed that nongingival lesions were present more frequently (55% of cases) and desquamative gingivitis was noted in less than a third of the cases.[65] These data are consistent with previous reports of site-specific oral mucosal involvement of PV.[63,66,67]

Diagnosis and Assessment

The extent of involvement of mucosal and skin lesions should be assessed along with the disease-related damage and functional impairment, as part of the physical examination. Nikolsky sign, a perilesional mechanical manipulation leading to the formation of a new vesicle, is commonly positive. Although this test is only moderately sensitive, it has been reported to show high specificity for the diagnosis of PV.[68,69]

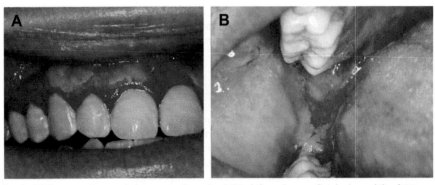

Fig. 4. Diffuse erosion and desquamative gingivitis (*A*) and superficial ulcers (*B*) of PV.

Histopathology and immunofluorescence

A biopsy of a vesicle that was first noted less than 24 hours before the visit or of the perilesional mucosa is recommended. Suprabasilar clefting and acantholysis with Tzanck cells within the cleft are characteristic of PV (**Fig. 5**). Variable degrees of chronic inflammation may be noted.

In addition to routine histologic analysis, DIF studies should be submitted from lesional/perilesional tissue. In PV, these show intercellular deposits of IgG in a meshlike pattern; IgA may also be noted (**Fig. 6**). In patients with positive DIF, serologic studies can further support the diagnosis. Indirect immunofluorescence (IIF) microscopy uses monkey esophagus to detect the presence of autoantibodies to intracellular structural proteins of keratinocytes.[70] ELISA (enzyme-linked immunosorbent assay) can also help confirm the presence of IgG autoantibodies and is positive in more than 90% of cases.[71,72] Because the levels of circulating autoantibodies frequently correlate with the course of disease, IIF and ELISA aid with monitoring disease activity and response to treatment. However, active disease may infrequently occur in the absence of detectable IgG autoantibodies[73]; in contrast, up to 40% of patients in clinical remission may have detectable levels of antibodies.[74,75]

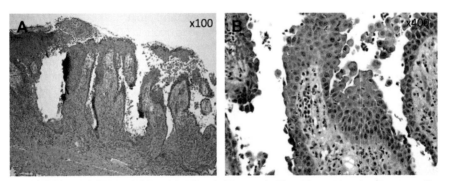

Fig. 5. PV histopathology. (*A*) Suprabasilar clefting and villouslike connective tissue papillae with acantholytic cells (original magnification ×100). (*B*) Rounded acantholytic (Tzanck) cells protruding into the cleft with scattered acute and chronic inflammatory cells (original magnification ×400).

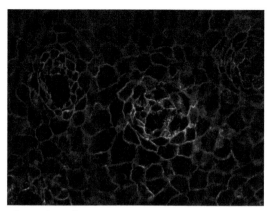

Fig. 6. Intercellular deposition of IgG in PV.

PNP (paraneoplastic autoimmune multiorgan syndrome [PAMS]), a rare variant of pemphigus associated with malignancy, may present with similar oral findings to PV. Differentiation can be facilitated by the identification of clinical features such as highly symptomatic, therapy-refractory hemorrhagic mucositis of the lip and tongue mucosa (**Fig. 7**). The reported cohort is of patients in the fourth to seventh decades, with both sexes affected equally.[76–78] Extensive mucocutaneous involvement is common, often with a heterogeneous clinical course and presentation. It is crucial for a thorough diagnostic work-up to rule out an occult malignancy.[78] In addition to developing the characteristic IgG autoantibodies to Dsg1 and/or Dsg3, other antigens from the plakin family have also been implicated.[76,79] A severe complication of PNP/PAMS is the development of bronchiolitis obliterans, related to the disease-associated cytotoxic T-cell activity.[80,81]

Treatment

Therapy in patients with PV is designed to produce symptomatic improvement either via direct reduction of serum autoantibodies or immunosuppression. Similar to OLP, topical corticosteroids may be considered if the oral findings are localized (see **Table 3**).

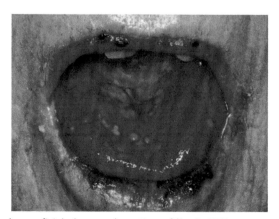

Fig. 7. Widespread superficial ulcers and crusting of lips in PNP.

Because the first priority during the initial phase of therapy is to attain rapid disease control, systemic corticosteroids are often used in addition to or instead of topical agents, with a starting dosage of prednisone of 0.5 to 1.5 mg/kg/d[82] This treatment can be supplemented with steroid-sparing, immunosuppressive adjuvants, particularly in patients with the risk of developing complications associated with therapy or prolonged corticosteroid use.[69] The first-line corticosteroid-sparing immunosuppressive agents, azathioprine and mycophenolate mofetil, show relative safety and efficacy.[83] More recent add-ons to first-line treatment are anti-CD20 monoclonal antibodies, rituximab and ofatumumab. Introduction of rituximab in a patient's therapeutic regimen is warranted in patients with moderate to severe disease and in cases without successful clinical remission with systemic corticosteroids and immunosuppressive therapy. In long-term follow-up studies, up to 45% of patients who were treated with rituximab remained in remission even when taken off of systemic therapy.[84–86]

Other steroid-sparing agents currently used include intravenous Ig (IVIG) administered at 2 g/kg over 2 to 5 days per month. Patients receive IVIG in combination with first-line systemic corticosteroids and/or immunosuppressive agents. Although the significant cost of IVIG has been cited as a concern to patients and physicians, it is cost-effective when considering the reduction in side effects associated with conventional immunosuppressive therapy.[87] Cyclophosphamide and other modalities, such as immunoadsorption, are used as the last resort if all other options fail.[69]

Prognosis

Until the introduction of corticosteroids as first-line therapy for patients with pemphigus, the mortalities were as high as 90%, but have since drastically reduced to between 5% and 10%.[88–90] The use of corticosteroids has associated comorbidities such as Cushing syndrome/hypercortisolism, osteoporosis, and adrenal insufficiency.[90] With the introduction of other first-line therapies, these are seen less often.

The ultimate goal for PV management is long-term remission after the discontinuation of therapy. With the use of immunosuppressive adjuvants and the addition of rituximab to the treatment arsenal, complete remission off therapy is achievable. The outcomes vary vastly based on the treatment modalities used.

MUCOUS MEMBRANE PEMPHIGOID
Epidemiology

MMP is an uncommon autoimmune subepithelial blistering disorder that belongs to the group of pemphigoid diseases, along with at least 7 other distinct entities.[91] Although the epidemiology of MMP is unclear, some studies estimate the incidence to be around 1.3 to 2.0 per million people, and the prevalence is almost twice in women.[92–94] Most patients with MMP are in the fifth to seventh decades of life at the time of diagnosis.[94,95]

Pathobiology

The most widely accepted theory for the development of MMP is based on the development of circulating antibodies in response to altered immunologic tolerance to structural proteins located in the basement membrane of epithelium/epidermis.[96] At least 6 target antigens have been identified and include BP180, laminin 332, laminin 311, BP230, both subunits of α6β4 integrin, and type VII collagen.[91] Specifically, IgG and IgA autoantibodies were found most commonly against BP180 in patients with MMP (50%–75%) and patients with ocular lesions presented with reactivity to β4 integrin (>85%).[97] The binding of autoantibodies to BMZ antigens leads to the weakening of the attachment of the hemidesmosomes to the basement membrane and ultimately the development of a subepithelial cleft. A potential contributing factor, increased prevalence of *HLA-DQB1*0301*, has been reported in patients with MMP.[98]

Clinical Presentation

The hallmark feature of MMP is the presence of clinically evident bullae, erosions, and secondary scarring of the mucosa and, less often, the skin.[99] However, the oral mucosa tends to be spared from the scarring effects of the disease process.[91] The clinical severity is extremely variable and can present as a discrete bulla, widespread lesions, or desquamative gingivitis. Lesions present most frequently in the oral cavity (85%), followed by other mucosal sites such as conjunctiva (65%), nasal cavity (20%–40%), anogenital area (20%), pharynx (20%), and larynx (5%–10%).[91]

Oral MMP typically presents with erythematous patches and erosions with/without a pseudomembrane.[99] The detection of intact vesicles or bullae is uncommon because they tend to quickly rupture, leaving irregularly shaped erosions. The most common presentation of oral lesions in MMP is that of desquamative gingivitis (84% of cases; **Fig. 8**), and extragingival lesions are noted in less than 10% of cases.[65,100]

Diagnosis and Assessment

The diagnosis of MMP must be rendered based on a combination of the clinical presentation, histopathology, and immunofluorescence studies.[99] The occurrence of desquamative gingivitis in a patient should prompt the physician to include MMP in the list of differentials (see **Box 2**).[29] Although unreliable and not included as a diagnostic criterion, Nikolsky sign may be positive in oral MMP.[99,101]

Histopathology and immunofluorescence

A biopsy of an intact blister or perilesional tissue in proximity to the erosion is obtained and submitted for routine H&E and DIF studies.[102] A subepithelial cleft or detached fragments of epithelium showing intact basal cells are characteristically noted. Variable epithelial thickness and inflammation may be present (**Fig. 9**). DIF studies of MMP show linear deposition of IgG, C,3 and IgA in the BMZ (**Fig. 10**). IIF is rarely used because circulating antibodies are rarely detectable in patients (5%–25%) with MMP.

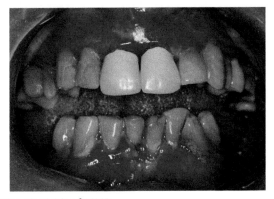

Fig. 8. Desquamative gingivitis of MMP.

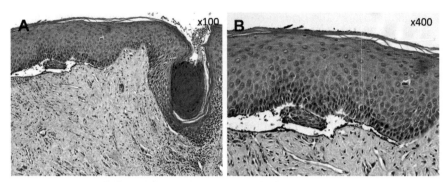

Fig. 9. MMP histopathology. (*A*) Hyperkeratosis, variable epithelial hyperplasia, a subepithelial cleft and scattered inflammatory cells (original magnification ×100). (*B*) Subepithelial clefting with preservation of basal cells (original magnification ×400).

Treatment

Therapy for oral MMP includes a combination of topical and systemic agents designed to reduce disease severity and symptoms without tipping the balance in favor of immunosuppression. Patients are stratified as high or low risk to help guide therapeutic decisions. The classification is based on the site of disease involvement, severity, and progression of disease, and indicates the risk of developing sequelae from scarring.[99] Involvement of the oral mucosa, with or without the skin, renders the patient low risk and a more conservative approach is indicated.

Topical corticosteroids are first-line therapy for localized disease (see **Table 3**). An occlusive tray is recommended for gingival disease. Alternatively, gauze may be used to help keep the medication in close contact with the lesions. Topical tacrolimus 0.1% ointment also may be used in refractory cases.

Systemic therapy primarily comprises corticosteroids and steroid-sparing agents and is administered to high-risk patients with MMP and low-risk patients who fail topical therapeutics (**Table 4**). Other systemic agents have been reported to be used for treatment of oral MMP and include tetracycline, nicotinamide, and

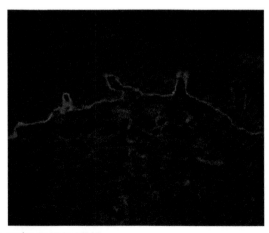

Fig. 10. Linear C3 at the BMZ in MMP.

Table 4
Mucous membrane pemphigoid: risk stratification

Risk Class	Criteria	Treatment
Low	Oral mucosa/oral mucosa and limited skin	Moderate-dose to high-dose topical corticosteroids (see **Table 3**)

High	• Ocular, genital, nasopharyngeal, esophageal, and/or laryngeal mucosae; or
	• Rapid disease progression
		Mild disease
		• Dapsone (50–200 mg/d) or
		• Sulfamethoxypyridazine (0.5–1 g/d) or
		• Sulfapyridine (0.25–1 g/d)
		Severe disease
		• Prednisone (0.5–1.5 mg/kg/d)
		  Adjuvant therapies:
		  • Cyclophosphamide (1–2 mg/kg/d) or
		  • Azathioprine (1–2 mg/kg/d) or
		  • Mycophenolate mofetil (1–2 g/d in divided doses)

Data from McMillan R, Taylor J, Shephard M, et al. World Workshop on Oral Medicine VI: a systematic review of the treatment of mucocutaneous pemphigus vulgaris. Oral surgery, oral medicine, oral pathology and oral radiology. 2015;120(2):132–42.e161; and Chan LS, Ahmed AR, Anhalt GJ, et al. The first international consensus on mucous membrane pemphigoid: definition, diagnostic criteria, pathogenic factors, medical treatment, and prognostic indicators. Arch Dermatol. 2002;138(3):370–9.

methotrexate.[103] IVIG and rituximab have also been used to treat ocular MMP successfully; large studies are yet to be published on therapeutic protocols for these agents in oral MMP.[82,91]

Prognosis

MMP may result in debilitating or life-threatening disease in the absence of treatment. However, even with treatment, prognosis is unpredictable because response differs among individuals and relapse is common. Based on clinical evidence gathered over the past several decades, prognostic predictors are now recognized for MMP and serve as a guide for therapeutics and patient counseling. The site of involvement, presence and titers of dual isotypes of autoantibodies (IgG and IgA), and the antigen-specific autoantibodies are prognostic indicators of disease severity.[99]

ERYTHEMA MULTIFORME
Epidemiology

Erythema multiforme (EM) is an acute, self-limiting, immune-mediated disorder affecting the skin and/or mucosal surfaces. The oral mucosa is the most frequently involved mucosal site, with a reported frequency of up to 70%.[104,105] EM usually occurs in healthy young adults with a peak age at onset in the 3rd to 4th decades of life, although up to 20% of cases occur in children.[106,107] While epidemiological data is scarce, the annual incidence of EM is estimated to be far less than 1 percent.[106] Most cases are transient and resolve without long-term sequelae, but a subset of patients experience repeated episodes over many years, leading to recurrent EM.[104,107]

Pathobiology

A hypersensitivity reaction, EM is primarily triggered by infectious agents (approximately 90% of cases), with herpes simplex virus (HSV) most frequently implicated, followed by *Mycoplasma pneumonia* (PM) which is also the major cause of EM in children.[108,107] Drugs are the second most frequently suspected cause of EM.[109,110] Implicated medications include sulfonamides, NSAIDs, and penicillins.

The underlying pathogenesis of HSV-related EM is the most studied and is thought to involve a cell-mediated immune reaction against HSV DNA fragments in the skin or mucosa.[111–113] Following a recurrent HSV infection, the virus is present in the blood and phagocytosed by circulating mononuclear cells, particularly circulating CD34+ Langerhans cell precursors. The engulfed viral DNA is then transported to the epithelium, where the expression of HSV DNA fragments, notably the viral *pol* gene, leads to activation of HSV-specific T cells and production of effector cytokines. This step initiates an inflammatory cascade that promotes the lysis of HSV-infected cells and recruitment of autoreactive T cells. The specific immune response to the viral *Pol* protein, which is synthetized and expressed for only a few days, may explain the transient nature of EM lesions.

Clinical presentation

EM is characterized by acute targetoid erythematous lesions with symmetric, acral distribution and can be classified into isolated cutaneous (EM minor, EMm) and mucocutaneous forms (EM major, EMM). Mucosal involvement alone is rare.[109,110] Typical targetoid lesions are regular, well-defined round papules or plaques consisting of at least three concentric zones: a central disk, a peripheral pale ring, and an erythematous halo.[114] Lesions generally measure less than 3 cm in diameter. Atypical raised target lesions may also appear, manifesting as elevated, palpable lesions with only two zones and/or an ill-defined border. By definition, less than 10% body surface area (BSA) is affected in EM. Lesions are generally asymptomatic, although burning or itching may be reported, and persist for one week or longer before healing without scarring.

Oral involvement is primarily seen in EMM, whereas the lips alone may be involved in EMm. The lips tend to become swollen and show pathognomonic hemorrhagic crusting.[115,116] Intraorally, diffuse areas of erythema and/or superficial ulcerations typically affect the lingual, buccal, and labial mucosa, particularly in the anterior parts of the mouth. Occasional intact vesicles may be seen. Lesions are painful, compromising speech and alimentation. They usually occur simultaneously with skin lesions, and, similarly, heal without scarring.[117]

Diagnosis and assessment

The diagnosis of EM is based on clinical presentation. Patients' history should be reviewed for evidence of a triggering factor, with special emphasis on a recent HSV infection.[110,114,118] Laboratory work up is not required, as there are no specific diagnostic tests for EM, however aids in identification of causal agents and exclusion of other disorders.

Stevens-Johnson syndrome (SJS) can be differentiated from EMM primarily based on clinical appearance (**Table 5**).[115,119,120] Painful, predominantly macular atypical target lesions are characteristic. Other differentiating criteria include constitutional symptoms, distribution of lesions, and clinical severity, with SJS considered a life-threatening reaction.

Confirmation of active HSV infection in HSV-associated EM can be achieved using viral culture, cytology, or direct fluorescent antibody (DFA) testing. In cases where a clear relationship to HSV is not supported by history and clinical examination, serology for HSV antibodies excludes HSV-associated EM when negative. Positive serology coupled with molecular testing (polymerase chain reaction [PCR] or in-situ hybridization) for HSV on tissue specimens indicates subclinical HSV reactivation, and possible

Table 5
Erythema multiforme major versus Stevens-Johnson syndrome: different diseases with distinct features

	Cause	Prodromal Symptoms	Cutaneous Lesions	Mucosal Involvement
EMM	Likely infectious	Usually absent	• Distribution: localized, acral; <10% BSA • Pattern: typical targets, raised atypical targets • Nikolsky sign: negative	Often limited to oral mucosa: erythema, ulceration, and hemorrhagic crusting
SJS	Likely drugs	Common, flu-like	• Distribution: widespread, including central trunk; <10% BSA • Pattern: flat atypical targets, macules • Nikolsky sign: positive	• At least two sites involved • Oral cavity almost always affected: extensive ulceration with hemorrhagic crusts

Abbreviations: BSA, body surface area; EMM, erythema multiforme major; SJS, Stevens-Johnson syndrome.

HSV-associated EM. In patients with respiratory symptoms, molecular or serologic testing for M. pneumoniae infection are indicated to support a diagnosis of M. pneumoniae-related EM. Finally, tissue biopsy and immunofluorescent studies allow to differentiate EM from other vesiculobullous disorders.

Histopathology and immunofluorescence
Histological features are often nonspecific and if a biopsy is mandated, the epithelium shows spongiosis, keratinocyte apoptosis and necrosis, lymphocyte satellitosis and degeneration of basal cells. Variable chronic inflammation is noted, and eosinophils are often present. As mentioned earlier, the diagnosis is primarily based on clinical findings and a biopsy may be performed in order to rule out a vesiculobullous disorder.

Treatment
The goals of treatment are two-fold: 1) to reduce the duration of acute EM and prevent complications, and 2) to prevent or reduce the frequency and severity of recurrences. Thus, the management of EM depends on the severity of the disease and its course, as well as the underlying cause. Evidence to support the various treatments derives primarily from retrospective series or small controlled trials.[114,121]

In suspected drug-induced EM, the first measure is to discontinue the offending drug and avoid re-exposure. Mild disease, manifesting with only cutaneous involvement or nondisabling, limited oral mucosal involvement, is managed with focus on symptomatic relief. Topical corticosteroids serve as first-line therapy (**Table 3**) alongside topical anesthetics, as needed. Short-term systemic corticosteroids are often used in severe cases with extensive oral mucosal involvement and risk of dysphagia, although controlled studies are lacking. Hospitalization for nutrition and pain control may be required.

In cases of recurrent HSV-associated EM, continuous antiviral therapy with systemic acyclovir, valacyclovir, or famciclovir is effective at suppressing attacks.[104,105,122] Prophylactic antiviral therapy should also be considered in patients with idiopathic recurrent EM, when subclinical HSV infection cannot be excluded. Evidence is lacking to support specific recommendations for treatment duration in cases with favorable response. For patients with recurrent EM resistant to continuous antiviral therapy, second-line therapies include azathioprine, mycophenolate mofetil, or dapsone.[114,121]

Prognosis

Acute EM is usually self-limiting, with complete resolution within weeks without significant sequelae. Some patients, however, experience recurrences. The severity and frequency of attacks is highly variable and unpredictable. In a large case series, Schofield et al. reported an average of six attacks per year, and an overall mean duration of disease of 9.5 years.[105] Several features have been associated with a less favorable prognosis for disease control in patients with recurrent EM.[104] These include severe oral involvement, inability to identify a specific cause, lack of improvement with continuous antiviral therapy, extensive corticosteroid therapy, and immunosuppressive therapy with two or more agents.

SUMMARY

Oral lesions may be the first and occasionally the only manifestation of mucocutaneous diseases. As such, oral health practitioners are integral members of the multidisciplinary team caring for patients with mucocutaneous disease. Early and proper diagnosis is crucial to prevent systemic progression and to ameliorate outcomes. Although some oral features are pathognomonic for the specific condition, others are nonspecific, making diagnosis difficult to achieve based on clinical examination only. Aside from the routine histologic examination, diagnostic tools such as immunofluorescence and serologic testing aid in achieving an accurate diagnosis.

REFERENCES

1. Eisen D. The evaluation of cutaneous, genital, scalp, nail, esophageal, and ocular involvement in patients with oral lichen planus. Oral Surg Oral Med Oral Pathol Oral Radiol Endod 1999;88(4):431–6.
2. Le Cleach L, Chosidow O. Lichen planus. N Engl J Med 2012;366(8):723–32.
3. Carbone M, Arduino PG, Carrozzo M, et al. Course of oral lichen planus: a retrospective study of 808 northern Italian patients. Oral Dis 2009;15(3):235–43.
4. McCartan BE, Healy CM. The reported prevalence of oral lichen planus: a review and critique. J Oral Pathol Med 2008;37(8):447–53.
5. Thornhill MH. Immune mechanisms in oral lichen planus. Acta Odontol Scand 2001;59(3):174–7.
6. Lodi G, Scully C, Carrozzo M, et al. Current controversies in oral lichen planus: report of an international consensus meeting. Part 1. Viral infections and etiopathogenesis. Oral Surg Oral Med Oral Pathol Oral Radiol Endod 2005;100(1): 40–51.
7. Lehman JS, Tollefson MM, Gibson LE. Lichen planus. Int J Dermatol 2009;48(7): 682–94.
8. Farhi D, Dupin N. Pathophysiology, etiologic factors, and clinical management of oral lichen planus, part I: facts and controversies. Clin Dermatol 2010; 28(1):100–8.
9. Payeras MR, Cherubini K, Figueiredo MA, et al. Oral lichen planus: focus on etiopathogenesis. Arch Oral Biol 2013;58(9):1057–69.
10. Kurago ZB. Etiology and pathogenesis of oral lichen planus: an overview. Oral Surg Oral Med Oral Pathol Oral Radiol 2016;122(1):72–80.

11. Rojo-Moreno JL, Bagan JV, Rojo-Moreno J, et al. Psychologic factors and oral lichen planus. A psychometric evaluation of 100 cases. Oral Surg Oral Med Oral Pathol Oral Radiol Endod 1998;86(6):687–91.
12. Pippi R, Romeo U, Santoro M, et al. Psychological disorders and oral lichen planus: matched case-control study and literature review. Oral Dis 2016;22(3): 226–34.
13. Issa Y, Duxbury AJ, Macfarlane TV, et al. Oral lichenoid lesions related to dental restorative materials. Br Dent J 2005;198(6):361–6 [disussion: 549]; [quiz: 372].
14. Khudhur AS, Di Zenzo G, Carrozzo M. Oral lichenoid tissue reactions: diagnosis and classification. Expert Rev Mol Diagn 2014;14(2):169–84.
15. Cheng YS, Gould A, Kurago Z, et al. Diagnosis of oral lichen planus: a position paper of the American Academy of Oral and Maxillofacial Pathology. Oral Surg Oral Med Oral Pathol Oral Radiol 2016;122(3):332–54.
16. Muller S. Oral lichenoid lesions: distinguishing the benign from the deadly. Mod Pathol 2017;30(s1):S54–s67.
17. Halevy S, Shai A. Lichenoid drug eruptions. J Am Acad Dermatol 1993;29(2 Pt 1):249–55.
18. Carrozzo M, Pellicano R. Lichen planus and hepatitis C virus infection: an updated critical review. Minerva Gastroenterol Dietol 2008;54(1):65–74.
19. Lodi G, Pellicano R, Carrozzo M. Hepatitis C virus infection and lichen planus: a systematic review with meta-analysis. Oral Dis 2010;16(7):601–12.
20. Alaizari NA, Al-Maweri SA, Al-Shamiri HM, et al. Hepatitis C virus infections in oral lichen planus: a systematic review and meta-analysis. Aust Dent J 2016; 61(3):282–7.
21. Harden D, Skelton H, Smith KJ. Lichen planus associated with hepatitis C virus: no viral transcripts are found in the lichen planus, and effective therapy for hepatitis C virus does not clear lichen planus. J Am Acad Dermatol 2003;49(5): 847–52.
22. Tziotzios C, Lee JYW, Brier T, et al. Lichen planus and lichenoid dermatoses: Clinical overview and molecular basis. J Am Acad Dermatol 2018;79(5): 789–804.
23. Eisen D, Carrozzo M, Bagan Sebastian JV, et al. Number V oral lichen planus: clinical features and management. Oral Dis 2005;11(6):338–49.
24. Thornhill MH, Sankar V, Xu XJ, et al. The role of histopathological characteristics in distinguishing amalgam-associated oral lichenoid reactions and oral lichen planus. J Oral Pathol Med 2006;35(4):233–40.
25. Montebugnoli L, Venturi M, Gissi DB, et al. Clinical and histologic healing of lichenoid oral lesions following amalgam removal: a prospective study. Oral Surg Oral Med Oral Pathol Oral Radiol 2012;113(6):766–72.
26. Andreasen JO. Oral lichen planus. 1. A clinical evaluation of 115 cases. Oral Surg Oral Med Oral Pathol 1968;25(1):31–42.
27. Eisen D. The clinical manifestations and treatment of oral lichen planus. Dermatol Clin 2003;21(1):79–89.
28. Lo Russo L, Fedele S, Guiglia R, et al. Diagnostic pathways and clinical significance of desquamative gingivitis. J Periodontol 2008;79(1):4–24.
29. Maderal AD, Lee Salisbury P 3rd, Jorizzo JL. Desquamative gingivitis: clinical findings and diseases. J Am Acad Dermatol 2018;78(5):839–48.
30. van der Meij EH, van der Waal I. Lack of clinicopathologic correlation in the diagnosis of oral lichen planus based on the presently available diagnostic criteria and suggestions for modifications. J Oral Pathol Med 2003;32(9): 507–12.

31. Suresh L, Neiders ME. Definitive and differential diagnosis of desquamative gingivitis through direct immunofluorescence studies. J Periodontol 2012; 83(10):1270–8.

32. Sultan A, Stojanov IJ, Lerman MA, et al. Oral lichen planus pemphigoides: a series of four cases. Oral Surg Oral Med Oral Pathol Oral Radiol 2015;120(1): 58–68.

33. Al-Hashimi I, Schifter M, Lockhart PB, et al. Oral lichen planus and oral lichenoid lesions: diagnostic and therapeutic considerations. Oral Surg Oral Med Oral Pathol Oral Radiol Endod 2007;103(Suppl):S25.e21-12.

34. Lodi G, Carrozzo M, Furness S, et al. Interventions for treating oral lichen planus: a systematic review. Br J Dermatol 2012;166(5):938–47.

35. Davari P, Hsiao HH, Fazel N. Mucosal lichen planus: an evidence-based treatment update. Am J Clin Dermatol 2014;15(3):181–95.

36. Tziotzios C, Brier T, Lee JYW, et al. Lichen planus and lichenoid dermatoses: Conventional and emerging therapeutic strategies. J Am Acad Dermatol 2018;79(5):807–18.

37. Tejani S, Sultan A, Stojanov I, et al. Candidal carriage predicts candidiasis during topical immunosuppressive therapy: a preliminary retrospective cohort study. Oral Surg Oral Med Oral Pathol Oral Radiol 2016;122(4):448–54.

38. Lodi G, Scully C, Carrozzo M, et al. Current controversies in oral lichen planus: report of an international consensus meeting. Part 2. Clinical management and malignant transformation. Oral Surg Oral Med Oral Pathol Oral Radiol Endod 2005;100(2):164–78.

39. Eisen D. Hydroxychloroquine sulfate (Plaquenil) improves oral lichen planus: an open trial. J Am Acad Dermatol 1993;28(4):609–12.

40. Lear JT, English JS. Erosive and generalized lichen planus responsive to azathioprine. Clin Exp Dermatol 1996;21(1):56–7.

41. Silverman S Jr, Gorsky M, Lozada-Nur F, et al. A prospective study of findings and management in 214 patients with oral lichen planus. Oral Surg Oral Med Oral Pathol 1991;72(6):665–70.

42. Wee JS, Shirlaw PJ, Challacombe SJ, et al. Efficacy of mycophenolate mofetil in severe mucocutaneous lichen planus: a retrospective review of 10 patients. Br J Dermatol 2012;167(1):36–43.

43. van der Meij EH, Schepman KP, Smeele LE, et al. A review of the recent literature regarding malignant transformation of oral lichen planus. Oral Surg Oral Med Oral Pathol Oral Radiol Endod 1999;88(3):307–10.

44. Aghbari SMH, Abushouk AI, Attia A, et al. Malignant transformation of oral lichen planus and oral lichenoid lesions: a meta-analysis of 20095 patient data. Oral Oncol 2017;68:92–102.

45. Amagai M. Pemphigus. In: Bolognia J, Jorizzo J, Schaffer J, editors. Dermatology, vol. 1. Elsevier; 2012. p. 461–74.

46. Kasperkiewicz M, Ellebrecht CT, Takahashi H, et al. Pemphigus. Nat Rev Dis Primers 2017;3:17026.

47. Alpsoy E, Akman-Karakas A, Uzun S. Geographic variations in epidemiology of two autoimmune bullous diseases: pemphigus and bullous pemphigoid. Arch Dermatol Res 2015;307(4):291–8.

48. Shah AA, Seiffert-Sinha K, Sirois D, et al. Development of a disease registry for autoimmune bullous diseases: initial analysis of the pemphigus vulgaris subset. Acta Derm Venereol 2015;95(1):86–90.

49. Simon DG, Krutchkoff D, Kaslow RA, et al. Pemphigus in Hartford County, Connecticut, from 1972 to 1977. Arch Dermatol 1980;116(9):1035–7.

50. Asilian A, Yoosefi A, Faghini G. Pemphigus vulgaris in Iran: epidemiology and clinical profile. Skinmed 2006;5(2):69–71.
51. Michailidou EZ, Belazi MA, Markopoulos AK, et al. Epidemiologic survey of pemphigus vulgaris with oral manifestations in northern Greece: retrospective study of 129 patients. Int J Dermatol 2007;46(4):356–61.
52. Meyer N, Misery L. Geoepidemiologic considerations of auto-immune pemphigus. Autoimmun Rev 2010;9(5):A379–82.
53. Yan L, Wang JM, Zeng K. Association between HLA-DRB1 polymorphisms and pemphigus vulgaris: a meta-analysis. Br J Dermatol 2012;167(4):768–77.
54. Sinha AA. The genetics of pemphigus. Dermatol Clin 2011;29(3):381–91, vii.
55. Amagai M, Klaus-Kovtun V, Stanley JR. Autoantibodies against a novel epithelial cadherin in pemphigus vulgaris, a disease of cell adhesion. Cell 1991;67(5): 869–77.
56. Stanley JR, Amagai M. Pemphigus, bullous impetigo, and the staphylococcal scalded-skin syndrome. N Engl J Med 2006;355(17):1800–10.
57. Koch PJ, Walsh MJ, Schmelz M, et al. Identification of desmoglein, a constitutive desmosomal glycoprotein, as a member of the cadherin family of cell adhesion molecules. Eur J Cell Biol 1990;53(1):1–12.
58. Mao X, Nagler AR, Farber SA, et al. Autoimmunity to desmocollin 3 in pemphigus vulgaris. Am J Pathol 2010;177(6):2724–30.
59. Grando SA. Pemphigus autoimmunity: hypotheses and realities. Autoimmunity 2012;45(1):7–35.
60. Schmidt E, Spindler V, Eming R, et al. Meeting report of the pathogenesis of pemphigus and pemphigoid meeting in Munich, September 2016. J Invest Dermatol 2017;137(6):1199–203.
61. Yoshida K, Takae Y, Saito H, et al. Cutaneous type pemphigus vulgaris: a rare clinical phenotype of pemphigus. J Am Acad Dermatol 2005;52(5):839–45.
62. Laskaris G, Sklavounou A, Stratigos J. Bullous pemphigoid, cicatricial pemphigoid, and pemphigus vulgaris. A comparative clinical survey of 278 cases. Oral Surg Oral Med Oral Pathol 1982;54(6):656–62.
63. Mignogna MD, Lo Muzio L, Bucci E. Clinical features of gingival pemphigus vulgaris. J Clin Periodontol 2001;28(5):489–93.
64. Santoro FA, Stoopler ET, Werth VP. Pemphigus. Dent Clin North Am 2013;57(4): 597–610.
65. Sultan AS, Villa A, Saavedra AP, et al. Oral mucous membrane pemphigoid and pemphigus vulgaris-a retrospective two-center cohort study. Oral Dis 2017; 23(4):498–504.
66. Shklar G, Frim S, Flynn E. Gingival lesions of pemphigus. J Periodontol 1978; 49(8):428–35.
67. Said S, Golitz L. Vesiculobullous eruptions of the oral cavity. Otolaryngol Clin North Am 2011;44(1):133–60, vi.
68. Uzun S, Durdu M. The specificity and sensitivity of Nikolskiy sign in the diagnosis of pemphigus. J Am Acad Dermatol 2006;54(3):411–5.
69. Murrell DF, Pena S, Joly P, et al. Diagnosis and management of pemphigus: recommendations by an international panel of experts. J Am Acad Dermatol 2018. [Epub ahead of print].
70. van Beek N, Rentzsch K, Probst C, et al. Serological diagnosis of autoimmune bullous skin diseases: prospective comparison of the BIOCHIP mosaic-based indirect immunofluorescence technique with the conventional multi-step single test strategy. Orphanet J Rare Dis 2012;7:49.

71. Amagai M, Komai A, Hashimoto T, et al. Usefulness of enzyme-linked immuno-sorbent assay using recombinant desmogleins 1 and 3 for serodiagnosis of pemphigus. Br J Dermatol 1999;140(2):351–7.
72. Schmidt E, Dahnrich C, Rosemann A, et al. Novel ELISA systems for antibodies to desmoglein 1 and 3: correlation of disease activity with serum autoantibody levels in individual pemphigus patients. Exp Dermatol 2010;19(5):458–63.
73. Schmidt E, Zillikens D. Modern diagnosis of autoimmune blistering skin diseases. Autoimmun Rev 2010;10(2):84–9.
74. Kwon EJ, Yamagami J, Nishikawa T, et al. Anti-desmoglein IgG autoantibodies in patients with pemphigus in remission. J Eur Acad Dermatol Venereol 2008; 22(9):1070–5.
75. Naseer SY, Seiffert-Sinha K, Sinha AA. Detailed profiling of anti-desmoglein autoantibodies identifies anti-Dsg1 reactivity as a key driver of disease activity and clinical expression in pemphigus vulgaris. Autoimmunity 2015;48(4):231–41.
76. Anhalt GJ, Kim SC, Stanley JR, et al. Paraneoplastic pemphigus. An autoimmune mucocutaneous disease associated with neoplasia. N Engl J Med 1990;323(25):1729–35.
77. Anhalt GJ. Paraneoplastic pemphigus. Adv Dermatol 1997;12:77–96 [discussion: 97].
78. Yong AA, Tey HL. Paraneoplastic pemphigus. Australas J Dermatol 2013;54(4): 241–50.
79. Schepens I, Jaunin F, Begre N, et al. The protease inhibitor alpha-2-macroglobulin-like-1 is the p170 antigen recognized by paraneoplastic pemphigus autoantibodies in human. PLoS One 2010;5(8):e12250.
80. Nousari HC, Deterding R, Wojtczack H, et al. The mechanism of respiratory failure in paraneoplastic pemphigus. N Engl J Med 1999;340(18):1406–10.
81. Hoffman MA, Qiao X, Anhalt GJ. CD8+ T lymphocytes in bronchiolitis obliterans, paraneoplastic pemphigus, and solitary Castleman's disease. N Engl J Med 2003;349(4):407–8.
82. McMillan R, Taylor J, Shephard M, et al. World workshop on oral medicine VI: a systematic review of the treatment of mucocutaneous pemphigus vulgaris. Oral Surg Oral Med Oral Pathol Oral Radiol 2015;120(2):132–42.e1.
83. Beissert S, Mimouni D, Kanwar AJ, et al. Treating pemphigus vulgaris with prednisone and mycophenolate mofetil: a multicenter, randomized, placebo-controlled trial. J Invest Dermatol 2010;130(8):2041–8.
84. Feldman RJ, Ahmed AR. Relevance of rituximab therapy in pemphigus vulgaris: analysis of current data and the immunologic basis for its observed responses. Expert Rev Clin Immunol 2011;7(4):529–41.
85. Colliou N, Picard D, Caillot F, et al. Long-term remissions of severe pemphigus after rituximab therapy are associated with prolonged failure of desmoglein B cell response. Sci Transl Med 2013;5(175):175ra130.
86. Wang HH, Liu CW, Li YC, et al. Efficacy of rituximab for pemphigus: a systematic review and meta-analysis of different regimens. Acta Derm Venereol 2015;95(8): 928–32.
87. Daoud YJ, Amin KG. Comparison of cost of immune globulin intravenous therapy to conventional immunosuppressive therapy in treating patients with autoimmune mucocutaneous blistering diseases. Int Immunopharmacol 2006;6(4): 600–6.
88. Langan SM, Smeeth L, Hubbard R, et al. Bullous pemphigoid and pemphigus vulgaris–incidence and mortality in the UK: population based cohort study. BMJ 2008;337:a180.

89. Huang YH, Kuo CF, Chen YH, et al. Incidence, mortality, and causes of death of patients with pemphigus in Taiwan: a nationwide population-based study. J Invest Dermatol 2012;132(1):92–7.

90. Hsu DY, Brieva J, Sinha AA, et al. Comorbidities and inpatient mortality for pemphigus in the U.S.A. Br J Dermatol 2016;174(6):1290–8.

91. Schmidt E, Zillikens D. Pemphigoid diseases. Lancet 2013;381(9863):320–32.

92. Bernard P, Vaillant L, Labeille B, et al. Incidence and distribution of subepidermal autoimmune bullous skin diseases in three French regions. Bullous Diseases French Study Group. Arch Dermatol 1995;131(1):48–52.

93. Bertram F, Brocker EB, Zillikens D, et al. Prospective analysis of the incidence of autoimmune bullous disorders in Lower Franconia, Germany. J Dtsch Dermatol Ges 2009;7(5):434–40.

94. Hubner F, Recke A, Zillikens D, et al. Prevalence and age distribution of pemphigus and pemphigoid diseases in Germany. J Invest Dermatol 2016; 136(12):2495–8.

95. Scully C, Lo Muzio L. Oral mucosal diseases: mucous membrane pemphigoid. Br J Oral Maxillofac Surg 2008;46(5):358–66.

96. Kourosh AS, Yancey KB. Pathogenesis of mucous membrane pemphigoid. Dermatol Clin 2011;29(3):479–84, x.

97. Oyama N, Setterfield JF, Powell AM, et al. Bullous pemphigoid antigen II (BP180) and its soluble extracellular domains are major autoantigens in mucous membrane pemphigoid: the pathogenic relevance to HLA class II alleles and disease severity. Br J Dermatol 2006;154(1):90–8.

98. Delgado JC, Turbay D, Yunis EJ, et al. A common major histocompatibility complex class II allele HLA-DQB1* 0301 is present in clinical variants of pemphigoid. Proc Natl Acad Sci U S A 1996;93(16):8569–71.

99. Chan LS, Ahmed AR, Anhalt GJ, et al. The first international consensus on mucous membrane pemphigoid: definition, diagnostic criteria, pathogenic factors, medical treatment, and prognostic indicators. Arch Dermatol 2002;138(3): 370–9.

100. Bagan J, Jimenez Y, Murillo J, et al. Oral mucous membrane pemphigoid: a clinical study of 100 low-risk cases. Oral Dis 2018;24(1–2):132–4.

101. Gallagher G, Shklar G. Oral involvement in mucous membrane pemphigoid. Clin Dermatol 1987;5(1):18–27.

102. Scully C, Carrozzo M, Gandolfo S, et al. Update on mucous membrane pemphigoid: a heterogeneous immune-mediated subepithelial blistering entity. Oral Surg Oral Med Oral Pathol Oral Radiol Endod 1999;88(1):56–68.

103. Xu HH, Werth VP, Parisi E, et al. Mucous membrane pemphigoid. Dent Clin North Am 2013;57(4):611–30.

104. Wetter DA, Davis MD. Recurrent erythema multiforme: clinical characteristics, etiologic associations, and treatment in a series of 48 patients at Mayo Clinic, 2000 to 2007. J Am Acad Dermatol 2010;62(1):45–53.

105. Schofield JK, Tatnall FM, Leigh IM. Recurrent erythema multiforme: clinical features and treatment in a large series of patients. Br J Dermatol 1993;128(5): 542–5.

106. Huff JC, Weston WL, Tonnesen MG. Erythema multiforme: a critical review of characteristics, diagnostic criteria, and causes. J Am Acad Dermatol 1983; 8(6):763–75.

107. Heinze A, Tollefson M, Holland KE, et al. Characteristics of pediatric recurrent erythema multiforme. Pediatr Dermatol 2018;35(1):97–103.

108. Howland WW, Golitz LE, Weston WL, et al. Erythema multiforme: clinical, histo-pathologic, and immunologic study. J Am Acad Dermatol 1984;10(3):438–46.
109. Lerch M, Mainetti C, Terziroli Beretta-Piccoli B, et al. Current perspectives on erythema multiforme. Clin Rev Allergy Immunol 2018;54(1):177–84.
110. Sokumbi O, Wetter DA. Clinical features, diagnosis, and treatment of erythema multiforme: a review for the practicing dermatologist. Int J Dermatol 2012;51(8):889–902.
111. Aurelian L, Kokuba H, Burnett JW. Understanding the pathogenesis of HSV-associated erythema multiforme. Dermatology 1998;197(3):219–22.
112. Ono F, Sharma BK, Smith CC, et al. CD34+ cells in the peripheral blood transport herpes simplex virus DNA fragments to the skin of patients with erythema multiforme (HAEM). J Invest Dermatol 2005;124(6):1215–24.
113. Aurelian L, Ono F, Burnett J. Herpes simplex virus (HSV)-associated erythema multiforme (HAEM): a viral disease with an autoimmune component. Dermatol Online J 2003;9(1):1.
114. Roujeau J-C, Mockenhaupt M. Erythema multiforme. Chapter 43. In: Kang S, Amagai M, Bruckner AL, et al, editors. Fitzpatrick's dermatology. 9th edition. McGraw-Hill Education; 2019.
115. Al-Johani KA, Fedele S, Porter SR. Erythema multiforme and related disorders. Oral Surg Oral Med Oral Pathol Oral Radiol Endod 2007;103(5):642–54.
116. Samim F, Auluck A, Zed C, et al. Erythema multiforme: a review of epidemiology, pathogenesis, clinical features, and treatment. Dent Clin North Am 2013;57(4):583–96.
117. Ayangco L, Rogers RS. Oral manifestations of erythema multiforme. Dermatol Clin 2003;21(1):195–205.
118. Scully C, Bagan J. Oral mucosal diseases: erythema multiforme. Br J Oral Maxillofac Surg 2008;46(2):90–5.
119. Auquier-Dunant A, Mockenhaupt M, Naldi L, et al. Correlations between clinical patterns and causes of erythema multiforme majus, Stevens-Johnson syndrome, and toxic epidermal necrolysis: results of an international prospective study. Arch Dermatol 2002;138(8):1019–24.
120. Assier H, Bastuji-Garin S, Revuz J, et al. Erythema multiforme with mucous membrane involvement and Stevens-Johnson syndrome are clinically different disorders with distinct causes. Arch Dermatol 1995;131(5):539–43.
121. de Risi-Pugliese T, Sbidian E, Ingen-Housz-Oro S, et al. Interventions for erythema multiforme: a systematic review. J Eur Acad Dermatol Venereol 2019;33(5):842–9.
122. Tatnall FM, Schofield JK, Leigh IM. A double-blind, placebo-controlled trial of continuous acyclovir therapy in recurrent erythema multiforme. Br J Dermatol 1995;132(2):267–70.

Differential Diagnosis of Periapical Radiopacities and Radiolucencies

Mel Mupparapu, DMD, MDS[a],*, Katherine Jie Shi, DMD[b], Eugene Ko, DMD, MS[a]

KEYWORDS

- Radiolucency • Radiopacity • Cyst • Granuloma • Dentoalveolar abscess
- Benign tumor • Malignant tumor • Metastases

KEY POINTS

- Periapical radiolucencies are most commonly odontogenic. Nonodontogenic radiolucencies tend to be not localized and span across the mandible or maxilla within the alveolus and sometimes extend inter-radicularly.
- Periapical radiopacities can be solitary or generalized. Solitary radiopacities can be attached to either a tooth or several teeth at the lamina dura. Occasionally, solitary opacifications, such as a cementoblastoma, mask the apical portion of the tooth due to cemental proliferation.
- Apical lesions can be mixed where both radiolucencies and opacities can be interspersed, as seen in disorders of fibro-osseous nature, specifically the periapical osseous dysplasia, focal, or florid osseous dysplasia.
- Large expansile radiolucencies, both septate and nonseptate, are described separately as a group because their characteristics are much different from the commonly occurring periapical lucencies that are of pulpal origin.

INTRODUCTION

Radiographic examination is the most important investigation method in general dental practice for the evaluation of dental and jaw lesions. Periapical [PA] radiographs often have an advantage to view the changes over teeth and its adjacent bone in detail. PA radiographs cannot be used, however, when a lesion is larger than 3 cm. An extraoral radiographic method, panoramic radiograph, is widely used in general

Disclosure Statement: The authors have nothing to disclose.
[a] Department of Oral Medicine, Robert Schattner Center, University of Pennsylvania School of Dental Medicine, 240 South 40th Street, Philadelphia, PA 19104, USA; [b] Department of Endodontics, Tufts University School of Dental Medicine, 1 Kneeland Street, Boston, MA 02111, USA
* Corresponding author.
E-mail address: mmd@upenn.edu

Dent Clin N Am 64 (2020) 163–189
https://doi.org/10.1016/j.cden.2019.08.010
0011-8532/20/© 2019 Elsevier Inc. All rights reserved.

dental practice to visualize the larger lesions. PA radiopacities/radiolucencies are the changes observed at the apex of the tooth. Dentists must carefully interpret these changes, however, because PA radiological observations are due to not only tooth-related pathologies but also the pathologies adjacent to the tooth/bone, which may be seen at the apex of the tooth. The most common PA pathologies can be diagnosed based on the vitality responses from the teeth. Ruling out the tooth-associated pathologies is an important step in securing a diagnosis from differential diagnosis panel of PA radiolucencies. When formulating radiological differential diagnosis, features should be evaluated carefully, such as (1) location, (2) locularity, (3) relation to dentition (4) density of lesion, (5) margin, (6) type of radiological change (radiolucent/radiopaque/mixed), (7) periosteal reaction, (8) cortical integrity, and (9) clinical presentation. This article aims to discuss dental/jaw conditions associated with radiolucent and radiopaque defects of PA region of tooth (see the list in **Box 1**).

PERIAPICAL RADIOPAQUE LESIONS
Developmental Conditions

Hypercementosis
Definition: Hypercementosis is a non-neoplastic deposition of excessive cementum along the roots of 1 or multiple teeth.[1] Hypercementosis can be idiopathic or associated with local and/or systemic factors, such as PA inflammation, trauma, developmental disorders, vitamin A deficiency, and Paget disease of bone.[2] A recent study has linked hypercementosis with mutations in ENPP1 and GACI.[3]

Epidemiology: predominantly found in adults and frequency increases with age.[1] Mandibular molars are the most frequently affected teeth, followed by mandibular and maxillary second premolars.[4]

Clinical findings: asymptomatic and generally incidentally detected after radiographic examination.[4]

Radiographic findings: an affected tooth shows cemental thickening, often at the apical third of the root, with a normal periodontal ligament (PDL) space and intact lamina dura.[1] A majority of cases result in club-shaped hypercementosis due to diffuse cemental hyperplasia that may be mild, moderate, or severe[5,6] (**Fig. 1**). Presentations may be diverse, however, including focal hypercementosis with localized nodular enlargement, circular cementum hyperplasia hypercementosis with a shirt cuff shape, and presence of multiple cemental spikes.[6,7]

Management: no treatment is necessary[4] aside from periodic radiographic evaluation and follow-up.

Periapical cemento-osseous dysplasia
Definition: This is a rare, benign fibro-osseous dysplastic process distinct from other cemento-osseous dysplasias (CODs) by its distribution restricted to the apical region of vital anterior incisors, especially in the mandible.[8] Although the etiology of CODs is unknown, the lesions are suggested as originating from the PDL.[8] CODs are associated with a coexistence of simple bone cysts,[9] propensity for osteomyelitis when exposed to oral pathogens, no malignant association, and a lack of systematic manifestations.[10]

Epidemiology: demographics plays a key role in diagnosis with PA COD affecting predominantly black women above age 40 years.[11] Prevalence of PA COD is between 0.24% and 5.9%.[8] A new association has recently been published between PA COD and female patients with neurofibromatosis type 1.[12]

Clinical findings: CODs are associated with vital teeth or extraction sites and are primarily asymptomatic.[13,14] The hypovascular nature of the affected area is

Box 1
Periapical radiopacities and radiolucencies

PA radiopacities
  Developmental conditions
    Hypercementosis
    PA COD
    FCOD
    Florid COD
    Idiopathic osteosclerosis (enostosis, dense bone island, bone scar, focal PA osteopetrosis)
    FD
    Exostoses (tori)
  Inflammatory disorders
    Condensing osteitis (PA sclerosing osteitis, sclerosing osteitis, focal sclerosing osteitis, focal
    sclerosing osteomyelitis)
    Reactional osteogenesis
    PCO
    SCO (chronic suppurative osteomyelitis)
    Osteomyelitis with proliferative periostitis (Garre osteomyelitis, juvenile chronic
    osteomyelitis, periostitis ossificans, nonsuppurative ossifying periostitis)
  Benign tumors
    Cementoblastoma
    Osteoblastoma
    Osteoma
    Osteoid osteoma
    Cemento-ossifying fibroma
    Compound odontoma
    Complex odontoma
  Mimicking lesions as PA radio-opacities due to superimposition
  Malignant and metastatic lesions
    Supernumerary teeth
    Sialolith
    PA radiopacities
    Developmental
    Dentigerous cyst
    Lateral periodontal cyst
    Inflammatory lesions
    Apical periodontitis
    PA abscess

PA radiolucencies
  Developmental
    Dentigerous cyst
    Lateral periodontal cyst
  Inflammatory disorders
    Apical periodontitis
    PA abscess
  Cystic lesions
    PA cyst
    Odontogenic keratocyst
    Glandular odontogenic cyst
  Benign tumors
    Ameloblastoma
  Malignant tumors
    Ameloblastic carcinoma

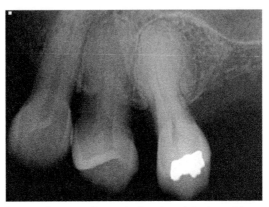

Fig. 1. Maxillary left premolar PA radiograph showing club-shaped hypercementosis of second premolar due to cemental deposition. Note the preservation of PDL space and lamina dura in the affected area.

predisposed to osteomyelitis and pathologic fracture, and, if infection is present, then symptoms can include dull pain, purulent mucosal discharge, and jaw expansion.[10]

Radiographic findings: all CODs present with 3 stages: (1) the osteolytic phase with radiolucent lesions, followed by (2) the cementoblast phase with mixed radiodensity lesions, and, finally, (3) the osteogenic phase with radiopaque lesions surrounded by a thin radiolucent peripheral halo.[15] Clinically, the most common stage is the second phase with mixed radiodensity lesions (**Figs. 2** and **3**).[13] With cone-beam computed tomography (CBCT) images, COD presents as well-defined lesions with no tooth displacement and may exhibit expansion and thinning on cortical plates.[13]

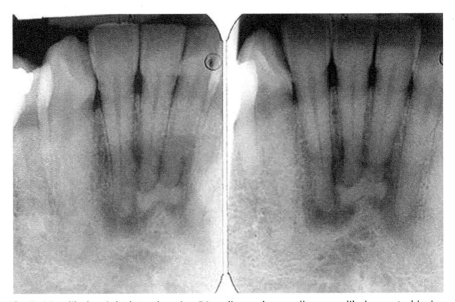

Fig. 2. Mandibular right lateral-canine PA radiograph as well as mandibular central incisor PA radiograph showing the mixed density masses apical to all the anterior teeth. The radio-pacities are surrounded by a radiolucent rim. The teeth are all vital. This is a typical presentation of PA COD.

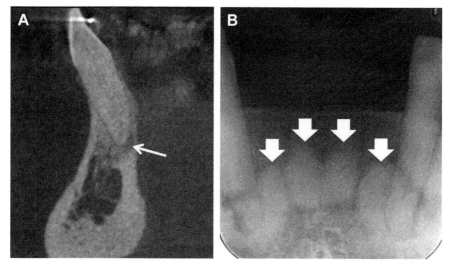

Fig. 3. CBCT orthogonal view of mandibular anterior region (*A*) showing changes at the PA region. Note the widened PDL as well as the opacities at the apex suggestive of the cemento-osseous changes. PCD-related radiopacities remain even after the extraction of the teeth as noted in the maxillary central incisor PA (*B*).

Management: unnecessary biopsy should be avoided to avoid risk of osteomyelitis.[10] And, surgical intervention should be avoided, such as extraction, periodontal surgery, and implant therapy.[8] No treatment is necessary for this self-limiting condition aside from periodic radiographic evaluation and follow-up.

Focal cemento-osseous dysplasia

Definition: This is a rare, benign fibro-osseous dysplastic process distinct from other CODs by its distribution restricted to the apical region of vital posterior teeth, especially in the mandible.[16] Although the etiology of CODs is unknown, the lesions are suggested to originate from the PDL.[8] CODs are associated with a coexistence of simple bone cysts,[9] propensity for osteomyelitis when exposed to oral pathogens, no malignant association, and a lack of systematic manifestations.[10]

Epidemiology: demographics plays a key role in diagnosis with focal COD (FCOD), affecting predominantly black women with a mean age in the mid-30s.[17] The 2 main populations at risk as defined by a systematic review in 2008 are those with East Asian and African descent.[18]

Clinical findings: clinical findings are similar to PA COD. Focal lesions are common in 1 or more posterior teeth (**Fig. 4**).

Radiographic findings: reference radiographic findings as PA COD.

Management: management is similar to PA COD.

Florid cemento-osseous dysplasia

Definition: rare, benign fibro-osseous dysplastic process distinct from other CODs by its distribution in multiple posterior quadrants of the maxilla and mandible in tooth-bearing areas.[10] Although the etiology of CODs is unknown, the lesions are suggested to originate from the PDL.[8] CODs are associated with a coexistence of simple bone cysts,[9] propensity for osteomyelitis when exposed to oral pathogens, no malignant association, and a lack of systematic manifestations.[10]

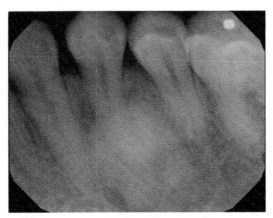

Fig. 4. FCOD. Mandibular left premolar PA radiograph showing a mixed density lesion in the vicinity of the first premolar, a vital tooth. A radiolucent rim is noted encompassing the radiopaque masses suggestive of a capsule. Radiographically, the lesions are consistent with FCOD.

Epidemiology: demographics plays a key role in diagnosis with florid COD affecting predominantly black women in their fourth to fifth decades of life. In a 2003 systematic literature review, 97% were female, 59% were black, 37% were Asian, and 3% were white.[19] Reports have documented autosomal dominant familial inheritance cases, but no underlying genetic cause has been identified.[10]

Clinical findings: clinical findings are similar to both PA COD and FCOD.

Radiographic findings: radiographic findings are similar to other COD lesions except that the lesions are seen in more than 2 quadrants (**Fig. 5**)

Management: management is similar to PA COD and FCOD.

Idiopathic osteosclerosis (enostosis, dense bone island, bone scar, and focal periapical osteopetrosis)

Definition: an increased bone production in the jaw with unknown etiology, considered a developmental variation of normal bone architecture, and without inflammatory or systemic disease.[20]

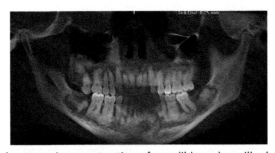

Fig. 5. CBCT-based panoramic reconstruction of mandible and maxilla showing radiodense masses interspersed with lytic areas that would appear on a regular panoramic image as mixed opaque-lucent areas in all quadrants. This is pathognomonic for a radiographic diagnosis of florid expansile COD. (*Courtesy of* Steven R. Singer, DDS, Rutgers School of Dental Medicine, Newark, NJ.)

Epidemiology: no significant demographic differences exist in relation to gender or age.[20] Incidence has been reported from 2.3% to 9.7%.[21] The most common location is at the first molar region of the mandible.[20]

Clinical findings: asymptomatic, nonexpansile, associated with a vital tooth, and generally found incidentally.[22]

Radiographic findings: well-defined radiopaque and varied in size and shape; may present as round, elliptical, or irregular and may be anywhere in size from 2 mm in diameter to the entire height of the mandible body (**Figs. 6** and **7**).[20] Most lesions occurred at root apices but also may present between roots or away from teeth[20]; 10% to 12% of cases present with external root resorption.[23]

Management: no treatment is needed aside from periodic radiographic evaluation and follow-up.[20]

Fibrous dysplasia

Definition: localized, non-neoplastic, benign fibro-osseous bone disorder with 3 presentations: (1) monostotic, (2) polyostotic, and (3) polyostotic with endocrinopathies.[24] Fibrous dysplasia (FD) is associated with a defect in stem cell differentiation with a somatic mutation in GNAS1 gene.[25] For the purpose of this section, the focus is on monostotic craniofacial FD in the initial stages limited to the apical region as a differential for PA lesions; 0.4% of FD is associated with malignant transformation, with the craniofacial region the most common site.[26]

Epidemiology: FD constitutes 2.5% of all bone lesions and 7% of all benign bone tumors and has an incidence of 1 in 4000 to 10,000.[26] Craniofacial FD is rare and presents in the posterior regions of the maxilla and mandible, in younger patients, and with no to slight female gender preference.[26,27]

Clinical findings: a characteristic finding is unilateral involvement with uninhibited physical expansion that can lead to severe deformity and asymmetry.[26] May be associated with bone pain and dental anomalies, such as malocclusion, crowding, or spacing.[24]

Radiographic findings: varied presentation depending on the stage; may appear lytic, mixed, or sclerotic.[26] Characteristic radiographic findings for FD of the jaws are poorly defined margins and presence of a ground-glass appearance

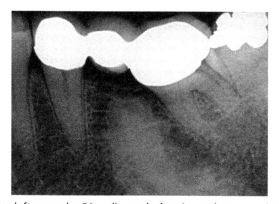

Fig. 6. Mandibular left premolar PA radiograph showing a dense opacity in the region of the missing second premolar. The density is similar to cortical bone and the opacity has well-defined borders that appear to merge with the surrounding bone. This is radiographically consistent with an idiopathic osteosclerosis or a dense bone island. The entire extent of the radiopacity is not captured in this PA radiograph.

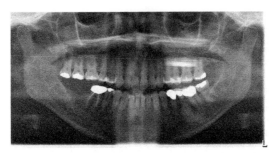

Fig. 7. Panoramic radiograph of the same area noted in **Fig. 6** shows the complete extent of the radiodensity which appears to extend inferiorly to the inferior cortex. This is radiographically consistent with an idiopathic osteosclerosis or dense bone island.

(**Fig. 8**).[24,25] In addition, associated teeth may be displaced and exhibit loss of lamina dura.[24]

Management: treatment options range from radical surgery with complex reconstruction to bone contouring with lifelong monitoring for recurrent disease.[27]

Exostoses (tori)

Definition: benign ectopic bone formation that is considered a variation of normal, including torus palatinus (TP) on the palate, torus mandibularis (TM) on the lingual side of the mandible unilaterally or bilaterally near the canine or premolar region, and buccal and palatal exostoses most commonly on the buccal of the maxilla.[28,29] The etiology is multifactorial with genetic, environmental, and systemic factors.[30] Bruxism often is reported in association; however, Bertazzo-Silveira and colleagues[30] conducted a 2017 systematic review showing lack of sufficient evidence.

Epidemiology: TP and TM are common, with a prevalence of 12% to 15% and present in early adulthood, whereas buccal and palatal exostoses are less common and associated with increasing age.[29] TP is 2 times more common in women, and TM and buccal and palatal exostoses are more common in men.[29]

Clinical findings: asymptomatic, hard, and nontender to palpation and usually diagnosed incidentally on clinical examination.[31]

Radiographic findings: radiopaque well-defined lesion that, although not associated with the PA region of teeth (**Fig. 9**), may radiographically mask by superimposition or mimic other existing lesions in the area in a 2-dimensional radiograph. Thus, CBCT imaging may be indicated.[32]

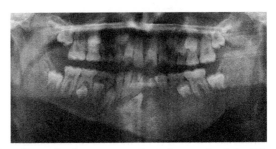

Fig. 8. Panoramic radiograph of a young patient shows mixed dentition and the inferior expansion of left mandible showing thinning of the cortex. Several erupting permanent teeth appear to have been caught in the process.

Management: no treatment is necessary; surgical removal may be performed if the lesion interferes with speech, mastication, or fabrication of a dental prosthesis, among other reasons.[31]

Inflammatory Disorders

Condensing osteitis (periapical sclerosing osteitis, sclerosing osteitis, focal sclerosing osteitis, and focal sclerosing osteomyelitis)

Definition: defined by the American Association of Endodontists *Glossary of Endodontic Terms* as a localized bony reaction secondary to low-grade inflammation and usually associated with apex of affected tooth.[33]

Epidemiology: most commonly reported radiopaque lesion of the jaws and occurs in 4% to 7% of the general population.[34] Predilections have been reported for women and the mandibular first molar region.[34,35]

Clinical findings: the lesion often is asymptomatic and nonexpansile.[17] An odontogenic infection or inflammatory association is essential to diagnosis[23]; thus, clinically may find evidence of deep caries and/or large restorations.

Radiographic findings: diffuse and uniform radiopaque lesion concentrically around the apex of the involved tooth (**Fig. 10**).[35]

Management: nonsurgical endodontic treatment is the first treatment of choice in which most cases demonstrate partial or complete regression.[23]

Reactional osteogenesis

Definition: inflammatory periosteal reaction in the maxillary sinus secondary to root canal infection in the PA regions of the posterior maxilla.[36] The bony dimension

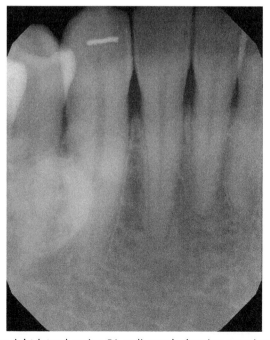

Fig. 9. Mandibular right lateral-canine PA radiograph showing superimposed mandibular tori over the apical two-thirds of the canine and first premolar roots. The radiopacity is distinct with defined borders. Although not common, in this instance, the PDL and lamina dura of both the canine and premolar are noted through the opacity.

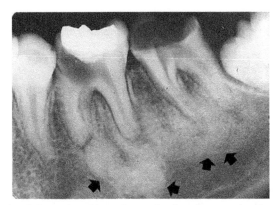

Fig. 10. Mandibular left molar PA radiograph showing condensing osteitis in relation to both first and second molar roots. Note that both the crowns show secondary caries. Root apices show widened PDL and rarefaction suggestive of PA rarefying osteitis.

between roots of teeth and maxillary sinus are significantly larger for teeth with apical pathology.[37]

Epidemiology: only 4 cases have been reported by Estrela and colleagues,[36] in 2015, in adult women with ages in the fifth and seventh decades. More cases are required to evaluate the true demographics of the lesion.

Clinical findings: often asymptomatic and incidentally detected on radiographic examination.[36]

Radiographic findings: radiopaque, well-defined localized lesions at the apex of involved teeth with varied size and shape from irregular to round to ovoid (**Fig. 11**).[36] CBCT is especially helpful in this evaluation with the ability to view the extent of involvement without the 2-dimensional superimposition of maxillary structures.

Management: the first line of treatment is nonsurgical root canal treatment, and, if unresolved, followed by surgical enucleation of the PA lesion.[36]

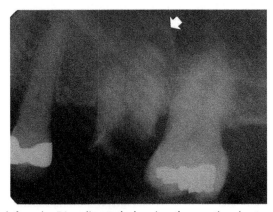

Fig. 11. Maxillary left molar PA radiograph showing the reactional osteogenesis in relation to the palatal root apex (*arrow*). The root is in close proximity to the maxillary sinus but is draped by the floor of the sinus.

Primary chronic osteomyelitis
Definition: nonodontogenic, nonsuppurative, and nonbacterial chronic inflammatory condition with unknown etiology and possible genetic, autoimmune, or lack of vascularity associations.[38]

Epidemiology: peak onset is in young patients between ages of 10 years and 20 years and older patients above age 50 years, with no determined gender preference.[38] Affects almost exclusively the mandible.[39]

Clinical findings: for more than 4 weeks and often lasting longer than 2 years, exhibiting chronic intermittent episodes of pain, swelling in lower jaw, trismus, paresthesia over lower lip and/or affected area, and enlarged regional lymph nodes.[38,39] In addition, there is an absence of history of trauma, radiation, or other predisposing factors; no pus, fistula, or sequestration; and no response to antibiotics.[38,39]

Radiographic findings: medullary sclerosis is the most prominent finding; generally variable presentations of sclerosis, osteolysis, and periosteal (onion-skin) reactions.[39]

Management: management is complex with difficult to understand etiology; proposed treatments vary with various surgical intervention and nonsurgical treatments, including anti-inflammatory drug therapy, antibiotics, hyperbaric oxygen, bisphosphonate treatment, and muscle relaxants.[40]

Secondary chronic osteomyelitis (chronic suppurative osteomyelitis)
Definition: more common than primary chronic osteomyelitis (PCO), secondary chronic osteomyelitis (SCO) is a suppurative chronic inflammatory condition with well-defined etiology of bacterial invasion from dental infection, trauma, and/or surgery to the affected area.[38] Note that SCO is the longer duration version of acute osteomyelitis.

Epidemiology: commonly affects the mandible and has no significant preference in age or gender.[41]

Clinical findings: for more than 4 weeks exhibiting chronic episodes of pus, abscess, fistula formation, and/or sequestration.[39] Unlike PCO, symptoms usually are resolved earlier than 2 years.[42] Pain and swelling were the most common complaints, followed by paresthesia and tooth mobility.[41]

Radiographic findings: varying presentations of lucent and sclerotic changes with osteolysis, bone sclerosis, sequestration, and/or periosteal reaction.[41,42]

Management: treatment of the etiology is important in SCO and usually leads to resolving the condition; treatment includes surgical débridement and antibiotics.[41]

Osteomyelitis with proliferative periostitis (garre osteomyelitis, juvenile chronic osteomyelitis, periostitis ossificans, and nonsuppurative ossifying periostitis)
Definition: special type of chronic nonsuppurative sclerosing osteomyelitis that is juvenile in nature, may be considered an early-onset form of PCO, and shows distinct thickening of the periosteum.[43] The etiology often is associated with an odontogenic infection leading to pulpal necrosis.[44]

Epidemiology: condition is seen almost exclusively in children and young adults with a mean age of 13 years, no gender preference, and more often affecting the mandible than maxilla.[43]

Clinical findings: common symptoms include facial asymmetry and swelling that is usually unilateral; other symptoms possible are pain, trismus, and malaise.[45]

Radiographic findings: CBCT aids in the understanding of the extent and etiology of the condition. Planar radiographs also show the onion-skin lamellated appearance due to periosteal new bone formation (**Fig. 12**), coarse trabecular bone with wide marrow spaces, and modified mature trabecular bone.[45]

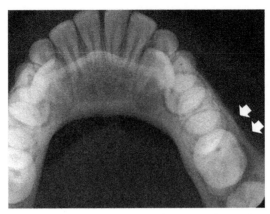

Fig. 12. Mandibular floor of the mouth occlusal radiograph shows the lamellar pattern of the periosteal reaction secondary to Garre osteomyelitis in relation to left permanent first molar infection.

Management: surgical resection is unnecessary; the goal is to eliminate the etiologic facture, which is frequently of odontogenic origin, and deliver antibiotics.[43]

Benign Tumors

Cementoblastoma

Definition: a benign neoplastic ectomesenchymal odontogenic tumor with unknown etiology and unlimited growth potential.[46]

Epidemiology: rare, accounting for less than 1% to 6.2% of all odontogenic tumors, and has no definitive gender preference.[47] There is a higher incidence in young adults before age of 30 years and most frequently involves mandibular molars and premolars, with half of cases affecting mandibular first molars.[1] Very rarely involves primary or impacted teeth.[48]

Clinical findings: symptoms of tenderness, pain, and swelling may occur along with cortical plate expansion, erosion, or perforation.[47] Teeth may remain vital.[48]

Radiographic findings: a well-circumscribed radiopaque mass continuous with root of tooth surrounded by a thin radiolucent line.[46] Additional signs include root resorption, disrupted lamina dura, and loss of root contour (**Fig. 13**).[1]

Management: gold standard treatment is the complete surgical extraction of affected teeth and calcified area.[1] Recurrence is common with curettage alone and with the incomplete removal of lesion.[48]

Osteoblastoma

Definition: a benign neoplastic primary bone tumor characterized by a proliferation of osteoblasts that often is slow growing with limited growth potential.[49] Aggressive variants exist and malignant transformation is rare.[50]

Epidemiology: rare, accounting for only approximately 1% of all primary bone tumors.[50] When involving the jaw, location is primarily in the mandibular premolar and molar region.[51] Preference for men, with a 2:1 male-to-female ratio and for patients younger than age 30 years, with a peak incidence in the second decade of life.[50]

Clinical findings: most common symptoms are a dull aching pain that is localized and often spontaneous, swelling that is tender to palpation, and cortical bone expansion buccally and/or lingually.[51] Pain may not be present in some cases.[51] If present,

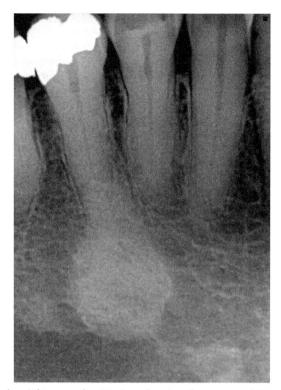

Fig. 13. Mandibular right premolar PA view showing the cementoblastoma noted at the root apex of the second premolar. The apical third of the root cannot be seen as it is surrounded by dense cementoblastoma.

pain is not relieved by aspirin as it does in osteoid osteoma.[52] Affected teeth often are vital but may become mobile and tender to percussion.[51]

Radiographic findings: highly variable radiographic appearance, resulting in no single pathognomonic feature; lesion often is larger than 2 cm, well-delineated, ranges in radiodensity from lucent to mixed to opaque, and may contain small calcifications.[50] Does not require tooth association but when associated is not fused to the cementum and may cause tooth displacement and/or mobility.[52]

Management: the treatment may include curettage, local excision, or complete resection with margins in normal tissues.[50,52] Aggressive cases may require additional radiotherapy and/or chemotherapy.[50]

Osteoma (central)

Definition: benign slow-growing neoplastic tumor with proliferation of mature cortical or cancellous bone and may be central (located within the cancellous bone) or peripheral (located on the outer surface of bone).[53] Osteomas generally are not associated with teeth and almost always associated with craniofacial bones; common areas of presentation include the walls of paranasal sinuses, posterior mandibular body, and condyle.[54] Note that multiple mandibular osteomas are a classic sign for Gardner syndrome.[53] The remainder of this section focuses on solitary central osteomas of the jaw.

Epidemiology: although osteomas are the most common benign sinonasal tumors,[55] solitary central osteomas of the jaw are rare, with only 14 cases reported as of December 2018, with 6 in the maxilla and 8 in the mandible.[54] Demographics for all osteomas include a slight male preference and wide range of ages, with a mean between the ages of 40 years and 65 years.[56]

Clinical findings: with the few cases, a majority of solitary jaw central osteomas clinically exhibit expansion, tooth displacement, and pain but may be asymptomatic.[53,54]

Radiographic findings: radiopaque well-defined homogenous sclerotic mass.[53] Without bony expansion, may not be able to differentiate from idiopathic osteosclerosis.[56] External root resorption is possible.[56]

Management: smaller asymptomatic central osteomas generally do not require treatment; surgical excision is recommended for symptomatic, large, and/or functionally impairing lesions.[57]

Osteoid osteoma

Definition: a rare benign neoplastic bone tumor with unknown etiology that is characterized by a central nidus surrounded by sclerotic bone.[58]

Epidemiology: 80% of cases occur in long bones and less than 1% occur in the jaws.[59] Generally, occurs in young patients under age of 30 years, slightly more in women, with a ratio to men of 1.2:1, and slightly more often in the posterior body of the mandible.[59]

Clinical findings: a key clinical symptom is severe pain and tenderness, often nocturnal, that is relieved partially or completely with salicylates and nonsteroidal anti-inflammatory drugs.[60,61]

Radiographic findings: usually smaller than 2 cm in size with a radiopaque nidus surrounded by new sclerotic bone formation.[50,59] When in the jaw, presents as a radiopaque mass that is generally cause root resorption or lead to tooth displacement[59] but not associated with roots of any tooth. An unusual presentation, however, involving roots of the tooth is described by Mohammed and colleagues.[58]

Management: recommended treatment is complete surgical excision and involved tooth if associated.[58,60]

Cemento-ossifying fibroma

Definition: classified by the World Health Organization (WHO) as a primary bone-forming tumor of the jaw.[62] A benign fibro-osseous tumor believed to arise from PDL with unknown etiology, but a majority of cases report history of trauma to the affected area.[62]

Epidemiology: affects predominantly women in the third and fourth decades; when present, is in the mandible 70% to 75% of the time; and does not show a close association with roots of the tooth.[63,64]

Clinical findings: slow-growing, painless bone expansion with possible facial asymmetry and tooth displacement.[63]

Radiographic findings: well-circumscribed unilocular lesions that are radiolucent with small radiopaque calcifications; a characteristic finding includes downward displacement of the inferior cortex.[64] May cause root divergence.[63]

Management: recommended treatment is curettage or enucleation, with a recurrence rate of less than 5%.[63]

Compound odontoma

Definition: slow-growing neoplastic mixed (epithelial and ectomesenchymal) odontogenic tumors that form multiple "odontoids" or "denticles," presenting as tiny teeth with well-formed and correctly arranged dental tissues.[65,66] Etiology is unknown but may be influenced by genetics, infection, and/or trauma.[65]

Epidemiology: most commonly diagnosed in the second and third decades of life with a preference for the anterior maxilla region.[66] No gender preference.[65,66]

Clinical findings: often asymptomatic and diagnosed incidentally when radiographically examining for unerupted teeth; patients may present with jaw expansion, pain from expansion, delayed eruption of permanent teeth, persistent primary teeth, devitalization, and/or swelling.[67]

Radiographic findings: radiopaque mass between 5 mm and 30 mm formed of on average 4 to 21 odontoids with same radiopacity as teeth that often surrounded by a radiolucent rim (**Fig. 14**).[66] May cause resorption of adjacent teeth.[67]

Management: treatment is complete surgical excision of the encapsulated tumor; the recommendation for tooth extraction increases with the age of the patient.[66,67]

Complex odontoma

Definition: slow-growing neoplastic mixed (epithelial and ectomesenchymal) odontogenic tumors that form an irregular and disordered mass of dental tissues.[66] Etiology is unknown but may be influenced by genetics, infection, and/or trauma.[65]

Epidemiology: more often in the posterior mandible, especially between the roots of erupted teeth in the area of the second and third mandibular molars.[65] Most commonly diagnosed in second and third decades and gender preference has been varied in reports without consensus.[65,66]

Clinical findings: often asymptomatic and diagnosed incidentally when radiographically examining for unerupted teeth; patients may present with delayed eruption of permanent teeth, persistent primary teeth, devitalization, pain, and/or swelling.[67]

Radiographic findings: radiopaque mass that may be irregular, single or multiple, and of varying radiopacities (**Fig. 15**).[65] May cause resorption of adjacent teeth.[67]

Management: treatment is complete surgical excision of the encapsulated tumor; the recommendation for tooth extraction increases with the age of the patient.[66,67]

Malignant and Metastatic Lesions Appearing as Periapical Radiopacities

Definition: metastatic lesions occurring from a prior primary malignancy elsewhere (breast, prostate, and so froth) can mimic both osteolytic areas periapically and also

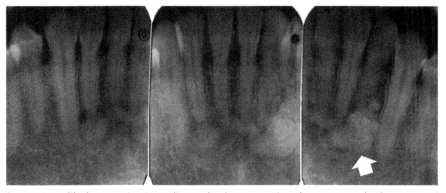

Fig. 14. Mandibular anterior PA radiographs demonstrating the compound odontoma apical to the left lateral incisor, retained primary canine and the permanent canine. Incidentally, the patient also demonstrates apical lesions consistent with PA COD. (*Courtesy of* Steven R. Singer, DDS, Rutgers School of Dental Medicine, Newark, NJ.)

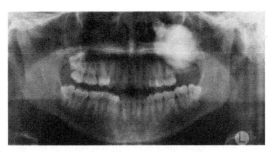

Fig. 15. Panoramic radiograph showing a large complex odontoma in the left maxilla noted in the molar region. Also note the impacted molar at the level of the maxillary sinus. A CBCT scan was recommended for localization of the area of interest and the relationship of the complex odontoma to the maxillary sinus. (*Courtesy of* Steven R. Singer, DDS, Rutgers School of Dental Medicine, Newark, NJ).

osteogenic areas within the radiolucencies. These are primarily irregular and ill-defined appearing lesions on intraoral and panoramic radiographs as well as computed tomography (CT) scans and light up on fludeoxyglucose F 18 (FDG)-PET or sodium fluoride F 18–PET scans. Detection of intraosseous malignancy of the mandible from a distant malignancy using FDG-PET/CT was reported by Asaka and colleagues.[68]

Clinical findings: jaw lesions are detected incidentally on radiographic examinations and on occasion; clinical examination reveals an ulcerated area or a mass intraorally. Lymph node involvement is another positive finding on clinical examination. Biopsy is required for confirmation of diagnosis.

Radiographic findings: irregular radiolucent areas on planar and tomograms. CT or CBCT scans show irregular lytic areas sometimes interspersed with dense opacifications.

Management: as with any malignant lesion, this has to be evaluated by a head and neck oncology team. Surgery often is the first line of treatment of the metastatic lesions followed by either chemotherapy or radiation therapy.

Supernumerary teeth

Definition and epidemiology: conditions, such as supernumerary teeth, both anterior maxillary (mesiodens) and posterior maxillary and mandibular, can mimic PA pathoses due to their superimposition in the vicinity of the root apices. Albert and Mupparapu[69] reviewed the literature on mesiodens and reported a classification system based on their position and appearance on radiographs.

Clinical findings: usually none, because they are incidental findings on radiographic examinations. Once seen, relevant radiographic examinations can be done.

Radiographic findings: on intraoral radiographs, they appear as PA dense opacifications but the presence of follicular space usually gives up the diagnosis unless the tooth is malformed or smaller like a mesiodens (**Fig. 16**). In those cases, a small-volume CBCT is recommended for accurate diagnosis as well as localization of the tooth in question.

Mesiodens, once formed in the anterior maxillary area, can be noted within the alveolar bone, or sometimes seen within the nasopalatine canal or at the level of the floor of the nasal fossa. In such cases, the teeth are inverted and hence the eruption is toward the floor of the nasal fossa. These are relatively rare occurrences.

Management: once identified and localized, the teeth are surgically removed.

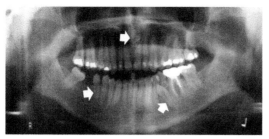

Fig. 16. Panoramic radiograph showing a mesiodens at the level of the floor of the nasal fossa between the root apices of maxillary central incisors. There are 2 supernumerary teeth, o1ne on either side in the mandible. The supernumerary tooth on the right mandible has erupted whereas the supernumerary tooth on the left mandible is still unerupted.

Sialolith

Definition and epidemiology: conditions, such as submandibular sialoliths, are superimposed on mandibular anterior and posterior radiographs and mimic pathology.

Clinical findings: detailed history and clinical examination might give a clue to the presence of a sialolith but it may be completely asymptomatic, in which case it is an incidental finding.

Radiographic findings: if PA radiographs show a round opacity near the apex of a tooth, the type of opacification need to be studied. If teeth are vital, then the possibility that it is a superimposed structure is taken in to consideration. Generally, the sialoliths can be concentric or round opacifications with smooth borders and vary in sizes depending on the degree of calcification (**Fig. 17**). When suspected, a radiograph at right angles to the PA radiograph (for eg, an occlusal radiograph) shows the sialolith. Because occlusal radiographs are not available as a technique since the advent of digital radiography, an alternative is to use small field-of-view CBCT of the mandible on the side in question.[70] This shows the presence of the radiopaque structure that was noted on a PA radiograph. On occasion, this also is a calcified lymph node or another dystrophic calcification in the floor of the mandible.

Management: once identified and localized via specialized techniques like sialography (if the salivary gland is not inflamed) or sialendoscopy, the sialolith is surgically removed via lithotripsy or other surgical approaches.

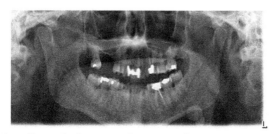

Fig. 17. Panoramic radiograph showing a large opacification superimposed over the left body of the mandible in the vicinity of the submandibular fossa suspected to be a large sialolith and possibly calcification within the submandibular gland. Large sialoliths usually are seen at the junction of the Wharton duct and the gland itself.

PERIAPICAL RADIOLUCENCIES
Developmental

Lateral periodontal cyst
Definition: lateral periodontal cysts are cystic lesions that tend to occur on the lateral aspect of vital teeth.

Epidemiology: lateral periodontal cysts account for fewer than 1% of the reported cases of odontogenic cysts.[71]

Clinical findings: most lateral periodontal cysts area located in the mandibular incisor-canine-premolar area.[71]

Radiographic findings: radiographically, lateral periodontal cysts present as a unilocular radiolucent lesion between the roots of teeth or associated with the lateral aspect of a tooth (**Fig. 18**).[72]

Management: surgical enucleation with preservation of involved teeth is an appropriate treatment of lateral periodontal cysts. Recurrence is rare.[73] The multiloculated variant called botryoid odontogenic cysts has been reported to demonstrate a higher recurrence rate than its unilocular counterpart.[71]

Inflammatory Lesions

Apical periodontitis, periapical abscess
Definition: spectrum of inflammation involving the PA area of teeth that results from pulpal infection by microorganisms.

Epidemiology: apical periodontitis is the most frequent inflammatory lesion related to teeth in the jaws.[74]

Clinical findings: apical periodontitis can be classified as either asymptomatic or symptomatic; clinical examination of percussion and palpation of the tooth yields negative results in the former and usually positive results in the latter. The results

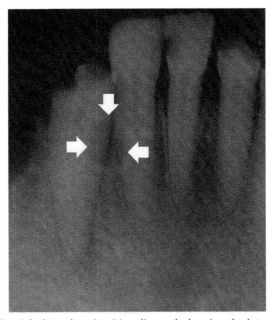

Fig. 18. Mandibular right lateral-canine PA radiograph showing the lateral periodontal cyst in the inter-radicular area of the lateral incisor and the canine (*arrows*).

of pulp sensitivity tests for both conditions, however, are negative.[75] In the early stage of PA inflammation, the PA PDL can exhibit acute inflammation without abscess formation. This localized alteration may or may not proceed to abscess formation.[76]

Radiographic findings: in apical periodontitis, radiographs may show a thickened PDL space (**Fig. 19**). If an abscess develops after a long-standing apical periodontitis, radiographs reveal a radiolucent area around the root apex.[75]

Management: apical periodontitis is an inflammatory disease caused by a persistent infection of the root canal system.[77] The recommended treatment is the removal of the dead nerve and bacteria either through extraction of the tooth or root canal treatment. Antibiotics are recommended only when there is severe infection that has spread from the tooth into the surrounding tissues[78] (**Fig. 20**).

Cystic Lesions

Periapical (radicular) cyst
Definition: radicular cyst is a cyst of inflammatory origin associated with a nonvital tooth.

Epidemiology: radicular cysts represent the most common odontogenic cyst.[79] Radicular cysts are most commonly associated with at the tooth apex, but a lateral radicular cyst can be associated with a lateral root canal.[80]

Clinical findings: radicular cysts are always associated with a nonvital tooth, and this is an important criterion for diagnosis.[80]

Radiographic findings: radiographs often show a well-defined radiolucent lesion at the apex of a tooth (**Fig. 21**). Radicular cysts can displace or resorb the roots of adjacent teeth.[81]

Management: the treatment of radicular cysts can include nonsurgical root canal therapy to surgical treatment, such as apicoectomy.

Odontogenic keratocyst
Definition: an odontogenic cystic lesion with distinctive histologic features. Recently reclassified back into a cystic category in the recent 2017 *WHO Classification of*

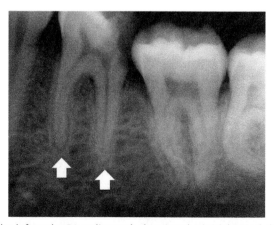

Fig. 19. Mandibular left molar PA radiograph showing the initial apical changes in relation to the first molar secondary to a symptomatic gross carious lesion. If the offending causes remain, this will continue to an apical osteitis, resulting in loss of trabecular bone and possibly even cortical bone before it shows up radiographically.

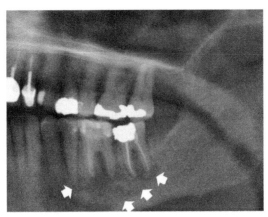

Fig. 20. Cropped panoramic radiograph showing localized osteomyelitis secondary to PA infection in relation to the mandibular left first and second molars (*arrows*).

Head and Neck Tumours. Current evidence seemed lacking to justify the continuation of classifying it as a tumor.[82]

Epidemiology: odontogenic keratocysts are the third most common cyst of the jaws.[79]

Clinical findings: most common location of odontogenic keratocysts is the mandibular molar region.[83,84]

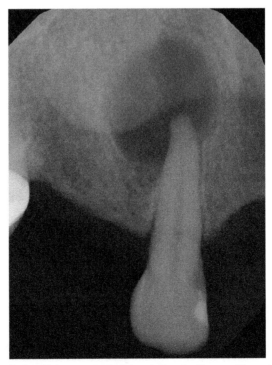

Fig. 21. A large apical radiolucency noted in relation to the maxillary right lateral incisor tooth on this maxillary right lateral-canine PA radiograph.

Radiographic findings: odontogenic keratocyst size can be variable, ranging from a unilocular radiolucent lesion surrounding the crown of an unerupted tooth (**Fig. 22**), resembling a dentigerous cyst, to a large size that results in facial deformity and destruction of surrounding structures.[83] Lesions tend to grow in a posteroanterior direction, however, that results in a lack of cortical expansion.[84]

Management: odontogenic keratocysts tend to be more aggressive in its growth pattern with a higher recurrence rate than other odontogenic cysts.[85] Recurrence may be due, however, to incomplete removal or the presence of satellite (daughter) cysts.[86] Treatment includes enucleation (with or without peripheral ostectomy, treatment with Carnoy solution), marsupialization, or resection.[84]

Glandular odontogenic cyst

Definition: a developmental cyst with features that resemble glandular differentiation.

Epidemiology: glandular odontogenic cysts represent less than 1% of odontogenic cysts.[85,86]

Clinical findings: there is a predilection for the mandible.[87] But in the maxilla, the canine seems commonly involved. Swelling and expansion were the most common presenting complaints.[88]

Radiographic findings: radiographically, glandular odontogenic cysts present as a well-defined unilocular or multilocular radiolucency associated with the roots of teeth; association with impacted teeth is rare.[80]

Management: glandular odontogenic cysts have a tendency to recur especially when lesions are removed with simple enucleation.[87]

Benign Tumors

Ameloblastoma

Definition: benign, slow-growing epithelial odontogenic neoplasm with unmitigated growth potential.

Epidemiology: ameloblastomas are the most common odontogenic tumors, excluding odontomas.[89] In the United States, African Americans seem to have an overall 5-fold increase risk of disease compared with whites.[90]

Clinical findings: tumor often presents as an asymptomatic swelling of the posterior mandible and can be associated with an unerupted tooth. Buccal and lingual expansion often is observed.[80]

Radiographic findings: radiographs commonly show corticated multilocular (soap-bubble) radiolucency (**Fig. 23**).[90]

Management: the unmitigated growth potential and tendency to recur require operative management involving segmental or marginal resection. When treated by enucleation alone, much higher rates of recurrence are reported.[91,92]

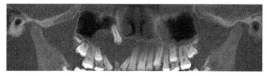

Fig. 22. CBCT panoramic reconstruction of maxilla showing a large well-defined lytic area coronal to the impacted right canine. Histologically confirmed as an odontogenic keratocyst. (*Courtesy of* Steven R. Singer, DDS, Rutgers School of Dental Medicine, Newark, NJ.)

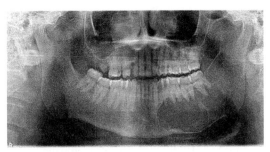

Fig. 23. Panoramic radiograph showing a large well-defined, multilocular radiolucency extending from the area of first molar on the left into the ramus area. Note the expansion and thinning of the cortices. Ameloblastoma was confirmed histologically.

Malignant Tumors

Ameloblastic carcinoma

Definition: a rare, malignant counterpart for ameloblastoma. Not to be confused with metastasizing ameloblastoma, this is a histologically benign ameloblastoma metastasizing to distant sites. In the recent *WHO Classification of Head and Neck Tumours*, metastasizing ameloblastoma has been separated from ameloblastic carcinoma and included as a type of conventional ameloblastoma.[80]

Epidemiology: incidence rate was 1.79 per 10 million person/year with male and black population predominance. The overall survival is 17.6 years.[93]

Clinical findings: the most common site is the posterior mandible. Often, pain and expansion are the first clinical manifestations. Most cases arise de novo, but some arise in preexisting ameloblastomas.[80]

Radiographic findings: radiographically, ameloblastic carcinomas can present as poorly defined, irregular radiolucencies consistent with a malignancy, or indistinguishable from a benign radiolucency.[80,94]

Management: generally considered radio-resistant tumor, radical surgical resection is the first line of treatment.

SUMMARY

The PA radiolucent and radiopaque defects of bone not only are alterations due to carious pathology but also could be resultant of benign, malignant, or developmental defects. Misdiagnosis of peraipcial radiolucencies are likely to be more common than PA radiopacities due to higher prevalence of endodontic pathologies in general dental practice. Misdiagnosis of noncarious, that is, nonendodontic PA, lesions may lead to oral conditions as undiagnosed at that stage; this might be uneventful when malignant conditions are underlying cause of radiolucent/radiopaque defect. Vitality testing remains key for differentiating endodontic versus nonendodontic PA radiolucencies. Hence, dentists require a sound knowledge on clinicoradiological concepts on conditions that show PA changes in dentition.

REFERENCES

1. Pinto ASB, Carvalho MS, Farias ALC, et al. Hypercementosis: diagnostic imaging by radiograph, cone-beam computed tomography, and magnetic resonance imaging. J Oral Maxillofac Radiol 2017;5(3):90–3.

2. Eren Y, Erdai O, Serdar B, et al. Evaluation of the frequency and characteristics of hypercementosis in the turkish population with cone-beam computed tomography. Niger J Clin Pract 2017;20(6):724–8.
3. Thumbigere-Math V, Alqadi A, Chalmers NI, et al. Hypercementosis associated with ENPP1 mutations and GACI. J Dent Res 2018;97(4):432–41.
4. Shoor H, Sujir N, Mutalik S, et al. Hypercementosis: a rare finding in a patient with systemic lupus erythematosus. BMJ Case Rep 2014;2014 [pii:bcr2013202370].
5. Consolaro A, Consolaro RB, Francischone LA. Cementum, apical morphology and hypercementosis: a probably adaptive response of the periodontal support tissues and potential orthodontic implications. Dental Press J Orthod 2012;17(1): 21–30.
6. Pinheiro BC, Pinheiro TN, Capelozza AL, et al. A scanning electron microscopic study of hypercementosis. J Appl Oral Sci 2008;16(6):380–4.
7. Jeddy N, T R, C K, et al. Localized multiple cemental excrescenses: a rare presentation of hypercementosis. J Clin Diagn Res 2014;8(5):16–7.
8. Senia ES, Sarao MS. Periapical cemento-osseous dysplasia: a case report with twelve-year follow up and review of literature. Int Endod J 2014;48(11):1086–99.
9. Mupparapu M, Singer SR, Milles M, et al. Simultaneous presentation of focal cemento-osseous dysplasia and simple bone cyst of the mandible masquerading as a multilocular radiolucency. Dentomaxillofac Radiol 2005;34(1):39–43.
10. Fenerty S, Shaw W, Verma R, et al. Florid cemento-osseous dysplasia: review of an uncommon fibro-osseous lesion of the jaw with important clinical implications. Skeletal Radiol 2017;46(5):581–90.
11. Roghi M, Scapparone C, Crippa R, et al. Periapical cemento-osseous dysplasia: clinicopathological features. Anticancer Res 2014;34(5):2533–6.
12. Visnapuu V, Peltonen S, Ellilia T, et al. Periapical cemental dysplasia is common in women with NF1. Eur J Med Genet 2007;50(4):274–80.
13. Cavalcanti PHP, Cascimento EHL, Pontual MLA, et al. Cemento-osseous dysplasia: Imaging features based on cone beam computed tomography scans. Braz Dent J 2018;29(1):99–104.
14. Aiuto R, Gucciardino F, Rapetti R, et al. Management of symptomatic florid cemento-osseous dysplasia: literature review and a case report. J Clin Exp Dent 2018;10(3):e291–5.
15. Delai D, Bernardi A, Felippe GS, et al. Florid cemento-osseous dysplasia: a case of misdiagnosis. J Endod 2015;41(11):1923–6.
16. Rao GS, Kamalapur MG, Acharya S. Focal cemento-osseous dysplasia masquerading as benign cementoblastoma: a diagnostic dilemma. J Oral Maxillofac Pathol 2014;18(1):150.
17. Cankaya AB, Erdem MA, Logac V, et al. Focal cemento-osseous dysplasia of mandible. BMJ Case Rep 2012;1–4 [pii:bcr2012006432].
18. MacDonald-Jankowski DS. Focal cemento-osseous dysplasia: a systematic review. Dentomaxillofac Radiol 2008;37(6):350–60.
19. MacDonald-Jankowski DS. Florid cemento-osseous dysplasia: a systematic review. Dentomaxillofac Radiol 2003;32(3):141–9.
20. Sisman Y, Ertas ET, Ertas H, et al. The frequency and distribution of idiopathic osteosclerosis of the jaw. Eur J Dent 2011;5(4):409–14.
21. Halse A, Molven O. Idiopathic osteosclerosis of the jaws followed through a period of 20-27 years. Int Endod J 2002;35(9):747–51.
22. Bsoul SA, Samer A, Alborz S, et al. Idiopathic osteosclerosis (enostosis, dense bone silands, focal periapical osteopetrosis). Quintessence Int 2004;35(7):590–9.

23. Mainville GN, Lalumiere C, Turgeon D, et al. Asymptomatic, nonexpansile radio-paity of the jaw associated with external root resorption: a diagnostic dilemma. Gen Dent 2016;64(1):32–5.

24. Burke A, Collins MT, Boyce AM. Fibrous dysplasia of bone: craniofacial and dental implications. Oral Dis 2017;23(6):697–708.

25. MacDonald-Jankowski DS. Fibrous dysplasia: a systematic review. Dentomaxillofac Radiol 2009;38(4):196–215.

26. Menon S, Venkatswamy S, Ramu V, et al. Craniofacial fibrous dysplasia: surgery and literature review. Ann Maxillofac Surg 2013;3(1):66–71.

27. De Melo WM, Sonoda CK, Hochuli-Vieira E. Monostotic fibrous dysplasia of the mandible. J Craniofac Surg 2012;23(5):e452–4.

28. Mermod M, Hoarau R. Mandibular tori. CMAJ 2015;187(11):826.

29. Brierley DJ, Crane H, Hunter KD. Lumps and bumps of the gingiva: a pathological miscellany. Head Neck Pathol 2019;13(1):103–13.

30. Bertazzo-Silveira E, Stuginski-Barbosa J, Porporatti AL, et al. Association between signs and symptoms of bruxism and presence of tori: a systematic review. Clin Oral Investig 2017;21(9):2789–99.

31. Morrison MD, Tamimi F. Oral tori are associated with local mechanical and systemic factors: a case-control study. J Oral Maxillofac Surg 2013;71(1):14–22.

32. Krishnan U, Maslamani MA, Moule AJ. Cone beam CT as an aid to diagnosing mixed radiopaque radiolucent lesions in the mandibular incisor region. BMJ Case Rep 2015;2015 [pii:bcr2014207617].

33. AAE. Glossary of endodontic terms. 9th edition. AAE; 2015.

34. Yeh H, Chen C, Chen P, et al. Frequency and distribution of mandibular condensing osteitis lesions in a Taiwanese population. J Dent Sci 2015;10(3):291–5.

35. Green TL, Walton RE, Clark JM, et al. Histologic examination of condensing osteitis in cadaver specimens. J Endod 2013;39(8):977–9.

36. Estrela C, Porto OC, Costa NL, et al. Large reactional osteogenesis in maxillary sinus associated with secondary root canal infection detected using cone-beam computed tomography. J Endod 2015;41(12):2068–78.

37. Bornstein MM, Wasmer J, Sendi P, et al. Characteristics and dimensions of the schneiderian membrane and apical bone in maxillary molars referred for apical surgery: a comparative radiographic analysis using limited cone beam computed tomography. J Endod 2012;38(1):51–7.

38. Berglund C, Ekstromer K, Abtahi J. Primary chronic osteomyelitis of the jaws in children: an update on pathophysiology, radiological findings, treatment strategies, and prospective analysis of two cases. Case Rep Dent 2015;2015:152717.

39. Baltensperger M, Gratz K, Bruder E, et al. Is primary chronic osteomyelitis a uniform disease? Proposal of a classification based on a retrospective analysis of patients treated in the past 30 years. J Craniomaxillofac Surg 2004;32(1):43–50.

40. Bevin CR, Inwards CY, Keller EE. Surgical management of primary chronic osteomyelitis: a long-term retrospective analysis. J Oral Maxillofac Surg 2008;66(10):2073–85.

41. Haeffs TH, Scott CA, Campbell TH, et al. Acute and chronic suppurative osteomyelitis of the jaws: a 10 year review and assessment of treatment outcome. J Oral Maxillofac Surg 2018;76(12):2551–8.

42. Amand MJS, Sigaux N, Gleizal A, et al. Chronic osteomyelitis of the mandible: A comparative study of 10 cases with primary chronic osteomyelitis and 12 cases with secondary chronic osteomyelitis. J Stomatol Oral Maxillofac Surg 2017;118(6):342–8.

43. Fukuda M, Inoue K, Sakashita H. Periostitis Ossificans arising in the mandibular bone of a young patient: report of an unusual case and review of the literature. J Oral Maxillofac Surg 2017;75(9):1834.e1-8.
44. Brazao-Silva MT, Pinheiro TN. The So-called Garrè's osteomyelitis of jaws and the pivotal utility of computed tomography scan. Contemp Clin Dent 2017;8:645–6.
45. Kadom N, Eglof A, Obleid G, et al. Juvenile mandibular chronic osteomyelitis: multimodality imaging findings. Oral Surg Oral Med Oral Pathol Oral Radiol Endod 2011;111(3):e38–43.
46. Borges DC, Rogerio de Faria P, Junior HM, et al. Conservative treatment of a periapical cementoblastoma: a case report. J Oral Maxillofac Surg 2019;77(2):272.e1-7.
47. Teixeira LR, Santos JL, Almeida LY, et al. Residual cementoblastoma: an unusual presentation of a rare odontogenic tumor. J Oral Maxillofac Surg Med Pathol 2018;30(2):187–90.
48. Huber AR, Fold GS. Cementoblastoma. Head Neck Pathol 2009;3(2):133–5.
49. Angiero F, Mellone P, Baldi A, et al. Osteoblastoma of the jaw: report of two cases and review of the literature. In Vivo 2006;20(5):665–70.
50. Wozniak AW, Nowaczyk MT, Osmola K, et al. Malignant transformation of an osteoblastoma of the mandible: case report and review of the literature. Eur Arch Otorhinolaryngol 2010;267(6):845–9.
51. Bsoul SA, Gharaibeh TM, Terezhalmy GT, et al. Osteoblastoma. Quintessence Int 2004;35(2):164–5.
52. Abdelkarim A. An osteoblastoma of the mandible: a case study. J Calif Dent Assoc 2016;44(12):737–40.
53. Kaplan I, Nicolaou Z, Hatuel D, et al. Solitary central osteoma of the jaws: a diagnostic dilemma. Oral Surg Oral Med Oral Pathol Oral Radiol Endod 2008;106(3):e22–9.
54. Bhatt G, Gupta S, Ghosh S, et al. Central osteoma of maxilla associated with an impacted tooth: report of a rare case with literature review. Head Neck Pathol 2018. [Epub ahead of print].
55. Halawi AM, Maley JE, Robinson RA, et al. Craniofacial osteoma: clinical presentation and patterns of growth. Am J Rhinol Allergy 2013;27(2):128–33.
56. Saha A, Breik O, Simpson I, et al. Large pediatric central osteoma with osteoblastoma-like features in the mandible. Head Neck Pathol 2019;13(2):264–9.
57. Nilesh K, Bhujbal RB, Nayak AG. Solitary central osteoma of mandible in a geriatric patient: report and review. J Clin Exp Dent 2016;8(2):e219–22.
58. Mohammed I, Jannan NA, Elrmali A. Osteoid osteoma associated with the teeth: unusual presentation. Int J Oral Maxillofac Surg 2013;42(2):298–302.
59. Singh A, Solomon MC. Osteoid osteoma of the mandible: a case report with review of the literature. J Dent Sci 2017;12(2):185–9.
60. Karpik M, Wojnar J, Skowronski J, et al. Osteoid osteoma – diagnostic and therapeutic difficulties. A single-centre experience. Ortop Traumatol Rehabil 2016;18(2):131–40.
61. Infante-Cossio P, Restoy-Lozano A, Espin-Galvez F, et al. Mandibular osteoid osteoma. J Emerg Med 2017;52(3):e83–4.
62. Wright JM, Tekkesin MS. Odontogenic tumors: where are we in 2017? J Istanb Univ Fac Dent 2017;51(3 Suppl 1):S10–30.
63. Woo S. Central cemento-ossifying fibroma: primary odontogenic or osseous neoplasm? J Oral Maxillofac Surg 2015;73(12):S87–93.

64. MacDonald-Jankowski DS. Ossifying fibroma: a systematic review. Dentomaxillo-fac Radiol 2000;38(8):495–513.
65. Bereket C, Cakir-Ozkan N, Sener I, et al. Complex and compound odontomas: analysis of 69 cases and a rare case of erupted compound odontoma. Niger J Clin Pract 2015;18(6):726–30.
66. Tuczynska A, Bartosik D, Abu-Fillat Y, et al. Compound odontoma in the mandible – case study and literature review. Dev Period Med 2015;19(4):484–9.
67. Kammerer PW, Schneider D, Schiegnitz E, et al. Clinical parameter of odontoma with special emphasis on treatment of impacted teeth-a retrospective multicentre study and literature review. Clin Oral Investig 2016;20(7):1827–35.
68. Asaka T, Kitagawa Y, Yamazaki Y, et al. Differential diagnosis of intraosseous ma-lignancies of the mandible by FDG-PET/CT. J Nucl Med 2013;54:1528.
69. Albert A, Mupparapu M. Cone beam computed tomography review and classifi-cation of mesiodens: report of a case in the nasal fossa and nasal septum. Quin-tessence Int 2018;49:413–7.
70. Rzymska-Grala I, Stopa Z, Grala B, et al. Salivary gland calculi-contemporary methods of imaging. Pol J Radiol 2010;75:25–37.
71. Chrcanovic BR, Gomez RS. Gingival cyst of the adult, lateral periodontal cyst, and botryoid odontogenic cyst: an updated systematic review. Oral Dis 2019; 25:26–33.
72. Rasmusson LG, Magnusson BC, Borrmanol H. The lateral periodontal cyst: a his-topathological and radiographic study of 32 cases. Br J Oral Maxillofac Surg 1991;29(1):54–7.
73. de Andrade M, Pantosi Silva AP, de Moraes Ramos-Perez FM, et al. Lateral peri-odontal cyst: report of case and review of the literature. Oral Maxillofac Surg 2012;16(1):83–7.
74. Braz-Silva PH, Bergamini ML, Mardegan AP, et al. Inflammatory profile of chronic apical periodontitis: a literature review. Acta Odontol Scand 2019;77:173–80.
75. Rotstein I, Ingle JI. Ingle's endodontics. 7th edition. Raleigh (NC): PMPH USA, Ltd; 2019.
76. Nair PNR. On the causes of persistent apical periodontitis: a review. Int Endod J 2006;39:249–81.
77. Neville BW, Damm DD, Allen AM, et al. Oral and maxillofacial pathology. 4th edi-tion. St Louis (MO): Saunders Elsevier; 2016.
78. Cope AL, Francis N, Wood F, et al. Systemic antibiotics for symptomatic apical periodontiits and acute apical abscess in adults. Cochrane Database Syst Rev 2018;(9):CD010136.
79. Johnson NR, Gannon OM, Savage NW, et al. Frequency of odontogenic cysts and tumors: a systematic review. J Investig Clin Dent 2014;5(1):9–14.
80. El-Naggar AK, Chan JKC, Grandis JR, et al, editors. WHO classification of head and tumors. 4th edition. Lyon (France): IARC; 2017.
81. Scarfe WC, Toghyani S, Azevedo B. Imaging of benign odontogenic lesions. Ra-diol Clin North Am 2018;56:45–62.
82. Wright JM, Vered M. Update from the 4th edition of the World Health Organization Classification of Head and Neck: odontogenic and maxillofacial bone tumors. Head Neck Pathol 2017;11:68–77.
83. Jones AV, Craig GT, Franklin CD. Range and demographics of odontogenic cysts diagnosed in a UK population over a 30-year period. J Oral Pathol Med 2006;35: 500–7.
84. Bilodeau EA, Collins BM. Odontogenic cysts and neoplasms. Surg Pathol Clin 2017;10:177–222.

85. Morgan TA, Burton CC, Qian F. A retrospective review of treatment of the odontogenic keratocyst. J Oral Maxillofac Surg 2005;63:635–9.
86. Kaplan I, Anavi Y, Hirshberg A. Glandular odonotogenic cyst: a challenge in diagnosis and treatment. Oral Dis 2008;14:575–81.
87. Chrcanovic BR, Gomez RS. Glandular odontogenic cyst: an updated analysis of 169 cases reported in the literature. Oral Dis 2018;24:717–24.
88. Fowler CB, Brannon RB, Kessler HP, et al. Glandular odontogenic cyst: analysis of 46 cases with special emphasis on microscopic criteria for diagnosis. Head Neck Pathol 2011;5:364–75.
89. Buchner A, Merrell PW, Carpenter WM. Relative frequency of central odontogenic tumors: a study of 1088 cases from Northern California and comparison to studies from other parts of the world. J Oral Maxillofac Surg 2006;64:1343–52.
90. McClary AC, West RB, McClary AC, et al. Ameloblastoma: a clinical review and trends in management. Eur Arch Otorhinolaryngol 2016;273:1649–61.
91. Effiom OA, Ogundana OM, Akinshipo AO, et al. Ameloblastoma: current etiopathological concepts and management. Oral Dis 2018;24:307–16.
92. Peacock ZS. Controversies in oral and maxillofacial pathology. Oral Maxillofacial Surg Clin N Am 2017;29:475–86.
93. Rizzitelli A, Smoll NR, Chae MP, et al. Incidence and overall survival management of malignant ameloblastoma. PLoS One 2015;10(2):e0117789.
94. White SM. Malignant lesions in the dentomaxillofacial complex. Radiol Clin North Am 2018;56:63–76.

Oral Manifestation of Systemic Diseases

Natasha Bhalla, DDS*, Yoav Nudell, DDS, Jaykrishna Thakkar, DDS, Harry Dym, DDS

KEYWORDS

• Oral • Dental • Systemic • Symptoms

KEY POINTS

• The US Surgeon General's report *Oral Health in America* highlighted ways in which oral health and systemic conditions are associated with each other.
• Oral examination can reveal signs and symptoms associated with systemic conditions.
• Multiple systemic diseases and associated oral symptoms are discussed.

In 2000, the US Surgeon General's report *Oral Health in America* highlighted ways in which oral health and systemic conditions are associated with each other. An oral examination can reveal signs and symptoms associated with immunologic diseases, endocrinopathies, hematologic conditions, systemic infections, and nutritional disorders. In this article, multiple systemic diseases and associated oral symptoms are discussed.

SICKLE CELL ANEMIA

A single point mutation to the β-globin gene can alter the structure of hemoglobin, shifting the molecule's tendency to aggregate and subvert the biconcavity of the red blood cell (RBC) into a sickled cell, with the potential to reap profound morbidity and mortality.

Sickle cell disease (SCD) describes syndromes that produce sickled RBCs. The molecular genetic etiologies of SCD can vary. For instance, the homozygous inheritance of the point mutation (a missense, glu-val) that results in sickle hemoglobin causes sickle cell anemia (SCA). Alternatively, a coinherited sickle β-hemoglobin with alleles that render it genetically dominant, such as sickle β-thalassemia, hemoglobin SC, hemoglobin SD, and hemoglobin SE, can also cause SCD.[1]

Disclosure Statement: The authors have nothing to disclose.
Oral and Maxillofacial Surgery, The Brooklyn Hospital Center, 121 Dekalb Avenue, Brooklyn, NY 11201, USA
* Corresponding author.
E-mail address: natashaa95@gmail.com

Hemolytic anemia and vaso-occlusion drive the diverse and varied clinical manifestations of SCD. Acute features include chest syndrome, stroke, infection, asplenia, bone pain, and priapism. Chronic features can include bone necrosis, nephropathy, heart, lungs, and skin disorders.

Hemolytic anemia of SCA, when severe, can cause pallor of mucous membranes, specifically and most commonly observed in the palpebral conjunctiva and oral mucosa.[2-5]

Hemolytic anemia can cause an elevation in serum bilirubin, resulting in jaundice, a diffuse and generalized yellowish color change to skin and mucosa. The degree of color change is dependent on the serum level of bilirubin and tissue composition. Elastin fibers bind well to bilirubin. Sclera, lingual frenum, and soft palate have a high concentration of elastin and, therefore, are sites of prominent color change.[2,6,7]

The craniofacial morphologies attributed to SCD are variable and controversial. Most consistently reported is a protruding maxilla, skeletal class II malocclusion. Other abnormalities include overjet, overbite, and retrusion of the mandible.[8,9] It is hypothesized that the some morphologic changes are caused by hyperplasia, and expansion of the bone marrow occurs to compensate for the short half-life of RBCs maintaining larger volumes of hematopoietically active marrow.[9,10]

Radiographic findings in the sickle cell patient include hair-on-end appearance of the diploic space of the cranial vault,[11,12] coarse trabecular pattern, loss of alveolar bone height, pronounced lamina dura[13] (as seen **Fig. 1**A), generalized osteoporotic appearance due to bone marrow hyperplasia, and radiopaque lesions corresponding to areas of vaso-occlusive phenomena and infarctions.[14] Bone pain from vaso-occlusive, hypoxia-inducing attacks are more common in the posterior mandible.[14,15]

Individuals with SCA are at risk for systemic osteomyelitis, head and neck osteomyelitis is less common. When osteomyelitis does occur, it occurs most frequently in the posterior mandible.[16,17]

Other possible manifestations of SCA include mucosal damage due to anemia, papillary atrophy of the tongue, and fungal infections due to multiple antibiotic therapies often prescribed to SCA patients.[15] Additionally, loss of sensation to the lips, chin, and teeth has been observed and is thought to be caused by infarction to the vasculature supporting branches of the inferior alveolar nerve. Loss of sensitivity is often coincident with sickle cell crisis; the duration of neuropathy has been reported to be temporary or permanent.[15,18,19]

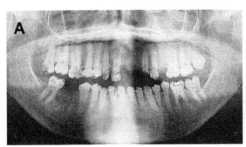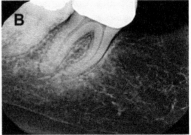

Fig. 1. (*A*) Panoramic radiograph showing enamel hypomineralization, cavitated teeth, missing teeth, and decreased trabeculation of bone. (*B*) Periapical radiograph tooth showing trabeculation of bone. (*From [A, B]* Kawar N, Alrayyes S, Aljewari H. Sickle cell disease: an overview of orofacial and dental manifestations. Dis Mon. 2018;64(6):293; with permission.)

Dental findings can include delayed tooth eruption, hypomaturation and hypomineralization of enamel and dentin (**Fig. 1**), hypercementosis, and pulp stones[15,20]; high frequency of caries has been observed.[21] A high frequency of dental malocclusions have been reported in SCD populations; however, causality is inconclusive.[9,22,23] Symptomatic or asymptomatic necrosis, possibly the result of abnormal pupil perfusion sickle cells, have been observed in pulp vasculature possibly obstruction blood flow.[18,21,24]

PLUMMER-VINSON SYNDROME

Plummer-Vinson syndrome (PVS), also known as Paterson-Kelly syndrome, is a rare condition with a triad of findings, including iron deficiency anemia (IDA), dysphagia, and cervical esophageal web formation. Historically, a majority of patients with PVS have been women of Scandinavian or Northern European descent in their third to fifth decades of life.[2,25–27] The etiology and pathogenesis has not been definitively elucidated. IDA plays an important role, along with other possible contributing factors, including genetic predisposition, autoimmunity, and malnutrition.[26]

There has been a decline in reported cases of PVS; this decline is thought to be due to improvements in nutrition, hygiene, and iron supplementation and a reduction in parasitic infestations.[28]

Dysphagia in PVS has a gradual onset, on the order of multiple years; it is usually painless and intermittent. Anemia precipitates fatigue, exertional dyspnea, weakness, tachycardia, and pallor.[25] When visualized with gastrointestinal endoscopy, esophageal webs appear in the proximal part of the esophagus—they are smooth, thin, and gray, with eccentric or central lumen.[26]

The mucosa of the oral cavity is commonly pale, consistent with IDA. Tongue findings include glossitis, atrophy of the fungiform, and filiform papillae. Other findings include angular cheilitis (**Fig. 2**), dryness of the mouth; stomatitis[29], atrophic mucosa of the oral cavity, hypopharynx, and the esophagus[29,30] and enlargement of the thyroid.[26]

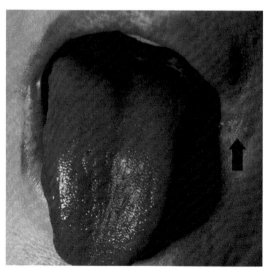

Fig. 2. An example of atrophic glossitis with angular cheilitis (*arrow*). (*From* McCord C, Johnson L. Oral manifestations of hematologic disease. Atlas Oral Maxillofac Surg Clin North Am. 2017;25(2):155; with permission.)

PVS is considered a premalignant condition predisposing patients to oral, esophageal, or pharyngeal squamous cell carcinoma.[2,31–33] Therefore, it is critical to be aware of the symptoms indicative of malignancy—for example, odynophagia, change in voice, nasal regurgitation of ingested solids and liquids, anorexia, and weight loss.[25]

SCURVY

Scurvy is a nutritional disease caused by a deficiency of L-ascorbic acid (vitamin C). Ascorbic acid is an essential nutrient that is involved in many processes critical for healthy physiology, such as collagen synthesis, fatty acid transport, neurotransmitter formation, wound healing, and immunity. If left untreated, this deficiency can lead to death.[2]

Today scurvy is uncommon in developed nations; however, there remain populations at risk for an altered nutritional status that may lead to scurvy, for example, populations with low socioeconomic status, isolated elderly persons, alcoholics with poor nutrition, diet faddists, those with unusual dietary habits, and those with psychiatric illness.[2,34,35]

Children at risk for scurvy typically have predisposing factors, including neurodevelopmental disabilities, autism spectrum disorder, intellectual disability, selective eating, and dietary insufficiency.[36] Within the special needs population, dental/oral pain and limitations in oral motor function can lead to dietary limitations, likely increasing their risk for nutritional deficiencies.[36–38]

The clinical signs of scurvy are primarily due to defective collagen synthesis. With a collagen deficiency, walls of the body's vasculature become weak and thus underlie spontaneous petechial hemorrhage and ecchymosis.[2,39,40] Additional findings include impaired wound healing, gingivitis, perifollicular hemorrhages,[41] petechiae, purpura, follicular hyperkeratosis, and corkscrew-shaped hairs on the lower limbs. Symptoms include weakness, fatigue, and depression.[34] Scurvy can also resemble rheumatologic disorders, such as pseudovasculitis or chronic arthritis, arthralgia, and mild to severe bone pain.[36]

The oral manifestations of scurvy can include generalized gingival swelling, gingival hypertrophy and gingival friability, spontaneous gingival hemorrhage, intraoral ulceration, tooth mobility, increased severity of periodontal infection and periodontal bone loss, halitosis, and loss of teeth, as seen in **Fig. 3**. Scorbutic gingivitis is the term used to describe the gingival lesions specific to patients with scurvy.[2,34,42]

Treatment of scurvy involves the supplementation of L-ascorbic acid. On supplementation, the prognosis for this condition is good. Additional steps, possibly with the help of allied health professionals, may need to be taken in specific at risk populations, such as children, the elderly, and those with special needs, involving diet modification and education for the individuals, their caretakers, and others responsible for the health of the patient.[36]

PEUTZ-JEGHERS SYNDROME

Peutz-Jeghers syndrome (PJS) is an autosomal dominant genetic condition. The STK11(LKB1) gene encodes a serine/threonine kinase and mutation of this gene is responsible for most cases of PJS. PJS has a prevalence of approximately 1 in 50,000 to 200,000 births.[43]

PJS is characterized by melanotic macules of the hands, perioral skin, and oral mucosa, in conjunction with multiple gastrointestinal hamartomatous polyps and predisposition for affected individuals to develop various neoplasms.[2]

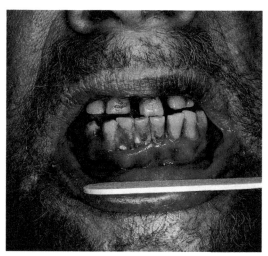

Fig. 3. Scurvy, gingivitis. (*From* James WD, Elston DM, Treat J, et al. Nutritional diseases. In: Andrews' diseases of the skin. 13th ed. Philadelphia: Elsevier; 2020. p. 475–84.e2; with permission.)

In early childhood, the melanotic macules of PJS typically develop around the orifices of the body in areas, such as oral, nasal, anal, genital regions. In approximately half of patients, the skin of the peripheral extremities exhibits melanotic macules.

The intestinal polyps can be found most commonly in the jejunum and ileum. Polyps can cause intestinal obstruction with intussusception. The polyps' role in cancer development is controversial[1]; however, it is estimated that that gastrointestinal cancer can developed in 9% to 14% of individuals by the age of 40 and 33% to 42% by the age of 60.[2,44]

Other tumors may develop in other tissues, including pancreas, gallbladder, bronchi, genital tract, breast, and ovary, among others.[2,43]

Mucocutaneous pigmented lesions in and around the oral cavity can be found in approximately 95% of patient with PJS.[43] They range in size from approximately 1 mm to 4 mm in diameter; they can be brown to blue-gray; they localize around the vermilion border, as seen in **Fig. 4**; and they can be found on the buccal mucosa

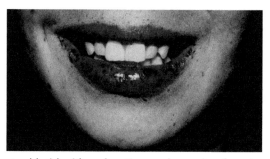

Fig. 4. PJS. A 12-year-old girl with melanotic macules on her face, in particular her lips. Melanotic macules were also present on her extremities, trunk, and mucous membranes. (*From* Mavropoulos JC, Cohen BA. Disorders of pigmentation. In: Cohen BA, editor. Pediatric dermatology. 4th ed. Philadelphia: Saunders/Elsevier; 2013. p. 148–68; with permission.)

(as seen in **Fig. 4**), labial mucosa, and the tongue. The number, distribution, and color can vary.[2] Mucocutaneous lesions may fade after puberty but often persist in the buccal mucosa. The histology of the pigmented lesions reveals basal cells with increased melanin possibly due to disrupted melanin migration from melanocyte to keratinocyte. Improvement in the appearance of mucocutaneous pigmented lesions has been reported using intense pulse light (590-nm), Q-switched ruby laser, and CO_2-based laser therapies.[43]

ADDISON DISEASE (HYPOADRENOCORTICISM)

Addison disease, also known as hypoadrenocorticism, is a disorder of the adrenal glands caused by the destruction of the adrenal cortex that results in the underproduction of adrenal corticosteroid hormones.

The incidence of new cases is approximately 110 to 140 per million population per year in the western hemisphere. The underlying causes of the adrenal cortex destruction are varied and include autoimmune destruction, infections, and trauma. Other rarer causes include metastatic tumors, sarcoidosis, hemochromatosis, and amyloidosis, among others.[2,45]

A related disorder, secondary hypoadrenocorticism, can develop if the pituitary gland is dysfunctional, causing decreased production of adrenocorticotropic hormone, the hormone that regulates serum levels of cortisol.[2]

The clinical features include fatigue, irritability, depression, weakness, and hypotension and can occur over a time period of months. As serum corticosteroid levels drop, this induces the production of corticotropin and α-melanoctye stimulating hormone (MSH). α-MSH is thought to directly stimulate melanocytes and increase melanin production, causing the mucocutaneous hyperpigmentation; on the skin it is described as bronzing.[45]

Symptoms may include gastrointestinal upset with anorexia, nausea, vomiting, diarrhea, weight loss, salt cravings, hypotension, easy bruising, fatigue, mood swings, depression, and weakness.[45]

In the oral cavity, the hyperpigmentation can manifest as diffuse or patchy, brown, macular pigmentation of the oral mucosa. The oral mucosal changes can be the earliest manifestation of the disease; skin hyperpigmentation can present as a late finding.[45] Sites of hyperpigmentation include areas of friction, recent scars, and the vermilion border of the lips. The buccal mucosa, periodontal soft tissues (**Fig. 5**A), and tongue (**Fig. 5**B) can also exhibit patchy macular areas of hyperpigmentation (**Fig. 5**C).[46]

Addison disease is treated with corticosteroid replacement therapy. The body may need additional corticosteroid hormones during stressful events, such as surgery. Without treatment, this condition can be fatal. With treatment this condition has a good prognosis.[2]

GARDNER SYNDROME

Gardner syndrome (GS), or familial colorectal polyposis, is an autosomal dominant disorder.[2] The incidence of GS ranges between 1 in 4000 and 1 in 12,000, depending on the region.[2] Multiple polyps in the colon along with tumors outside the colon characterize the disorder.[2] The tumors outside the colon may include osteomas of the skull, epidermoid cysts, fibromas, and thyroid cancer.[2]

There is a high association between GS and familial adenomatous polyposis. This association may manifest as aggressive fibromatosis (desmoid tumors).[2] The numerous polyps in the colon predispose the individual to colon cancer (adenocarcinomas).[2] Removal of the colon decreases the likelihood of developing colon cancer.[2]

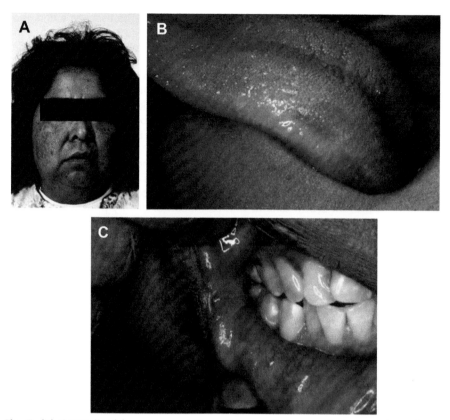

Fig. 5. (*A*) Generalized hyperpigmentation of face with increased pigmentation of acne scars and lips. (*B*) Tongue—patchy macular areas of hyperpigmentation. (*C*) Periodontal and buccal mucosal hyperpigmentation. (*From* [*A, C*] Nieman LK, Chanco Turner ML. Addison's disease. Clin Dermatol. 2006;24:278, with permission; and [*B*] Nieman LK, Chanco Turner ML. Addison's disease. Clin Dermatol. 2006;24:279; with permission.)

GS can be identified based on head, neck, and oral findings, including many impacted teeth, multiple supernumerary teeth, odontomas, osteomas of maxilla and mandible, causing a radiographic cotton-wool appearance.[2] There also is a congenital hypertrophy of the retinal pigment epithelium.[2]

Osteomas typically are asymptomatic, presenting without pain, and these lesions can cause expansile facial asymmetry and are radiographically radiopaque.[2] The osteomas often are observed during puberty and this can be prior to the gastrointestinal symptoms of bowel polyps. Indication for removal of jaw osteomas and epidermoid cysts is for cosmetic reasons.[2] The prognosis for the patient depends on the behavior of the bowel adenocarcinomas.[2]

BROWN TUMORS OF RENAL OSTEODYSTROPHY

Renal osteodystrophy can result in brown tumors.[2] The brown tumors are linked to secondary hyperparathyroidism in patients with chronic renal failure.[2] The rate of brown tumors in patients with secondary hyperparathyroidism related to chronic kidney disease ranges from 1.5% to greater than 13%.[2] The brown tumors derive its name from the color of the tissue on gross dissection.[2] The tissue is a dark red-brown, thought to be due to hemorrhage and hemosiderin found within the tumor.[2] Radiographically, these lesions are well defined as unilocular or multilocular radiolucencies.[2]

The brown tumors are brought about through breakdown of a focus of bone. The most common locations relate to areas where bone resorption is common and rapid.[2] A cycle of hemorrhage followed by infiltration with granulation tissue containing multi-nucleated giant cells that eventually displaced the healthy bone marrow, resulting in a brown tumor.[2] The lesions often are expansible and often affect the mandible, clavicles, ribs, and pelvis.[2]

Browns tumor is more likely to be found in the mandible compared with the maxilla.[2] The locations of the tumors can vary; patients present typically without pain; however, pain has been reported.[2] Patients with secondary hyperparathyroidism can help prevent brown tumors with restriction of dietary phosphate binders and vitamin D; surgical removal of the brown tumor mass sometimes may be required.[2]

HERPES SIMPLEX

Herpes simplex is caused by the herpes simplex virus (HSV). HSV-1 causes infection above the waist in areas, including perioral, and HSV-2 causes infection to the genital areas.[47] HSV-1 is primarily transmitted through infected oral secretions and is highly contagious in closed community settings, like daycare.[47]

HSV-1 spreads by infecting oral mucosal cells.[47] It can cause cell death of those cells and consequently the clinical symptoms appear.[47] Subsequently, HSV1 enters sensory nerve endings and establishes its latency here.[47]

Acute herpetic gingivostomatitis is the primary infection, as seen in **Fig. 6**A. Children generally get infected between ages of 6 months and 3 years.[47] The virus is latent for the first 2 days to 12 days.[47] Accompanying symptoms of cold, fever, and cough may occur. One day to 3 days later, clinical lesions begin as blisters of 1 mm to 2 mm in diameter that rupture and coalesce to ulcers. They are seen on the lips, tongue, gingiva, buccal mucosa, and palate.[4] These ulcers heal in 10 days to 14 days without scarring. Infected patients also can have a fever of greater than 38°C, enlarged cervical lymph nodes, increased salivary secretions, dehydration, and bad breath.[47]

Recurrent infections are associated with exposure to sunlight, stress, fatigue, cold, spicy food, menstruation, and orofacial trauma.[47] The recurrent herpes simplex virus

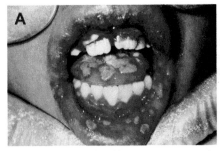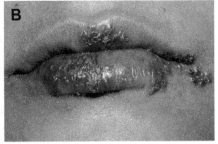

Fig. 6. (A) Acute herpetic gingivostomatitis. (B) Herpes labialis. (From [A, B] Neville BW, Damm DD, Allen CM, et al. Viral infections. In: Oral and maxillofacial pathology. 4th ed. St. Louis: Elsevier; 2016. p. 218–58; with permission.)

affects the lips, as seen in **Fig. 6**B, commissures, and perioral skin.[47] It is termed, *recurrent herpes labialis*. Preceding the lesions, patients can experience burning, tingling, soreness, and swelling at the sites where the lesions will occur.[47] Six hours later, the lesions appear as red macules, which become ulcers. The lesions tend to heal in 10 days without scarring.[47] Recurrent herpes simplex also can occur on the palate and gingival mucosa.[47]

Treatment includes acyclovir and valaciclovir.[47] If the course of disease is more than 5 days, antiviral drugs are not recommended. Acyclovir eye drops can be used on herpes labialis.[47]

HERPES ZOSTER

Varicella-zoster virus (VZV) can cause varicella and herpes zoster.[47] The initial infection is varicella and a reactivation is herpes zoster.[47] After primary infection, VZV maintains a latency in the sensory ganglia at a subclinical stage.[47] During aging or immunosuppression, however, VZV is reactivated.[47]

Varicella has an incubation period of 14 days to 16 days.[47] After this, pruritic erythematous lesions form on the scalp, face, and trunk with systemic symptoms of fever, fatigue, and anorexia.[47] Then, the maculopapular phase progresses to a vesicular phase, during which small fluid-filled vesicles occur with a range in number from 100 lesions to 300 lesions, as seen in **Fig. 7**A.[47] The crusting phase begins after this. Hypopigmentation is common and scarring is rare during healing.[47] The cutaneous rash is centripetally distributed, starting with the face and following with the trunk and limbs.[47] Ulcerative and painful lesions appear on mucous membranes, such as the oropharynx and conjunctivae.[47]

Herpes zoster is characterized by a rash in the skin that corresponds to the affected nerve.[47] The rash is unilateral and does not cross the midline.[47] Trigeminal herpes zoster is common4. Localized sensations range from mild itching to severe pain that precedes the development of the skin lesions.[47] As the cutaneous disease progresses, vesicles coalesce into larger fluid-filled lesions followed by scabbing, as seen in **Fig. 7**B.[47] The lesions usually heal within 2 weeks to 4 weeks.[47]

Treatment includes antiviral drugs, immunomodulatory drugs, painkillers, and neurotrophic drugs. Acyclovir, valaciclovir, and famciclovir are all effective

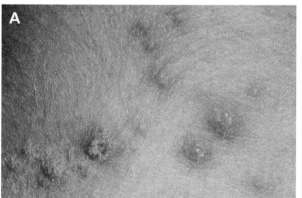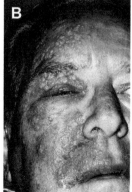

Fig. 7. (*A*) Varicella. (*B*) Herpes zoster. (*From* [*A, B*] Neville BW, Damm DD, Allen CM, et al. Viral infections. In: Oral and maxillofacial pathology. 4th ed. St. Louis: Elsevier; 2016. p. 218–58; with permission.)

drugs for treating herpes zoster.[47] Zostavax is a concentrated formulation of varivax that the US Food and Drug Administration has approved to prevent herpes zoster and its complications in immunocompetent adults ages greater than or equal to 60 years.[47] Additionally, the vaccine is recommended to prevent varicella in all children and adults who are seronegative for antibodies to the VZV.[47]

HUMAN IMMUNODEFICIENCY VIRUS

AIDS is caused by the human immunodeficiency virus (HIV).[4] This virus selectively invades CD4 cells.[47] HIV is able to fuse to the surface of the CD4 cell and consequently destroy the cell. CD4 plays a key role in the immune response and this destruction causes a decline in the immune function of the patients.[47]

HIV can be spread through unprotected sexual intercourse with an HIV-infected partner; sharing injectors, blood, or blood products polluted by HIV; artificial insemination; skin and organ transplantation; and maternal-fetal transmission.[47]

Several oral lesions have particular importance because of their strong association with HIV infection or their relationship to prognosis.[28] These lesions include oral candidiasis, oral hairy leukoplakia (OHL), and Kaposi sarcoma (KS).[28] A low threshold for HIV testing is recommended when a patient consults for these oral conditions.[48] Of importance, the features discussed previously are present in 50% of patients with HIV infection and 80% in patients with AIDS.[49]

HIV infection should be considered in young adults with these mentioned oral lesions, especially accompanied by recent weight loss, chronic diarrhea/cough for more than 1 month, or intermittent or persistent fever for more than 1 month.[47] The gold standard for the clinical diagnosis is enzyme-linked immunosorbent assay and Western blotting.[47]

ORAL CANDIDIASIS

In patients infected with HIV, the most common opportunistic infection seen is candidiasis caused by C albicans.[49] There are 4 forms of candidial infections: pseudomembranous candidiasis, erythematous candidiasis, hyperplastic candidiasis, and angular cheilitis. In patients infected with HIV, erythematous candidiasis tends to be the most prevalent whereas in patient with AIDS, pseudomembranous candidiasis tends to be the most prevalent.[49]

Angular cheilitis is present in the corners of the mouth. It can present as erythema or as fissuring.[49] Pseudomembranous candidiasis manifests like a whitish creamy curdlike plaques, which can occur in any oral mucosal surfaces but the most common area includes buccal mucosa and tongue, as seen in **Fig. 8**.[49] These plaques can be wiped away and leave an erythematous or bleeding underlying mucosa.[49] Hyperplastic candidiasis is also characterized by white plaques; however, they tend to present on the buccal mucosa and they do not scrape off.[49] Last, erythematous candidiasis is characterized by flat red lesions seen on the dorsal aspect of tongue or the hard or soft palate.[49] Patient complains of burning sensation while eating hot or spicy foods and drinking acid beverages.[49]

The candidal organism can be identified by doing exfoliative cytology or biopsy and can be seen microscopically.[49] The commonly used topical application depends on the severity of the disease.[49] In mild to moderate cases, nystatin oral suspension, clotrimazole troches, and nystatin pastilles can be used. In moderate to severe cases, systemic drug fluconazole is used.[49]

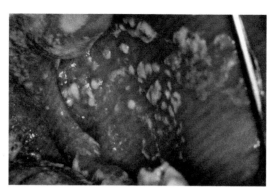

Fig. 8. HIV-associated candidiasis. (*From* Neville BW, Damm DD, Allen CM, et al. Viral infections. In: Oral and maxillofacial pathology. 4th ed. St. Louis: Elsevier; 2016. p. 218–58; with permission.)

ORAL HAIRY LEUKOPLAKIA

OHL is caused by the Epstein-Barr virus. The prevalence of OHL is reported as 9% to 25% in HIV seropositive patients.[28] The presence of OHL is a strong indication that a patient has been infected with HIV and/or that their immune status is worsening. Greenspan and colleagues[28] reported that 47% of the seropositive patients who developed hairy leukoplakia progressed to AIDS within 2 years; 67% of these patients developed AIDS within 4 years.

OHL manifests as white patches on the lateral border of the tongue, unilaterally or bilaterally, as seen in **Fig. 9**. It is usually asymptomatic but can cause a burning feeling. It can be differentiated from pseudomembranous candidiasis by the fact that it does not wipe off. Additionally, the use of antifungals does not treat OHL.[28] OHL is diagnosed clinically; however, a histopathologic sample demonstrates the Epstein-Barr virus in the basal epithelial cells.[28]

As discussed previously, OHL can present similarly, clinically, to pseudomembranous candidiasis; however, the administration of antifungals does not treat the OHL lesions.[50] In 80% of OHL lesions, the Candida organism is contained. OHL is not a premalignant lesion and hence does not convert to squamous cell carcinoma.[50] Patients generally, however, request treatment because the lesions can be unsightly.

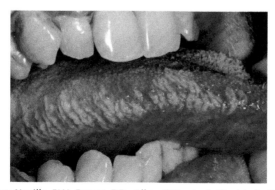

Fig. 9. OHL. (*From* Neville BW, Damm DD, Allen CM, et al. Viral infections. In: Oral and maxillofacial pathology. 4th ed. St. Louis: Elsevier; 2016. p. 218–58; with permission.)

Surgical treatment of the lesion is a possibility. The lesion can also be treated with acyclovir.[50]

KAPOSI SARCOMA

KS is a malignant systemic disease that arises from the vascular endothelium.[48] It is caused by human herpesvirus that is transmitted sexually or via the blood or saliva.[47] In patients with HIV, KS tends to manifest in the oral cavity first.[47]

Oral KS manifests as red or purple in color, may be macular or nodular, and may be ulcerated.[47] It can cause tissue destruction. Early lesions tend to be red and become darker over time.[47] The most common oral sites include the palate, attached gingiva of the alveolus, and the tongue, as seen in **Fig. 10.**[47] Alveolar involvement cause bone loss and consequently tooth loss. Biopsy is required for definitive diagnosis. The appearance of oral lesions is a sign of increasing mortality.[50] Therefore, any patient who develops oral KS should follow closely with a primary care provider, because this may indicate more serious progression of disease.[50] If a patient is not on highly active antiretroviral therapy (The terminology has evolved to combination antiretroviral therapy; it refers to the combinations of drugs that are used to keep HIV infections under control. Usually, they contain 3 or more different drugs.), the treatment of KS is to initiate it. Additionally, surgical excision, intralesional or systemic chemotherapy, sclerotherapy, or radiation is a treatment option.[50]

IMMUNE-MEDIATED CONDITIONS

In direct immunofluorescence, human immunoglobulin is inoculated in a goat. This creates antibodies against human immunoglobulin. These antibodies are harvested and tagged with fluorescein, which is a dye that glows under UV light. A frozen section of a patient's tissue is then placed on a slide and incubated with the goat antihuman antibodies that were dyed with fluorescein. The antibodies bind to any tissue where there is human immunoglobulin present. Excess is washed off and the section is viewed under the microscope.[51]

In indirect immunofluorescence, a frozen section of tissue that is similar to oral mucosa is placed on a slide and incubated with the patient's serum. The autoantibodies attach to the epithelial attachment on the frozen section. Excess is washed off and fluorescein-conjugated goat antihuman antibody is incubated with the section. Excess is washed off and UV light is used to visualize autoantibodies.[51]

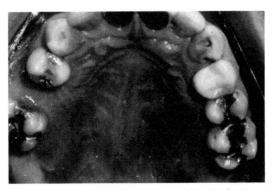

Fig. 10. KS. (*From* Neville BW, Damm DD, Allen CM, et al. Viral infections. In: Oral and maxillofacial pathology. 4th ed. St. Louis: Elsevier; 2016. p. 218–58; with permission.)

PEMPHIGUS VULGARIS

As the name pemphigus vulgaris describes, *vulgaris* being Latin for *common*, it is the most common immunobullous disease. One case to 5 cases of 1 million cases are diagnosed per year. If left untreated, this condition may cause death in the patient. The manifestation of this disease starts as oral lesions prior to forming cutaneous and genital lesions. The oral manifestation is described as "the first to show, and the last to go."

Pmphigus vulgaris is seen in adults at an average age of 50 years, is found equally in men and women, and is most common in people of Mediterranean, South Asian, and Jewish heritage. Prior to today's treatment modalities, 60% to 90% of patients died as a result of this disease modality. Today, with the use of long-term steroid therapy, the mortality rate has decreased to 5% to 10%.[51]

Microscopically, the epidermis is composed of epithelial cells that are combined to form a complex with the assistance of glycoproteins. Desmoglein 1 and desmoglein 3 are the glycoproteins that make up desmosomes, the fundamental binding force between cells. The autoantibodies that are prevalent in this autoimmune disorder are selective for these glycoproteins. Their interaction causes disruption of the structural stability of desmosomes and inhibits their function. Clinically, this inhibition causes formation of blisters.

Desmoglein 3 is found predominantly in the oral mucosa and the epidermis. Autoantibodies that direct toward desmoglein 3 causes pouching above the basal layer. Desmoglein 1 is found in the superficial portion of the epidermis and minimally in the oral mucosa. Thus, a similar pouching is found but rather in the epidermis.

Clinically, patients with this disease diagnosis first present with ulcerations on superficial oral mucosa, as seen in **Fig. 11**. Most of these lesions predominantly are found on the buccal mucosa, ventral tongue, and the gingiva. As described previously, patients present with oral lesions prior to skin lesions. These lesions appear as fluid-filled vesicular lesions that rupture and leave a painful erythematous surface.[51]

Ocular lesions may appear similar to bilateral conjunctivitis.[51] If a growing suspicion of pemphigus vulgaris is present, firm pressure on normal-appearing skin can induce formation of a fluid-filled vesicular lesion, termed *bullae*. This is termed positive Nikolsky sign.[51]

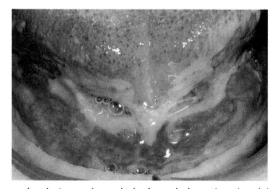

Fig. 11. Pemphigus vulgaris. Large, irregularly shaped ulcerations involving the floor of the mouth and ventral tongue. (*From* Neville BW, Damm DD, Allen CM, et al. Dermatologic diseases. In: Oral and maxillofacial pathology. 4th ed. St. Louis: Elsevier; 2016. p. 690–760; with permission.)

A biopsy should be performed to confirm diagnosis. Specimens show intraepithelial separation and/or complete separation from the basal layer, which appear to resemble a row of tombstones. This appearance is due to a rounded shape of the basal layer, called Tzanck cells, which helps confirm a final diagnosis.[51]

Direct immunofluorescence is used to make the final diagnosis. A tissue sample is submitted in Michel solution. IgG, IgM or complement 3 (C3) can be seen in the intercellular spaces between epithelial cells. Indirect immunofluorescence or ELISA can also show autoantibody circulation[51]

The nature of this disease is systemic, thus systemic corticosteroids in combination with other immunosuppressive drugs should be used. A systemic corticosteroid, such as prednisone, is started with supplementation with steroid-sparing agents, such as azathioprine. Topical corticosteroids are also used to treat this disease. Long-term side effects of systemic corticosteroids can cause diabetes mellitus, adrenal suppression, weight gain, osteoporosis, peptic ulcers, severe mood swings, and increased susceptibility to infections.[51]

To avoid such complications, physicians usually start early with a high dose of systemic corticosteroid to clear the lesions and then the patient is placed on a low dose of corticosteroids to control the condition. Even if pemphigus may undergo complete resolution, remission and exacerbations are common.[51]

BULLOUS PEMPHIGOID

Like pemphigus, bullous pemphigoid is characterized by formation of autoantibodies directed at the epithelium. This disease process involves inhibition of hemidesmosomes at the layer of the basement membrane and underlying connective tissue. The proteins that are targeted in hemidesmosomes are bullous pemphigoid antigens, BP180 and BP230. When antibodies bind to these complexes, it begins the complement cascade that causes the inflammatory response resulting in damage to the basement membrane and formulating bullae.[51]

Unlike pemphigus, bullous pemphigoid is not usually found in oral mucosa but rather superficial skin lesions. It is usually found in elderly individuals between the ages of 60 and 90. Patients may begin with inflammation of the skin prior to forming bullae. These vesicles eventually burst and form a superficial crust that does not scar.[51]

When viewing the epithelium under direct immunofluorescence, a linear band of IgG and C3 usually is visualized at the level of the basement membrane.[51]

As is performed with most autoimmune conditions, primarily this disease is managed with systemic corticosteroids along with other immunosuppressive agents. Most patients are started on prednisone and supplemented with azathioprine. The addition of multiple treatment therapies is based on severity of the disease process. Most patients have a good prognosis with remission after 2 years to 5 years.[51]

DIABETES MELLITUS

Diabetes mellitus is a metabolic disorder characterized by the presence of chronic hyperglycemia. Patients with diabetes have impaired function of polymorphonuclear leukocytes (leukocyte adhesion, chemotaxis, and phagocytosis), impaired bactericidal activity, altered response of exposure to antigens, and alteration to the function of T lymphocytes.[52] Frequently reported oral manifestations related to diabetes mellitus are salivary dysfunction—dry mouth, burning mouth syndrome, tooth decay, periodontal disease and gingivitis, oral candidiasis, taste disorders, delayed wound healing, increased incidence of infection, altered taste and other neurosensory disorders, and benign parotid hypertrophy.

SYSTEMIC LUPUS ERYTHEMATOSUS

Systemic lupus erythematosus (SLE) is a chronic autoimmune inflammatory disease, which involves the connective tissue. The condition is more common among women with an onset between 15 years and 40 years of age Common symptoms of SLE include fever, weight loss, glomerulonephritis, alopecia, rash, and vesiculobullous lesions Research shows that 25% of SLE patients have oral mucous membrane and lip involvement with possible petechiae. Oral manifestations of SLE are frequently encountered[53] and may include oral ulceration, honeycomb plaque, raised keratotic plaque, nonspecific erythema, purpura, petechiae, and cheilitis[54] Xerostomia/hyposalivation predispose patients with SLE to dental caries and recurrent noninfectious pharyngitis, candidiasis and oral ulcerations.

REFERENCES

1. Al-Salem A. Medical and surgical complications of sickle cell anemia. Heidelberg: Switzerland: Springer International Publishing; 2016.
2. Neville BW, Damm DD, Allen CM, et al. Oral and maxillofacial pathology. USA: Elsevier; 2016.
3. Mello SM, Paulo CAR, Alves C. Oral considerations in the management of sickle cell disease: a case report. Oral Health Dent Manag 2012;11:125–8.
4. Saint Clair de Velasquez Y, Rivera H. Sickle cell anemia oral manifestations in a Venezuelan population. Acta Odontol Latinoam 1997;10:101–10.
5. Messadi DV, Mirowski GW. Oral signs of hematologic disease. Springer Nature Switzerland AG; 2019.
6. Kayle M, Docherty SL, Sloane R, et al. Transition to adult care in sickle cell disease: a longitudinal study of clinical characteristics and disease severity. Pediatr Blood Cancer 2019;66:e27463.
7. Phore S, Panchal R. Dental implications of an adult jaundice patient: a rare case report. Med J DY Patil Vidyapeeth 2018;11:171–4.
8. Santos H, Barbosa IDS, de Oliveira TFL, et al. Evaluation of the maxillomandibular positioning in subjects with sickle-cell disease through 2- and 3-dimensional cephalometric analyses: a retrospective study. Medicine (Baltimore) 2018;97: e11052.
9. Costa CP, de Carvalho HL, Thomaz EB, et al. Craniofacial bone abnormalities and malocclusion in individuals with sickle cell anemia: a critical review of the literature. Rev Bras Hematol Hemoter 2012;34:60–3.
10. Elias EJ, Liao JH, Jara H, et al. Quantitative MRI analysis of craniofacial bone marrow in patients with sickle cell disease. AJNR Am J Neuroradiol 2013;34: 622–7.
11. Sebes JI, Diggs LW. Radiographic changes of the skull in sickle cell anemia. AJR Am J Roentgenol 1979;132:373–7.
12. Mnapo B, Shields M, Koop K. Hair-on-end. Am J Trop Med Hyg 2013;88:607.
13. Nowak A, Christensen J, Mabry T, et al. In: Nowak AJ, et al, editors. Pediatric dentistry. 6th edition; 2019. p. 66–76.e62. Content Repository Only!.
14. Kavadia-Tsatala S, Kolokytha O, Kaklamanos EG, et al. Mandibular lesions of vasoocclusive origin in sickle cell hemoglobinopathy. Odontology 2004;92:68–72.
15. Chekroun M, Chérifi H, Fournier B, et al. Oral manifestations of sickle cell disease. Br Dent J 2019;226:27–31.

16. Al-Ismaili H, Nasim O, Bakathir A. Jaw osteomyelitis as a complication of sickle cell anaemia in three omani patients: case reports and literature review. Sultan Qaboos Univ Med J 2017;17:e93–7.

17. Olaitan AA, Amuda JT, Adekeye EO. Osteomyelitis of the mandible in sickle cell disease. Br J Oral Maxillofac Surg 1997;35:190–2.

18. Kelleher M, Bishop K, Briggs P. Oral complications associated with sickle cell anemia: a review and case report. Oral Surg Oral Med Oral Pathol Oral Radiol Endod 1996;82:225–8.

19. Mendes PH, Fonseca NG, Martelli DR, et al. Orofacial manifestations in patients with sickle cell anemia. Quintessence Int 2011;42:701–9.

20. Soni NN. Microradiographic study of dental tissues in sickle-cell anaemia. Arch Oral Biol 1966;11:561–4.

21. Javed F, Correa FO, Nooh N, et al. Orofacial manifestations in patients with sickle cell disease. Am J Med Sci 2013;345:234–7.

22. Basyouni A, Almasoud NN, Al-Khalifa KS, et al. Malocclusion and craniofacial characteristics in Saudi adolescents with sickle cell disease. Saudi J Med Med Sci 2018;6:149–54.

23. Alves e Luna AC, Godoy F, de Menezes VA. Malocclusion and treatment need in children and adolescents with sickle cell disease. Angle Orthod 2014;84:467–72.

24. Demirbas Kaya A, Aktener BO, Unsal C. Pulpal necrosis with sickle cell anaemia. Int Endod J 2004;37:602–6.

25. Goel A, Bakshi SS, Soni N, et al. Iron deficiency anemia and Plummer-Vinson syndrome: current insights. J Blood Med 2017;8:175–84.

26. Novacek G. Plummer-Vinson syndrome. Orphanet J rare Dis 2006;1:36.

27. Chen TS, Chen PS. Rise and fall of the Plummer-Vinson syndrome. J Gastroenterol Hepatol 1994;9:654–8.

28. Grbic JT, Lamster IB. Oral manifestations of HIV infection. AIDS Patient Care STDS 1997;11(1):18–24.

29. Samad A, Mohan N, Balaji RVS, et al. Oral manifestations of plummer-vinson syndrome: a classic report with literature review. J Int Oral Health 2015;7:68–71.

30. Wynder EL, Hultberg S, Jacobsson F, et al. Environmental factors in cancer of the upper alimentary tract. A swedish study with special reference to plummer-vinson (Paterson-Kelly) syndrome. Cancer 1957;10:470–87.

31. Larsson LG, Sandström A, Westling P. Relationship of Plummer-Vinson disease to cancer of the upper alimentary tract in Sweden. Cancer Res 1975;35:3308–16.

32. Anderson SR, Sinacori JT. Plummer-Vinson syndrome heralded by postcricoid carcinoma. Am J Otolaryngol 2007;28:22–4. https://doi.org/10.1016/j.amjoto.2006.06.004.

33. Chisholm M. The association between webs, iron and post-cricoid carcinoma. Postgrad Med J 1974;50:215–9.

34. Stephen R, Utecht T. Scurvy identified in the emergency department: a case report. J Emerg Med 2001;21:235–7.

35. Halligan TJ, Russell NG, Dunn WJ, et al. Identification and treatment of scurvy: a case report. Oral Surg Oral Med Oral Pathol Oral Radiol Endod 2005;100:688–92.

36. Alqanatish JT, Alqahtani F, Alsewairi WM, et al. Childhood scurvy: an unusual cause of refusal to walk in a child. Pediatr Rheumatol Online J 2015;13:23.

37. Hahn T, Adams W, Williams K. Is vitamin C enough? A case report of scurvy in a five-year-old girl and review of the literature. BMC Pediatr 2019;19:74.

38. Aroojis AJ, Gajjar SM, Johari AN. Epiphyseal separations in spastic cerebral palsy. J Pediatr Orthop B 2007;16:170–4.

39. Lykkesfeldt J, Michels AJ, Frei B. Vitamin C. Adv Nutr 2014;5:16–8.

40. Varela-Lopez A, Navarro-Hortal MD, Giampieri F, et al. Nutraceuticals in periodontal health: a systematic review on the role of vitamins in periodontal health maintenance. Molecules 2018;23. https://doi.org/10.3390/molecules23051226.
41. James WD, Elston DM, Treat JR, et al. Andrews' diseases of the skin. Chapter 22. USA: Elsevier; 2016. p. 478–9.
42. Hodges RE, Hood J, Canham JE, et al. Clinical manifestations of ascorbic acid deficiency in man. Am J Clin Nutr 1971;24:432–43.
43. Beggs AD, Latchford AR, Vasen HF, et al. Peutz-Jeghers syndrome: a systematic review and recommendations for management. Gut 2010;59:975–86.
44. Hearle N, Schumacher V, Menko FH, et al. Frequency and spectrum of cancers in the Peutz-Jeghers syndrome. Clin Cancer Res 2006;12:3209–15.
45. Alawi F. Pigmented lesions of the oral cavity: an update. Dent Clin North Am 2013; 57:699–710.
46. Nieman LK, Chanco Turner ML. Addison's disease. Clin Dermatol 2006;24: 276–80.
47. Chen Q, Zeng X. Case based oral mucosal diseases. Singapore: Springer; 2018.
48. Parks ET, Lancaster H. Oral manifestations of systemic disease. Dermatol Clin 2003;21(1):171–82.
49. Warrier SA, Sathasivasubramanian S. Human immunodeficiency virus induced oral candidiasis. J Pharm Bioallied Sci 2015;7:812–4.
50. Smith JA. HIV and AIDS in the adolescent and adult: an update for the oral and maxillofacial surgeon. Oral Maxillofac Surg Clin North Am 2008;20(4):535–65.
51. Neville BW, Waldron CA, Herschraft EA. Oral & maxillofacial pathology. Philadelphia: Saunders; 1995.
52. Mauri-Obradors E, Estrugo-Devesa A, Jané-Salas E, et al. Oral manifestations of Diabetes Mellitus. A systematic review. Med Oral Patol Oral Cir Bucal 2017;22(5): e586–94.
53. Rutter-Locher Z, Smith TO, Giles I, et al. Association between systemic lupus erythematosus and periodontitis: a systematic review and meta-analysis. Front Immunol 2017;8:1295.
54. Chi AC, Neville BW, Krayer JW, et al. Oral manifestations of systemic disease. Am Fam Physician 2010;82(11):1381–8.

The Geriatric Syndrome and Oral Health

Navigating Oral Disease Treatment Strategies in the Elderly

Leslie R. Halpern, DDS, MD, PhD, MPH

KEYWORDS

- Geriatric syndrome • Frailty • Multimorbidity • Polypharmacy
- Oral and maxillofacial dysfunction

KEY POINTS

- Poor oral health in the geriatric population is being framed as a potentially new geriatric syndrome; an oral and maxillofacial geriatric syndrome.
- The article presents a roadmap approach using the concepts of the geriatric syndrome to apply therapeutic strategies for 5 common oral and maxillofacial dysfunctions seen in the elderly.
- The concept of the geriatric syndrome describes an innovative and well-tested approach in managing the interplay of age-related physiologic changes, chronic disease, functional stressors, and oral health in the elderly.

INTRODUCTION

The World Health Organization (WHO) has calculated that the global population is increasing at an annual rate of 1.7%, whereas those who are aged 65 years or older are increasing at a rate of 2.5%.[1] By the year 2050, 1 out of 5 persons in the United States will be aged 65 years or older.[2] These demographic projections will have a major impact on delivery of both general and oral health care, as well as how providers tailor treatment strategies within the elderly patient population. Oral and maxillofacial health affects systemic health, as well as different aspects of life with respect to social interaction, self-esteem, and the health-related quality of life for the geriatric population. Although many people aged 65 years or older remain healthy and visit medical/dental providers either infrequently or for health maintenance care, their cohorts experience increased rates of age-related physiologic changes in the oral cavity, changes

Disclosure: The author has nothing to disclose.
Oral and Maxillofacial Surgery, University of Utah, School of Dentistry, 530 South Wakara Way, Salt Lake City, UT 84108, USA
E-mail address: Leslie.halpern@hsc.utah.edu

Dent Clin N Am 64 (2020) 209–228
https://doi.org/10.1016/j.cden.2019.08.011
0011-8532/20/© 2019 Elsevier Inc. All rights reserved.

caused by the comorbidities of chronic illnesses and changes resulting from medications used to manage diseases.[3]

With an aging population, oral health care providers need to understand and apply the concepts of geriatrics to the delivery of oral health care. The concept of geriatric syndromes forms a framework for addressing the complex oral health needs of older adults and the managing of certain common geriatric oral syndromes, such as increased caries risk, periodontitis and its nexus with systemic disease, disorders in taste and swallowing, dysfunction in chewing and speaking (or mandibular dyskinesia/dystonia), and burning mouth syndrome (BMS).[1–3]

GERIATRIC SYNDROME/GERIATRIC 5MS/FRAILTY

Geriatric syndromes refer to "multifactorial health conditions that occur when the accumulated effects of impairments in multiple systems render [an older] person vulnerable to situational challenges."[3,4] The common geriatric syndromes, such as falls, functional decline, delirium, incontinence, polypharmacy, and frailty, are also described as "clinical conditions in older people that do not fit into discrete disease categories."[3,5,6] The geriatric provider's usage of the term syndrome emphasizes multiple causations of a unified manifestation. With this usage, the conceptualization of geriatric syndromes aligns itself well with the "the observable characteristics, at the physical, morphologic, or biochemical level, of an individual, as determined by the genotype and environment."[3,4] As such, it is multifactorial; that is, involving the interaction among stressors and age-related risk predictors that can have a devastating effect on multiple organ systems[4,7] (**Fig. 1**). Frailty is "a common and important geriatric syndrome associated with age-related declines in physiologic reserve/function across multi-organ systems."[5,7] The frailty phenotype is applied when 3 or more of

The Relationship Among Risk Factors, Geriatric Syndromes, and Poor Oral Health Outcomes

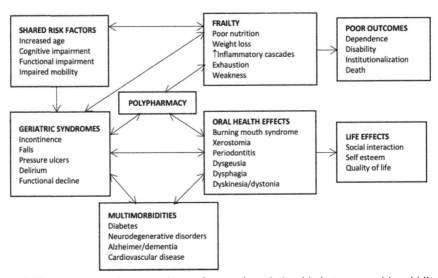

Fig. 1. The geriatric syndrome made up of a complex relationship between multimorbidity, polypharmacy, frailty, and poor oral health outcomes.

the following occur: weakness, a slow level of physical activity, poor endurance, breakdown in several inflammatory cascades, and weight loss.[3,5]

Although there is no single definition of polypharmacy, it consists of the use of several medications simultaneously to treat 1 or more diseases.[2] Studies in the United States showed that, out of 2500 female respondents older than ag 65 years, 23% took 5 or more medications and 12% took more than 10.[2] A study in the United Kingdom determined that 36% of geriatric patients more than 75 years of age used 4 or more prescription medications or nonprescription over-the-counter medications to cure or treat their oral cavity complaints.[7] In 2007 to 2008, more than 88% of Americans older than 60 years took at least 1 prescription medication, 76% used 2 or more prescription medications, and 37% used 5 or more.[8,9] Other studies suggest that the elderly use 2 to 4 nonprescription medications daily, most commonly nonsteroidal antiinflammatory drugs, antihistamines, antacids (H_2 blockers), laxatives, and sedatives.[8,9] However, these pharmacologic agents bind to other unwanted potential sites, causing side effects that affect the central nervous system (CNS) and/or the peripheral nervous system. CNS side effects may include confusion/disorientation, hallucinations, sleepiness, clumsiness or unsteadiness, convulsions, and mental status/behavior changes.[10,11] Peripheral side effects of medications can be salivary hypofunction, difficulty in speech and swallowing, mucous membrane dryness, blurred vision, increased breathing difficulty, difficulty urinating, and constipation.[11,12] Other problems related to polypharmacy include drug-drug interactions, increased expenses related to not only medications but also hospitalization, as well as adverse events from mistakes in dosing and type of medication given.[10–12] Dr Mark Beers crafted a set of criteria (Beer criteria) that identify medications that are potentially inappropriate for older adults because of increased risk of adverse events.[13]

As such, the concept of the geriatric syndrome describes an innovative and well-tested approach in managing the interplay between age-related physiologic changes, chronic disease, and functional stressors in the elderly and is now being applied across all health disciplines.[4,7] Over the last 3 decades, geriatricians have grappled with crafting a universal approach to inform health care educators of the value in training future providers to be competent in treating the elderly based on the complex causes of disease presentation. A recent keynote lecture at the Canadian Geriatrics Society Annual Meeting provided an algorithmic roadmap for the geriatric syndrome using the philosophy of the core competencies represented by the so-called geriatric 5Ms (mind, mobility, medications, multicomplexity, and matters most to me) (**Box 1**)[14] The health consequences of polypharmacy combined with multimorbidity of disease and their pathologic insults contribute to geriatric syndromes and frailty.[3] The association of frailty and polypharmacy is complex. Frailty is linked to the chronicity of disease (ie, multimorbidity), and this leads to polypharmacy. The relationship is bidirectional because polypharmacy leads to frailty based on the number of drugs administered, weight loss, poor nutrition caused by effects of drugs on oral cavity function, and ultimately the deterioration of health.[15] Other studies have suggested that both frailty and polypharmacy act as modulators for negative effects on health outcomes and that both act independently as risk factors for mortality.[12,15] The adverse reactions and their toxicities in older people can modify the goals of health care and influence decision making regarding medication delivery.

With these points in mind, the treatment of oral diseases in the elderly requires a comprehensive approach that combines the multimorbidity of diseases and polypharmacy in order to apply tailored therapeutic intervention for relief of age-related oral health consequences. This article presents a roadmap approach using the concepts of the geriatric syndrome, geriatric 5Ms, and frailty to evaluate symptoms and apply

Box 1	
The 5Ms of geriatrics	
Geriatric 5Ms	**Focus Areas**
Mind	Maintaining mental activity
	Helping manage dementia
	Helping to treat and prevent delirium
	Working to evaluate and treat depression
Mobility	Maintaining the ability to walk/balance
	Preventing falls
Medications	Reducing polypharmacy
	Deprescribing
	Prescribing treatment exactly for an older person's needs
	Helping to build awareness of harmful side effects
Multicomplexity	Helping older adults manage a variety of health conditions
	Assessing living conditions when they are affected by age, health, and social concerns
Matters most	Coordinating advance care plans
	Helping manage goals of care
	Making sure the patient's goals are reflected in the treatment plan

From Health in Aging Foundation. The 5Ms of geriatrics. Available at: https://www.healthinaging.org/tools-and-tips/5ms-geriatrics; with permission.

therapeutic strategies in 5 common oral and maxillofacial dysfunctions seen in every day practice. The article applies a comprehensive literature search using the search engines PubMed, Ovid, and Embassy. Publications only in English were chosen over a period of 23 years (1996–2019) using the following search terms: oral health in geriatrics, oral health and elderly, elderly, geriatric health oral health and systemic diseases, oral health related quality of life, polypharmacy, and oral health, and geriatric syndrome. Articles that were chosen also reflected systematic reviews, nonsystematic reviews, and observational and longitudinal studies.

MULTIMORBIDITY/POLYPHARMACY/ORAL AND MAXILLOFACIAL DYSFUNCTIONS

Oral health is part of overall health and well-being and, as such, requires dental practitioners to navigate through the multimorbidity/polypharmacy/chronic disease landscape in order to treat oral diseases that impede the health of their geriatric patients. The concepts of geriatric syndromes and frailty are applied later in this article to manage 5 common oral and maxillofacial dysfunctions associated with aging. Each oral disease entity is presented with respect to pathologic causation, associated multimorbidity of chronic disease, polypharmacy, and their contribution to these concepts.

ORAL AND MAXILLOFACIAL DYSFUNCTIONS
Xerostomia

Xerostomia (dry mouth) is a major oral health complaint in the elderly.[3,11,15] It can be either subjective, based on patient perception with or without diminished salivary flow, or objective, based on measurements of salivary flow. The prevalence rate for dry mouth in the geriatric population can vary from 25% to 30%.[16] There has been much debate about the role of aging on salivary function. Several investigators have supported the premise that aging of the major salivary glands causes a decreased ability to maintain their normal amount of salivary flow.[16] Vissink and colleagues[17] suggested that there is no significant age-related decrease in salivary gland function other than a slight decrease in acini cell number and increase in fatty tissue within the gland. Controversy still exists when the physiologic milieu of the glandular structure is evaluated because alterations in secretory product production at the protein level and other sialochemical electrolytes and immunoglobulins show fluctuations associated with aging.[16] The differences seen among studies may be caused by the type of collection methods used in sampling among patients.[16] There is agreement among all studies that the aging salivary glands, whether they are major or minor, show anatomic changes from secretory to fibrotic independent of the multimorbidity of disease and polypharmacy.[16–18]

Although several well-designed studies by Ship and colleagues[19] showed that parotid gland function remained stable across the age spectrum in healthy adults, xerostomia/diminished salivary function is a major consideration in the elderly, who frequently have multiple medical problems managed with medications. Diminished salivary function is significantly associated with age-related systemic conditions such as diabetes, autoimmune disease such as Sjögren syndrome, depression, polypharmacy, and other medical interventions such as radiation and chemotherapy for cancer and other tumors.[16] Many classes of drugs used for systemic illnesses have been linked to xerostomia, and the xerogenic effect increases with polypharmacy.[11,12] Studies equate xerostomia with subjective oral sensorial complaints (OSCs) and polypharmacy.[3,16] Nagler and Hershkovich[16] characterized relationships among age, drugs, OSCs, and salivary profiles using an age comparison study of healthy patients not hospitalized but living in a community. Patients who were on drugs showed a 50% greater tendency to have OSCs and xerostomia than those who were not on medications, and the total amount of salivary flow was reduced in the elderly compared with younger groups.[16] However, there were no differences in salivary flow rate when small samples of elderly patients on drugs were compared with their age-matched cohorts not on medications. The investigators concluded that there is a decreased rate of salivary flow in the elderly as well as the sialochemical makeup.[16]

Caries Risk and Salivary Hypofunction

Caries is a major oral health problem in the geriatric population because of the alterations of salivary function secondary to polypharmacy and periodontal compromise resulting in gingival recession.[15] Data from the National Institutes of Health, Section on Dental and Craniofacial Research, indicate that 93% of seniors 65 years of age and older have a history of dental caries in their permanent teeth and 18% of seniors 65 years of age and older have untreated caries.[20] Salivary biomolecules and proteins adhere to the tooth surface, establishing a stable protective shield against bacterial seeding and reducing the risk of caries by providing calcium, phosphorus, and fluoride ions, and essential minerals that maintain the highly calcified surface of the tooth. When hypofunction in salivary activity renders a loss of antimicrobial protection, the result may be an increase in cariogenic microorganism colonization.[21] Bacteria in the presence of fermentable carbohydrates become active in the production of acids that both demineralize the tooth surface and create an environment that selects for cariogenic microorganisms. This compromised microenvironment alters the homeostatic demineralization/remineralization cycle, resulting in an increase in caries. The effect is more profound for root caries because cementum and dentin dissolve at a higher pH than enamel.[11,21]

Treatment strategies: xerostomia and caries risk

Oral health care providers should evaluate patients for any oral and dental complications and then treat as needed based on acute or chronic symptoms. The multimorbidity and polypharmacy of xerostomia require reviewing the patient's medical and drug histories. After establishing a diagnosis, the clinician can suggest treatment options. All patients with xerostomia should be encouraged to hydrate while eliminating sugar sweeteners in foods and drinks, as well as various other sugar products, because of the increased risk of dental caries. Management of xerostomia is further divided into 2 categories based on the cause of dry mouth.

Local salivary stimulation The use of salivary substitutes locally in the oral cavity can help reduce the symptoms of xerostomia. Saliva substitutes are carboxymethylcellulose based and often short in relief duration.[11] Various water-soluble lubricants (K-Y Jelly, Taro-Gel, Biotene products) can be applied by foam brush or finger.[11] Although these measures are used with various success rates in many patients, their main disadvantage is limited effectiveness during the night when symptoms are most severe.[11,22] Sipping water on a frequent basis is a simple solution to providing relief for a dry mouth and is often more palatable to patients. Although salivary replacements may afford some relief, they do not deliver the physiologic constituents that give saliva its essential antimicrobial, lubricating, and demineralizing functions. A more effective strategy is to stimulate the production of saliva when glandular function remains. For instance, sugarless gums are an effective local stimulant because the chewing motion and the flavoring agents increase salivation.[11,22] Xylitol-based lozenges, sprays, and gum can stimulate the production of saliva, changing the osmotic gradients and improving pH and the buffering capacity. The increase in saliva has the potential to inhibit bacterial growth and metabolism in acidogenic species of *Streptococcus*.[11] Xylitol can also clear carbohydrate substrates, thereby reducing demineralization and increasing remineralization of hard tissues. Studies have shown a 10% reduction in caries in high-risk populations who are administered xylitol lozenges.[11,20,22] Alternative local measures include adhesive discs (eg, Oramoist, Ora-Coat, XyliMelts) that continuously release xylitol and a flavoring agent to stimulate the production of saliva.[11]

Systemic salivary stimulation Hypofunction of the major and minor salivary glands caused by polypharmacy is not an issue of physical damage to the salivary gland cells.[16] Studies report that 80% of the widely prescribed medicines cause xerostomia and more than 500 medicines lead to salivary gland dysfunction as a side effect without physical damage but by change in the flow rate of saliva.[16] The long-term use of tricyclic antidepressants, antihistamines, and antiarrhythmic and anticholinergic agents causes a decrease in both flow rate and amount of saliva.[8,9,11] Stimulation of saliva can be achieved using pharmacologic interventions. Drugs used to increase salivary flow are termed sialagogues. These medications are effective in increasing salivary secretions and have been shown to decrease xerostomia complaints in patients. Four main drugs are included in this category: pilocarpine, cevimeline, bethanechol chloride, and anethole trithione.[11] There are unwanted side effects of these sialagogues and so the dosages should be titrated up to their maximum amounts and spaced out over 3 months for a full effect (**Box 2** lists the dosing). Use for medication-induced xerostomia may be an off-label use.[11]

Caries risk Loss of saliva enhances the adherence of noxious microorganisms to the tooth surface. The use of supersaturated calcium and phosphate solutions may help to remineralize the hard tissue and decrease the potential for caries.[15] Fluoride salts are bactericidal and contribute to the action of calcium and phosphate in remineralizing the tooth surface. Fluoride varnishes should be considered at least twice per year for patients with high caries risk and 1.1% sodium fluoride can be prescribed for daily

Box 2
Pharmacologic agents for the treatment of xerostomia

Drug	Dose	Adverse Effects
Pilocarpine	3–5 mg 3 times per day	Sweating, nausea, dizziness Pulmonary secretions
Cevimeline	30 mg 3 times per day	Nausea, vomiting, diarrhea Rhinorrhea, sweating
Bethanechol chloride	10–50 mg 3–4 times per day	Miosis, sweating, GI upset
Anethole trithione	25 mg 3 times per day	Flatulence, abdominal pain GI upset

Abbreviation: GI, gastrointestinal.

From Ouanounou A. Xerostomia in the geriatric patient: causes, oral manifestations, and treatment. Compend Contin Educat Dent. 2016;37(5):306–11; with permission.

use to further enhance remineralization. Most important is the need for judicious follow-up of dental visits every 3 months. A careful evaluation of new caries and any soft tissue changes is paramount to assess new-onset inflammation and infection, as well as to monitor any changes caused by new or existing medication regimens.[6,11,15]

Periodontal disease
Periodontitis and multimorbidity of disease Periodontal disease is among the most prevalent oral manifestation seen in the geriatric dentate population both nationally and globally.[1,23,24] Studies have proposed that periodontitis in the elderly may not be considered a specific disease entity but a result of age-related changes in the periodontium caused by the length of time periodontal tissues are susceptible to bacterial exposure along with specific health problems of aging individuals.[23,24] Epidemiologic studies have shown that accumulation of plaque and consequent gingivitis/periodontitis become more severe as the patient ages (1.8% increasing to 3.3% after age 65 years).[6,23,24] With aging, the anatomy changes; gingiva and periodontal ligaments are weakened by decreased collagen. Atherosclerosis develops in alveolar bone and the vasculature of the ligaments becomes dysfunctional. The result is gingival recession and increase in crown length of the teeth with a subsequent risk of caries formation in the cementum exposed to the oral cavity. With aging, gingival epithelium becomes thinner and keratin tissue increases. In addition, increase is reported in the cellular density.[9,23,24]

At the biological level, changes in structure and function during aging can affect the host responses to the microorganisms responsible for plaque, and, as such, influence the rate of destruction of the periodontium.[21] Alterations in inflammatory cascades (discussed later) as a result of periodontal disease can then precipitate/exacerbate chronic diseases such as diabetes and cardiovascular disease (CVD) in the elderly.[21,25–27] Pena and colleagues[21] (2017) suggest that interaction of microbiota and aging of the immune system and motor systems contribute to exacerbation of chronic disease in the geriatric population. Over the past 2 decades, there has been a strong interest in the bidirectional relationship suggested earlier between systemic diseases and periodontitis in the geriatric population.[24,25] The bidirectionality is expressed through systemic disease that predisposes a person to periodontal disease. This periodontal-systemic connection is influenced by inflammatory mediators (interleukin-6; C-reactive protein), as well as endocrine deficiencies in insulin growth factor and dehydroepiandrosterone.[24,25] The resultant compromised immune system provides a breeding ground for infectious and opportunistic microbes that precipitate and exacerbate the chronic illnesses and chronic periodontitis that burden the elderly.[6,25,26]

Epidemiologic studies support valid evidence that periodontitis increases the risk of diabetes and CVD, both of which can serve as significant risk predictors for frailty.[27–30] Studies have shown that cohorts with diabetes mellitus are 2.8 times more likely to have periodontal disease and 4.2 times more likely to have alveolar bone loss compared with controls matched for age and sex.[25] Cronin[29] concluded that periodontal disease was a risk factor for CVD as well as osteoporosis among a community of older adults enrolled in a clinical trial over a 5-year period. The data also suggested that ethnicity was a significant risk predictor for osteoporosis and concomitant decline in periodontal status; it was greater in white people compared with African Americans.[25] Gender differences were also found and several studies suggested that CVD in women is not as significant as that seen in their male cohorts because of the effect of osteoporosis on dental disease (ie, less periodontitis because of earlier extractions and less caries).[26,30] As such, women may not reach the threshold of periodontal disease necessary for the vascular consequences and myocardial breakdown compared with their male cohorts.[30] Further studies are needed with larger cohorts to support this hypothesis.

Recent studies have focused on the relationship of periodontitis as a predisposing factor in dementia and Alzheimer disease.[6,28,31,32] This focus is not surprising because other studies have correlated the onset of neurodegenerative diseases with alterations in the ratio of several inflammatory mediators associated with periodontal disease, including C-reactive protein, tumor necrosis factors, and matrix metalloproteases.[28] Kamer and colleagues[31] suggested that oral diseases that alter inflammatory cascades influence the development or progression of Alzheimer disease and dementia by local and systemic inflammation that travel to the brain and cause vascular damage with subsequent neurodegeneration.[6] Chronic periodontitis and periapical lesions may also cause low-grade inflammation that can spread into the brain and secondarily provide a path for bacteria to penetrate the blood-brain barrier.[32] Causative bacteria for oral diseases, such as *Treponema denticola*, *Porphyromonas gingivalis*, and *Streptococcus mutans*, seem to have neuroinvasive properties.[32] Tiisanoja and colleagues[32] concluded that systemic inflammation can exert a burden on the CNS that may have the potential to alter cognitive function. Oral hygiene and good oral health may decrease the inflammatory burden, concomitant bacteremia, and susceptibility to dental caries, which may have the potential to prevent dementia and Alzheimer symptoms.[32] A complex balance of cofounding factors, such as biologically cognitive, psychological, and social interactions, may be significant contributors as well. However, interventional trials are still needed to support whether the so-called periosystemic connection precipitates/exacerbates dementia/Alzheimer disease, as well as other neurodegenerative disease sequelae. Further studies are needed to correlate mechanisms of altered inflammatory cascades in oral diseases and the development of neurodegenerative disorders.

Periodontitis and polypharmacy The impact of polypharmacy on periodontal disease according to Ciancio[2] can be separated into 4 main categories: (1) those affecting oral hygiene; (2) those affecting the ability to diagnose periodontitis; (3) those that affect gingival and oral mucosa; and (4) those affecting the alveolar bone.[2] In addition, the adverse effects of polypharmacy go beyond medicinal to include increased medical expenses, increased hospitalization, and mistakes in dosing of medicines in the elderly by the health care provider. Systemic illnesses being treated with polypharmacy can result in oral manifestations such as xerostomia and concomitant salivary gland dysfunction, the latter affecting periodontal health.[8,9] Groups of medications predisposing patients to xerostomia include cardiovascular (antihypertensive diuretics, angiotensin-converting enzyme inhibitors, and calcium channel blockers), antidepressants, anti-Parkinson medications, and antiallergy medications.[8,9,33] The effect of xerostomia predisposes pathologic invasion of bacteria and the excess plaque biofilm can cause caries, especially on root surfaces.

Medicinal agents such as ginger, fish oil, garlic, and ginseng can confound the diagnosis of gingivitis and periodontitis caused by anticoagulants, antiplatelet medications, nonsteroidal antiinflammatory drugs, aspirin, and herbal compounds.[10,33] Each can contribute to confusion with respect to causes of bleeding during the periodontal examination. Diseases of the oral mucosa, such as aphthous ulcers and lichenoid lesions, are often caused by antibiotics, antiseizure medications, and antipsychotic medications, which are often prescribed to the geriatric population. Other studies suggest that multiple medication regimens in elderly patients have the potential to affect clinical attachment levels and pocket depth.[33] The oral manifestations discussed earlier can impair health-related quality of life because of poor stability and mobility of removable prosthetic appliances causing speech and nutritional impairment. Natto and colleagues[33] suggest that clinical attachment level in the elderly may be associated with greater than 5 medications that are taken for chronic diseases, whereas other medications may decrease the risk of periodontal breakdown.

The effect of polypharmacy on alveolar bone is a topic that has gained much interest recently with the changes in treatment of osteoporosis and cancer therapies that are prolonging patients' lives. Medication-related osteonecrosis of the jaw, although an uncommon disease, is often of concern in patients who are exposed to bisphosphonates, antiresorptive medications, and antiangiogenic medications. Future studies are underway to discriminate whether drug combinations in varying numbers precipitate breakdown in the health of the geriatric periodontium (discussed later).

Treatment strategies: periodontal disease Oral hygiene in frail individuals, although poor, can be improved using an educational program or oral hygiene protocols administered by family members and skilled dental auxiliary/facility staff. A systematic review by Shanbhag and colleagues[34] (2012) suggests that nonsurgical debridement in the treatment of periodontitis provides moderate improvement in health-related quality of life among the elderly.[35] One of the major challenges for preventive care is to develop a plan for monitoring periodontal care because the basis for prevention is to diagnose disease at its earliest stages. Components for preventive strategies in the elderly with respect to periodontal disease are discussed next.

Plaque removal Mechanical plaque removal is a well-tested approach to decrease gingival inflammation and caries risk. Plaque retention in the elderly is often caused by gingival recession with root caries and large dental restorations. Poor diet also contributes to increased inflammation and concomitant gingival recession. The use of a soft tooth brush and the Bass technique allows minimal tooth abrasion. Patients with compromised manual dexterity from chronic diseases can be instructed with rotary brushing and specially designed toothbrushes that are easy to manipulate. Handles have been developed that are larger and easier to grasp if the handle of a regular toothbrush cannot be used.[1,35]

Mouth rinses The use of oral antimicrobial rinses is not new to oral health care. Okuda and colleagues[36] reviewed the use of Listerine as an antimicrobial that killed microbes in 30 seconds, many of which are significantly virulent (ie, *S mutans*,

Actinomyces viscosus, *Staphylococcus aureus*, *Candida albicans*, *Prevotella interme-dia*, and *P gingivalis*). There are an increasing number of elderly and medically compro-mised hosts who are potentially at risk for developing pneumonia because of silent aspiration of microbes in the oral cavity. As such, antimicrobial mouth rinse may be effective in preventing dental plaque accumulation when used in addition to the me-chanical control of plaque, because these patients tend to have difficulty in brushing teeth by themselves. The use of antimicrobial mouth rinse therefore has the potential to not only prevent bacterial pneumonia but also in improve patients' quality of life by preserving their oral health.[36] Chlorhexidine rinses have been well accepted for peri-odontal care and the treatment of plaque in the elderly.[1,34-36] The variety of therapeu-tic rinses now available are still beneficial to the hard and soft oral tissues, especially in the reduction of candidiasis and mucositis in patients who are undergoing chemotherapy.[1,34-36]

Tobacco use Numerous studies have supported the premise that smoking is a major factor associated with accelerated periodontal destruction.[35] Debate continues as to whether the progressive loss of periodontal support in later life is caused by excessive tobacco smoking in youth.[35] Several longitudinal studies suggest that 30 pack years is required to show an increased risk for severe periodontitis; however, several other risk predictors are required, such as low socioeconomic status, ethnic variation, and lack of regular visits to a dentist.[34,35] Other studies characterize a genetic link based on sin-gle nucleotide polymorphisms (SNPs) and smoking based on specific combinations of SNPs that must be present.[35] Studies are still underway and future directions include number of years of tobacco exposure, better genetic mapping, access to dental care, and coping mechanisms for stress.

Periodontal health and dental implants Systemic diseases, polypharmacy, and oral health imbalance can impede both the success of implant placement as well as their longevity. When older adults are compared with younger cohorts, implant survival seems constant over at least 3 to 5 years. However, bone loss over time seems sig-nificant in older patients.[35,37] A systematic review by Al-Fahd[37] concluded that dental implants in edentulous elderly patients are a predictable treatment option with minimal complications. However, practitioners must be cautious in their choice of patients because increased age is associated with increased risk for chronic disease. The latter can compromise the quantity and quality of bone and soft tissue required for implant survival and success. Further studies using randomized controlled trials and larger sample sizes are now underway to allow better prospective outcomes with respect to implant placement in the elderly.[37]

Although the literature with respect to periodontal therapy in the geriatric population is still under scrutiny, some consistencies remain. Gingival recession is a fact of aging and may be a sequela of periodontal pocketing earlier in life. An oral and maxillofacial geriatric syndrome is manifested by chronic illnesses and polypharmacy that impedes the periodontium's ability to heal. Significant challenges remain from the patients' perspective of oral maintenance and access to care. The practitioners' expectations for good oral hygiene depend on understanding how systemic diseases and their management affect the progression of periodontal disease.

Disorders in taste
Loss of taste in the geriatric population may result from physiologic changes in the cells initiating taste perception, a declining olfactory function, poor nutrition, certain diseases, medications, and inadequate dentition.[38-40] Alteration in the patient's perception of taste can significantly impede appetite, healthy food choices, and

health-related quality of life. Research has focused on food preferences and healthy nutrition in the elderly because of their declining perception of salty, bitter, and sour taste.[38–41] Studies in the detection and recognition of threshold levels of the 4 commonly tested tastes (sweet, salty, bitter, and sour) show modest age-related changes in healthy older people who take no medications. However, older adult cohorts with at least 1 medical condition and taking medications show a significant decline in taste perception.[39] As a whole, the preference seems to be for foods deficient in calcium, magnesium, iron, vitamin D, vitamin B_6, thiamin, retinol, and folic acid.[40] These deficiencies lend themselves to a subsequent shift to more unhealthy food choices and an increased risk of diet-related diseases such as obesity, cardiovascular dysfunction, and metabolic dysfunction, all of which potentiate adverse oral health in these patients.

Dysgeusia (altered sense of taste) is most often seen in the elderly as a result of chronic disease and polypharmacy, as well as the physiologic, psychosocial, and emotional stress that contribute to poor nutrition.[3,40] Dysgeusia is further potentiated by habits such as tobacco and alcohol use, both of which cause an alteration in salivary flow, with the resulting xerostomia potentially contributing to BMS and further loss of appetite (discussed elsewhere in relation to BMS). Toffannello and colleagues[41] compared loss of taste preferences in a cohort of hospitalized patients with the risk predictors of multimorbidity and polypharmacy with a healthy cohort matched for age. The ability to differentiate sour taste was significantly lower in hospitalized patients, as well as thresholds of sweet, bitter, and salty at diluted concentrations compared with other cohorts. The investigators concluded that elderly patients who are hospitalized and malnourished benefit from flavor-enhanced foods to increase their caloric intake and improve their health.

Treatment strategies: taste disorders The aging of the gustatory apparatus, as discussed earlier, and the multimorbidity of disease and its management with multiple medications become causative in clinical presentations of altered taste, loss of taste, metallic taste, and poor nutritional intake. As such, taste disorders are representative of an oral and maxillofacial geriatric syndrome. Taste disorders contribute to a vicious cycle of altered intake and a compromised nutritional status, which may in turn lead to further weakness and poor health outcomes contributing to frailty. Establishing treatment strategies to combat taste disorders in the elderly can therefore be challenging because of not only the multimorbidity of disease but also the polypharmacy administered. The latter contributes to a cascade of not only gustatory dysfunction but also weight loss, anorexia, muscle wasting, and malnutrition. Studies agree that although the need for medication is essential to combat systemic disease, taste perception can be reprogrammed so that the risk of malnutrition is reduced. Toffannello and colleagues,[41] in a cohort study, found that food choices, especially flavor-enhanced diets using artificial sweetener and monosodium glutamate, increased the elderly's perception of taste and diet preferences, increased salivary flow, increased grip strength, and decreased oral complaints. Future studies are underway to determine the relationship, if any, among physiologic, social, and psychological factors in the elderly's perception of taste and diet food choices.

Mastication/swallowing

Masticatory and swallowing disorders in the geriatric population are prevalent and together can be detrimental to everyday health and well-being. As patients age, mastication and swallowing serve as significant risk predictors for poor oral health and malnutrition. In addition, loss of teeth can serve as a good mortality predictor of elderly life impairment because of its direct influence on mastication and swallowing.[6,42,43] Prosthetic replacement of teeth can lead to adverse masticatory function if conditions such as palatal stomatitis or traumatic ulcers develop, and the outcome is worsened in the presence of poor oral hygiene and increased tobacco and alcohol use. In addition, the physiologic aging of mastication can be affected by socioeconomic status, degree of dependence on family support, and general state of health.[42,43] Chewing difficulties are more prevalent because of poor dentition, concomitant ill-fitting oral prostheses, and the increased incidence of chronic illnesses and neurodegenerative diseases that impede CNS control of gustatory function. Several studies have correlated tooth number with masticatory success in the elderly.[42,43] In patients with fewer than 21 teeth, there is a substantial alteration in choice of diet: a decrease in protein and an increase in carbohydrates and micronutrient consumption even if prosthetic rehabilitation is attempted.[42]

Dysphagia (disorders in swallowing) in the elderly is often associated with multimorbidity and polypharmacy, lack of saliva, and poor masticatory function, and can be considered as a geriatric syndrome.[44] Neuronal networks in the aging brain break down because of age-related physiologic changes associated with the biomechanics of swallowing, caused by neurologic diseases, gastrointestinal dysfunction, and/or tumors.[44–46] Various CNS illnesses, including Alzheimer disease, schizophrenia, and Parkinson disease, can contribute to a dyskinesia/dystonia of the musculature. Although there is no absolute prevalence rate for swallowing disorders, reported rates vary based on the anatomic location and type or stage of swallowing disorder (ie, oral, oropharyngeal, and esophageal).[43] The prevalence rate of oromandibular dystonia ranges from 0.52 to 30 per 100,000 in elderly patients based on meta-analyses.[45] **Box 3** lists causes of dysphagia in the elderly.

Long-term polypharmacy with sedatives, neuroleptics, anticholinergics, and opioids often leads to difficulty in swallowing caused by decreased salivary flow rate, as well as the quality of saliva secreted.[44] Drugs such as duloxetine, cetirizine, and amlodipine can cause tardive dyskinesia, which makes dental rehabilitation difficult and is detrimental to the overall health of patients. Specifically, these medications may elicit adverse head and neck motor events, including oromandibular dyskinesia

---

Box 3
Causes of dysphagia in the geriatric population

Oropharyngeal cause:
  Extrinsic: mechanical; goiter; cervical osteophytosis; neck cancer
  Intrinsic: postcricoid cartilage web; Zenker diverticulum
  Neurogenic: stroke; cerebral neoplasm; head injury; Alzheimer disease; Parkinson disease; multiple sclerosis, pseudobulbar palsy; medicine with CNS effects
  Neuromuscular junction: myasthenia gravis; Eaton-Lambert syndrome
  Muscular: myotonic dystrophy; polymyositis and dermatomyositis; hypothyroidism/hyperthyroidism; Cushing syndrome
  Abnormal relaxation of the upper esophageal sphincter: reflux esophagitis; medications with anticholinergic side effects

Esophageal:
  Intrinsic lesion: tumors: benign/malignant; webs and rings; strictures; foreign bodies
  Extrinsic: mediastinal tumor; aberrant subclavius; right atrial dilatation
  Neuromuscular (motility): achalasia; diffuse esophageal spasm; scleroderma; Chagas disease; diabetes mellitus; radiation esophagitis

Adapted from Lieu PK, Chong MS, Seshadri R. The impact of swallowing disorders in the elderly. Ann Acad Med Singapore 2001;30:148–54; with permission.

and dystonia. All of the adverse events mentioned earlier can result in aspiration, pneumonia, dehydration, malnutrition, and functional decline with an increased risk in morbidity and mortality.[46] There are several approaches in managing disorders of swallowing that can improve patients' nutrition and health-related quality of life (discussed later).

Treatment strategies: mastication and swallowing As described earlier, along with mastication, dysphagia is most often overlooked as a form of an oral geriatric syndrome that has the potential to exacerbate frailty. Treatment strategies begin with a proper work-up based on health history and clinical presentation because, in most cases, they are manifestations of chronic illness and polypharmacy (discussed earlier, and see **Box 3**). Patients often complain of food sticking in their throats, as well as problems with drinking fluids. A concomitant complaint of chest pain may suggest esophageal spasm and gastroesophageal reflux disease (GERD). Coughing is common, and patients may also have nasal regurgitation. Clinical testing of range of motion, laryngeal function, voice quality, and cranial nerves can help determine causes so that proper treatment can be rendered.[43,44] A positive gag reflex is common in 40% of the elderly and so it may be of little value in grading pharyngeal dysfunction.

Rehabilitation of patients who present with symptoms of dysphagia involves an interdisciplinary team effort. Speech therapists use numerous therapeutic approaches based on the cause of dysphagia presented. Patients who show this oral geriatric syndrome are often frail because of strokes, Parkinson disease, or dementia. Neurosensory stimulation, biofeedback modalities, endoscopy, and other physiologic techniques have had successful outcomes.[43–45] Although the neurologic deficits have cognitive symptoms, other approaches can help to overcome cognitive impairments (ie, diet modification, prosthetic devices, and surgical tracheostomy) (**Box 4**). Studies have also used pharmacologic management with nitrates, which improve oropharyngeal incompetence for stroke victims. In addition, chewing difficulties need to be assessed by both the dental practitioners and primary care physicians as part of a multidomain approach to treatment of geriatric syndromes other than those seen outside of the oral health arena. Oral health care providers play a critical role in maximizing masticatory function by supporting oral health maintenance and providing stable prosthetic replacement of missing teeth. With the appropriate work-up, these disorders can be managed to improve the health-related quality of life.

Box 4 Treatment options for dysphagia	
Condition	**Medical Management**
Achalasia	Soft diet; anticholinergics, calcium channel blockers, botulinum injections, myotomy
Diffuse esophageal spasm	Calcium channel blockers; nitrates; surgical dilatation; myotomy
Gastroesophageal reflux	H$_2$ blockers; proton pump inhibitors; domperidone; fundoplication
Infectious esophagitis	Antibiotics
Zenker diverticulum	Myotomy
Scleroderma	Antireflux treatment; medical management of scleroderma

Adapted from Lieu PK, Chong MS, Seshadri R. The impact of swallowing disorders in the elderly. Ann Acad Med Singapore 2001;30:148–54; with permission.

Burning mouth syndrome

BMS/glossodynia presents as burning sensations within the oral cavity (ie, tongue, lips, and oral mucosa) that are continuous and increase in intensity throughout the day. The epidemiology of BMS prevalence varies from 1% to 4.8% globally and although the BMS occurs in both men and women, more women are predisposed (6:1 female/male) to BMS during their perimenopausal to postmenopausal years.[47,48] The greatest frequency of BMS occurs on the anterior one-third of the tongue, followed by the gingiva and palate. Up to 50% of cases report concomitant xerostomia and dysgeusia, and the latter may be a result of a dysfunction of the sensory input to the tongue (ie, chorda tympani nerve).[47,48]

BMS is most often a diagnosis of exclusion, and several studies have classified it into 2 categories: (1) Primary/essential BMS, with an cause of central neuropathologic pathways; and (2) secondary BMS, arising as a result of local, systemic, or psychological factors.[47,48] BMS has been associated with fungal infections, geographic tongue, lichen planus, oral carcinomas, and microtrauma.[18,48] Infectious agents, such as *Streptococcus* species, can attach to the tooth surfaces and potentiate the growth of *Candida* spp, which provides an environment for opportunistic organisms to invade both hard and soft oral tissues. In addition, when *Candida* spp overgrow, they attach to the soft tissues such as tongue and mucosa, potentiating and exacerbating pseudomembranous cheilitis and angular cheilitis, which hinders the function of dental prosthetic rehabilitation.[9] Patients who have fissured tongues are especially at risk because of susceptibility to food trapping, inability to remove dead cells, and biofilm formation as a breeding ground for pathogenic microorganism, which further exacerbates poor wound healing from oral trauma.

Within the elderly population, BMS can manifest in a variety of systemic diseases (ie, GERD, diabetes, hypertension, and autoimmune diseases), and deficiencies in certain vitamins (ie, iron, vitamin B_{12}, and folic acid) can exacerbate BMS.[3,48] Multimorbidity and concomitant polypharmacy are critical risk factors that can precipitate/exacerbate BMS because both share common causal sequelae and pose significant challenges because most elderly with BMS present with systemic diseases and polypharmacy whose causes overlap.[47,48] Several studies have attempted to single out risk predictors for BMS in the geriatric population in the context of an oral and maxillofacial geriatric syndrome.[3,10] Pajukoski and colleagues[18] examined the prevalence of dry mouth and BMS in hospitalized versus outpatient elderly populations. Results suggested dry mouth and BMS did not differ between healthy and hospitalized patients except in patients with psychiatric diseases and number of medications used. Dentate status was associated with a decreased prevalence of BMS but not dry mouth in matched cohorts.[18] **Box 5** describes the symptoms of patients with BMS. Approaches for managing the symptoms of BMS can vary from topical agents to systemic medications (discussed later)

Treatment strategies: burning mouth syndrome BMS is a multifactorial disease and no single agent can result in a complete remission. As such, treatment planning should be specific for each patient because no single approach provides a gold standard for success. The multifactorial and complex causes of BMS are often associated with each oral dysfunction described earlier and necessitate both a systematic and interdisciplinary approach. Some investigators have coined the term primary BMS versus secondary BMS; an oral complaint caused by either a clinicopathologic entity or the result of a local/systemic pathologic state, respectively.[3,48] Studies have shown that management of BMS can be broadly classified by (1) topical medications; (2) systemic medications; and (3) behavioral therapy[12]

Box 5
Clinical presentation of patients with burning mouth syndrome

1. Pain can spread independently across all areas of the oral cavity

2. The pain can be spontaneous and spread

3. Pain does not occur when eating

4. Pain can worsen as the day progresses

5. Relief can occur from lozenges, candy, gum

6. Symptoms often associated with polypharmacy

7. Symptoms can continue over an extended period of time (ie, several months to years)

8. Pain sensitivity increases with spicy foods and drinks

9. Symptoms can increase during times of stress

10. Pharmacologic management with steroids, nonsteroidal antiinflammatory drugs, rinses are not effective to relieve pain

11. Dysgeusia, loss of taste, and metallic taste are some of the subjective complaints that are seen

12. Dry mouth often present

13. Mouth appears raw, rough, and patient complains of sticky symptoms

Adapted from Trang TH, Takenoshita M, Matsuoka H, et al. Current management strategies for the pain of elderly patients with burning mouth syndrome: a critical review. Biopsychosoc Med. 2019;13:1.

(**Box 6**). A therapeutic alliance is warranted for a supportive bridge toward a good patient-doctor relationship, because it is common for patients to show significant anxiety and fear about their symptoms.[48] Regardless of treatment strategy chosen, clinicians must be able to communicate with their patients because successful disease management cannot be achieved by only pharmacologic therapeutics. Favorable prognostic outcomes should be delineated and goals should be established so that patients feel motivated about therapy. Although there is no single cure in the treatment of BMS, both pharmacologic therapy and psychosocial support allow greater motivation and realistic expectations for relief of oral symptoms. Future directions include a more uniform definition with strict diagnostic criteria, as well as more definitive associations between BMS and systemic disorders. BMS strongly exemplifies the concept of an oral and maxillofacial geriatric syndrome in the arena of oral health care.

Geriatric oral and maxillofacial syndrome, frailty, and future directions This article applies the concept of the geriatric syndrome when evaluating 5 common oral and maxillofacial dysfunctions seen in the elderly patient population: xerostomia, the nexus of periodontal disease and systemic disease, disorders in taste, difficulties in mastication and swallowing, and BMS. The impact of multimorbidity and polypharmacy most often seen in the elderly can be confusing when these oral dysfunctions present to oral health care providers. Oral health status is further jeopardized by frailty, disability, care dependency, and limited access to professional oral health care. There is a necessity to evaluate the status of maxillofacial frailty and the geriatric syndrome in order to develop a diagnostic lens for better preventive and treatment modalities. The concept of frailty syndrome is especially relevant to vulnerable

---

Box 6
Medication therapeutics for pain management in patients with burning mouth syndrome

	Dosing
Topical Pain Management	
Capsaicin cream (0.025%)	3–4 times per day
Clonazepam	0.5 mg/d
Benzydamine hydrochloride (0.15%)	3 times per day
Systemic Medications	
Chlordiazepoxide	15–30 mg/d
Clonazepam	0.25-3 mg/d
Diazepam	2–5 mg/d
Amisulpride	50 mg/d
Paroxetine	20 mg/d
Sertraline	50–100 mg/d

Adapted from Scala A, Cheechi L, Montevecchi M, et al. Update on burning mouth syndrome: overview and patient management. Crit Rev Biol Med. 2003;14(4):286; with permission.

---

older patients with losses in 1 or more domains of function (ie, physical, psychological, and social function). Their adverse health outcomes may be exacerbated by poor oral health. The basic oral functions of mastication, speaking, swallowing, and intact salivary function all contribute to good physical and psychological health and are likely to deteriorate with frailty.

Providers must understand how to better integrate oral health care into general health care in order to improve the health status of this patient population both orally and systemically. Strategies to improve the oral health status of geriatric patients must begin by diagnosing the types of geriatric syndromes and risk of frailty in each patient (**Fig. 2**). Objective approaches to consider in the elderly include salivary flow rate measurements, oral mucosal pain testing, and tests for gustatory function. Subjective measurements include the Oral Health Impact Profile and the Geriatric Oral Health Assessment Index.[3,6] A well-focused oral health questionnaire that examines the degree of severity of each dysfunction can be crafted to aid in deciphering whether the complaints are related to a disease being treated or are de novo. Studies have hypothesized smartphone patient-generated health data platforms that can monitor oral and maxillofacial disorders so that elderly patients can be accurately examined and treated accordingly.[3,6] The Clinical Frailty Scale and Care Dependency Scale can enhance determination of the impact of frailty, care dependency, and disability on oral health maintenance so that appropriate treatment plans can be crafted and used as a baseline for successful outcomes.

The geriatric 5Ms (mind, mobility, medications, multicomplexity, and matters most) must also be considered because the principles of patient-centered care are paramount in successful treatment strategies. Oral health care providers are in a pivotal position to form a strong link in the interprofessional collaborative of geriatric health care by using the geriatric 5Ms. These elements already used by geriatric primary care, which include assessment of functional status, medication reviews, careful evaluation of risks and benefits of treatment, and assessment of goals of care and prognosis, must be part of the armamentarium of oral health care providers and their health teams. In oral health care, the 5Ms are essential to assessing and planning care for geriatric patients. Does the patient have the cognitive capacity to manage a prosthesis or follow a preventive regimen (mind)? Can the patient physically

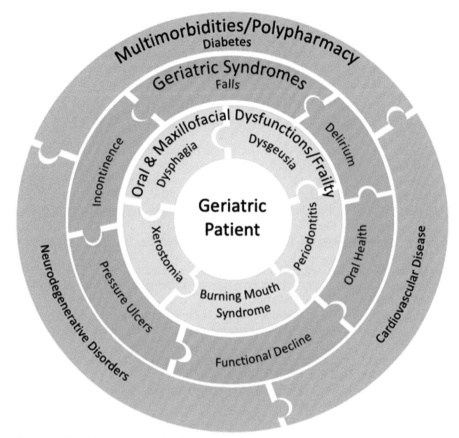

Fig. 2. Oral health care in the elderly is part of an oral and maxillofacial geriatric syndrome that is in a dynamic for overall health and well-being.

practice the mechanical biofilm removal required to maintain the dentition or physically gain access to dental services (mobility)? What contributes to oral geriatric syndromes and what can be mitigated (medications and multimorbidity)? What matters most to the patient?

Oral health care providers who are knowledgeable about the oral and maxillofacial geriatric syndromes must impart the concept to their colleagues so that recommendations for improvement in geriatric oral health can be tailored to individuals (see **Fig. 2**). Several types of approaches include implementing an oral health care guideline, domiciliary oral health care provisions with visiting dental hygienists, transforming oral health into medical oral health care, and revisiting the curricula of dental educational systems in order to develop oral physicians. Gaining a better understanding of oral, systemic, and social determinants of health and applying these effective methods of prevention and intervention will contribute to improving both the lifespan and health-related quality of life in the geriatric patient population. Providing appropriate oral health care to frail and medically compromised adults requires oral health care providers to be pivotal within an interprofessional collaborative to address the many diseases and conditions that can affect the oral and overall health of the geriatric patient population.

ACKNOWLEDGMENTS

The author thanks Lea Erickson, DDS, MSPH, Professor, Associate Dean of Student Affairs, University of Utah, School of Dentistry for reviewing the manuscript. The author thanks D4 student; Yuliya Petuckhova for the artwork in this manuscript.

REFERENCES

1. Razak PA, Richard KMJ, Thankachan RP, et al. Geriatric oral health: a review article. J Int Oral Health 2014;6(6):110–6.
2. Ciancio SG. Medications: a risk factor for periodontal disease diagnosis and treatment. J Periodontal 2005;76(Suppl):2061–5.
3. Nam Y, Kim N-H, Kho H-S. Geriatric oral and maxillofacial dysfunctions in the context of geriatric syndrome: review article. Oral Dis 2018;24:317–24.
4. Carlson C, Merel SE, Yukawa M. Geriatric syndromes and geriatric assessment for the generalist. Med Clin North Am 2015;99:263–79.
5. Chen X, Mao G, Leng SX. Frailty syndrome: an overview. Clin Interv Aging 2014; 9:433–41.
6. Gil-Montoya JA, Ferreira de Mello AL, Gonzalez-Moles MA, et al. Oral health in the elderly patient and its impact on general well-being: a nonsystematic review. Clinic Interv Aging 2015;10:461–7.
7. Inouye SK, Studenski S, Tinetti ME, et al. Geriatric syndromes: clinical, research, and policy implications of a core geriatric concept. J Am Geriatr Soc 2007;55: 780–91.
8. Abdulsamet T, Dogan MS, Fatih D, et al. Polypharmacy and oral health among the elderly. J Dent Oral Disord Ther 2016;4(1):1–5.
9. Singh ML, Papas A. Oral implications of polypharmacy in the elderly. Dent Clin North Am 2014;58:783–96.
10. Van der Putten GJ, de Baat C, Visschere LD, et al. Poor oral health, a potential new geriatric syndrome. Gerodontology 2014;31(Suppl 1):17–24.
11. Ouanounou A. Xerostomia in the geriatric patient: causes, oral manifestations and treatment. Compendium 2016;37(5):306–11.
12. Gutierrez-Valencia M, Izquierdo M, Cesari M, et al. the relationship between frailty and polypharmacy in older people: a systematic review. Br J Clin Pharmacol 2018;84:1432–44.
13. AGS Beers criteria for potentially inappropriate medication use in older adults. Available at: http://www.americangeriatrics.org/files/documents/beers/Printable BeersPocketCard.pdf. Accessed April 23, 2019.
14. Tinetti M, Huang A, Molnar F. The geriatric 5M's: a new way of communicating what we do. J Am Geriatr Soc 2017;65(9):2115.
15. Ghezzi EM. Developing pathways for oral care in elders: evidence-based interventions for dental caries prevention in dentate elders. Gerodontology 2014; 31(Suppl 1):31–6.
16. Nagler RM, Hershkovich O. Relationships between age, drugs, oral sensorial complaints and salivary profile. Arch Oral Biol 2005;50:7–16.
17. Vissink A, Spijkervet FK, Van Nieuw Amerongen A. Aging and saliva: a review of the literature. Spec Care Dentist 1996;16:95–103.
18. Pajukoski H, Meurmann JH, Odont D, et al. Prevalence of subjective dry mouth and burning mouth in hospitalized elderly patients and outpatients in relation to saliva, medication and systemic diseases. Oral Surg Oral Med Oral Pathol Oral Radiol Endod 2001;92:641–9.

19. Ship JA, Pillemer SR, Baum BJ. Xerostomia and the geriatric patient. J Am Geriatr Soc 2002;50:535–43.
20. NIDCR Caries risk in Seniors age 65 and over. Available at: https://www.nidcr.nih.gov/research/data-statistics/dental-caries/seniors. Accessed May, 2019.
21. Pena CG, Alvarez-Cisneros T, Quiroz-Baez R, et al. Microbiota and aging. A review and commentary. Arch Med Res 2017;48:681–9.
22. Tavares M, Lindfjeld CKA, San Martin L. Systemic diseases and oral health. Dent Clin North Am 2014;58(4):797–814.
23. Suresh R. Aging and periodontal disease. Prevention and treatment of age-related diseases. (the Netherlands): Springer; 2006. p. 193–200.
24. Lamster IB, Asadourian I, Del Carmen T, et al. The aging mouth: differentiating normal aging from disease. Periodontol 2000 2016;72:96–107.
25. Kim J, Amar S. Periodontal disease and systemic conditions: a bidirectional relationship. Odontology 2006;94(1):10–21.
26. Ozcaka O, Becerik S, Bicakci N, et al. Periodontal disease and systemic diseases in an older population. Arch Gerontol Geriatr 2014;59:474–9.
27. Meurman JH, Sanz M, Janket SJ. Oral health, atherosclerosis, and cardiovascular disease. Crit Rev Oral Biol Med 2004;15(6):403–13.
28. Persson GR. Dental geriatrics and periodontitis. Periodontol 2000 2017;74: 102–15.
29. Cronin A. Periodontal disease is a risk marker for coronary artery disease? Evid Based Dent 2009;10:22–5.
30. Desvarieux M, Schwahn C, V-Izke H, et al. Gender differences in the relationship between periodontal disease, tooth loss and atherosclerosis. Stroke 2004;35: 2029–35.
31. Kamer AR, Morse DE, Holm-Pedersen P, et al. Periodontal inflammation in relation to cognitive function in an older adult Danish population. J Alzheimers Dis 2012; 28(3):613–24.
32. Tiisanoja A, Syrjala A-M, Tertsonen M, et al. Oral diseases and inflammatory burden and Alzheimer's disease among subjects aged 75 or older. Spec Care Dentist 2019;39:158–65.
33. Natto ZS, Aladmawy M, Papas A. Is there a relationship between periodontal conditions and medications among the elderly? Ghana Med J 2016;50(1):9–15.
34. Shanbhag S, Dahaya M, Croucher R. The impact of periodontal therapy on oral health-related quality of life in adults: a systematic review. J Clin Periodontol 2012;39:725–35.
35. Persson GR. Rheumatoid arthritis and periodontitis – inflammatory and infectious connections. Review of the literature. J Oral Microbiol 2012;4:118–29.
36. Okuda K, Adachi M, Iijima K. The efficacy of antimicrobial mouth rinses in oral healthcare. Bull Tokyo Dent Coll 1998;39(1):7–14.
37. Al-Fahd AA. Old age alone may not be a risk factor for dental implant failure. J Evid Based Dent Pract 2016;16(3):176–8.
38. Sergi G, Bano G, Pizzato S, et al. Taste loss in the elderly: possible implications for dietary habits. Crit Rev Food Sci Nutr 2017;57(17):3684–9.
39. Schiffman SS. Taste and smell losses in normal aging and disease. JAMA 1997; 278:1357–62.
40. Pisano M, Hilas O. Zinc and taste disturbances in older adults: a review of the literature. Consult Pharm 2016;31:267–70.
41. Toffanello ED, Inelime EM, Imascopi A, et al. Taste loss in hospitalized multimorbid elderly subjects. Clin Interv Aging 2013;8:167–74.

42. Zhu Y, Hollis JH. Tooth loss and its association with dietary intake and diet quality in American adults. J Dent 2014;42(11):1428–35.
43. Lieu PK, Chong MS, Seshadri R. The impact of swallowing disorders in the elderly. Ann Acad Med Singapore 2001;30:148–54.
44. Baijens LWJ, Clave P, Cras P, et al. European society for Swallowing Disorders-European Union Geriatric Medicine society white paper: oropharyngeal dysphagia as a geriatric syndrome. Clin Interv Aging 2016;11:1403–28.
45. Sokoloff LG, Pavlakovic R. Neuroleptic-induced dysphagia. Dysphagia 1997;12:177–9.
46. Steeves TD, Day L, Dykeman J, et al. The prevalence of primary dystonia: a systematic review and meta-analysis. Mov Disord 2012;27:1789–96.
47. Trang TH, Takenoshita M, Matsuoka H, et al. Current management strategies for the pain of elderly patients with burning mouth syndrome: a critical review. Biopsychosoc Med 2019;13:1.
48. Scala A, Cheechi L, Montevecchi M, et al. update on burning mouth syndrome: overview and patient management. Crit Rev Oral Biol Med 2003;14:275–91.

Pediatric Oral Diseases

Sumitra S. Golikeri, DMD*, Jessica Grenfell, DDS, David Kim, DDS, Christopher Pae, DDS

KEYWORDS

- Pediatric dentistry • Oral diseases of the newborn • Measles • Herpes simplex virus
- Pediatric oral pathology

KEY POINTS

- This article educates dentists on some of the more common oral diseases seen in pediatric patients.
- This article reviews diseases that are easily overlooked by practitioners.
- This article provides guidance on possible treatment modalities for pediatric oral diseases.

INTRODUCTION

Dental caries, periodontal disease (gingivitis and periodontitis), malocclusions, and traumatic injuries of the teeth are frequent dental concerns from pediatric population. Whereas benign epithelial or soft tissue pathologies, lesions secondary to trauma, and oral signs and symptoms in systemic diseases are prevalent pathologies occurring in the oral tissues, malignant lesions in the pediatric age group are rare. The concern is that most oral pathologies correlate with definable age groups and their presentations may have an impact on the growth and development of oral structures. Jones and Franklin analyzed data on archived oral pathology specimens over a 30-year period and concluded that 10% of specimens were from children less than 16 years of age, many of them were benign, and only 1% of cases were malignant lesions.[1] Oral lesions presenting in the pediatric population do not generally require extensive surgical intervention because most are benign growths. Odontogenic tumors are relatively rare in the pediatric age group, except for adenomatoid odontogenic tumor and ameloblastoma. Ameloblastoma is discussed in Arvind Babu Rajendra Santosh and Orrett E. Ogle's article, "Odontogenic Tumors," in this issue. This article discusses the causes, clinical description, and treatment of common oral lesions in pediatric population (**Box 1**).

HYPERDONTIA

Hyperdontia is a dental developmental anomaly that causes patients to have an excess number of teeth. This is more commonly known as supernumerary teeth.

Disclosure Statement: The authors have nothing to disclose.
Woodhull Medical and Mental Health Center, 760 Broadway, Brooklyn, NY 11206, USA
* Corresponding author.
E-mail address: Sumitra.Golikeri@nychhc.org

Box 1
Pediatric oral lesions
Hyperdontia
Hypodontia
Measles
Gingival cyst of the newborn
Epstein's pearl
Bohn's nodules
Natal and neonatal teeth
Eruption cyst (eruption hematoma)
Epidermoid cyst
Dermoid cyst
Oropharyngeal candidiasis
Ankyloglossia
Parulis
Herpes simplex virus infection

These extra teeth can be classified in 2 different ways: supplemental or rudimentary. Usually, supernumerary teeth will present with normal morphology, which classifies them as supplemental. Rudimentary hyperdontia are when teeth differ from normal morphology and have conical, tuberculate, or molariform structures.[2]

Frequency and Prevalence

Supernumerary teeth are most commonly seen in the anterior maxilla of permanent dentition. A standard example of hyperdontia is the mesiodens, which occurs when a supernumerary tooth presents in between the central incisors (**Fig. 1**).[3] Males are more likely to display some form of hyperdontia than females.[2]

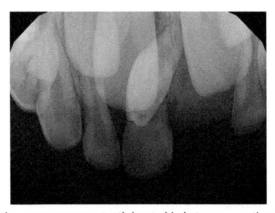

Fig. 1. Hyperdontia – supernumerary tooth located in between erupting teeth #8 and #9.

Etiology and Genetics

The exact process and genetics of hyperdontia is not well-understood. However, hyperdontia is often associated with a number of syndromes and conditions, such as (but not limited to) Apert syndrome, cleidocranial dysplasia, Gardner syndrome, and Crouzon syndrome.[2]

Treatment and Management

Management of supernumerary teeth differs based on severity. In many cases, hyperdontia may lead to crowding, impaction, root resorption, periodontal disease, and increased susceptibility to caries. Frequently, the recommended treatment is extraction to prevent future complications.[3]

HYPODONTIA, OLIGODONTIA, AND ANODONTIA

Hypodontia, oligodontia, and anodontia are developmental anomalies that indicate the absence of teeth with the difference being in the number of teeth missing. Hypodontia is used to classify the absence of fewer than 6 teeth, oligodontia for the absence of 6 or more teeth, and anodontia when all the teeth are missing.[4] Some of the more common terms that practitioners use to describe these conditions are tooth agenesis or congenitally missing teeth. Congenitally missing teeth is a result of disturbances during the early stages of development and is suggested as a mild dysplastic expression of the ectoderm (**Fig. 2**).[5]

Frequency and Relevance

Tooth agenesis in the deciduous dentition, although a rare finding, is often associated with maxillary lateral incisors or mandibular central incisors. Excluding third molars, the mandibular second premolar and the maxillary lateral incisors are the most commonly affected teeth in permanent dentition.[2] However, when a missing tooth is observed in the primary dentition, then an associated permanent tooth is likely to be absent.

Patients with hypodontia may have an association with other dental or oral anomalies. Hypodontia can be associated with syndromic conditions, such as (but not limited to) ectodermal dysplasia, Crouzon syndrome, Williams syndrome, achondroplasia, orofaciodigital syndrome I, and Rieger syndrome.[2] Furthermore, patients with hypodontia can have issues with other ectodermal organs, including salivary glands, skin, and sweat glands.

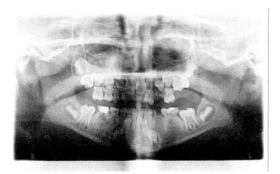

Fig. 2. Congenitally missing teeth is a result of disturbances during the early stages of development and is suggested as a mild dysplastic expression of the ectoderm.

Etiology and Genetics

Similar to hyperdontia, hypodontia has unclear genetic mechanisms. It is speculated that hypodontia may occur owing to tooth induction issues, lamina abnormalities, and obstructions during lamina formation.[4] Genetic mutations that could play a role in hypodontia are the PAX9, MSX1, and AXIN2 genes.[2]

Treatment and Management

Timing is a priority in the management of missing teeth in the pediatric population. A multidisciplinary approach is required and coordination of treatment with the pedodontist plays an important role in the management of missing teeth in a pediatric population with the aim to preserve space for permanent dentition. Interceptive and preventive orthodontic procedures assist in space management. Restoration with adhesive bridges or dentures are treatment options, depending on the severity of the missing teeth.

MEASLES
Frequency and Prevalence

In 2000, the United States reported that measles has been eliminated. However, a resurgence of measles has occurred as of early 2019 with more than 600 reported cases and rising.[6] Transmission occurs through respiratory droplets, aerosols, and close contact. The main reservoir of measles are humans and nonhuman primates.[7]

Etiology

Measles is caused by the single-stranded, negative-sense RNA virus called rubeola. It is a highly contagious disease where management levels vary based on each country's immunization rates. The primary receptor for the measles virus is CD150 expressed on various lymphocytes and nectin-4 on epithelial cells. Owing to the mode of transmission for the virus, the respiratory tract is usually the first place of infection. The lymphocytes that are affected eventually reach lymphoid tissues where replication occurs and dissemination follows.[8]

Description

Symptoms of measles usually begin with a rising fever associated with the 3 Cs: cough, coryza, and conjunctivitis. These symptoms gradually intensify for 2 to 4 days before a maculopapular rash can be seen. The onset of the maculopapular rash typically begins in the head and neck region and can spread generally throughout the body. Preceding the initial rash appearance, small raised white lesions called Koplik spots may be seen on the buccal mucosa and soft palate.[9] Koplik spots are not visible in all cases, but are pathognomonic for measles infection. Owing to the primary target of rubeola being lymphocytes, measles may even cause immunosuppression in individuals. This condition leads to secondary bacterial infections and increases the risk of morbidity.[7]

Measles may cause a variety of complications in different organ systems depending on the severity. The most commonly affected organ systems are the respiratory, gastrointestinal, and ocular tracts. Pneumonia can occur owing to the measles infection itself or from secondary infection from induced immunosuppression. In already immunocompromised patients, progressive pneumonia is the leading cause of death from measles. Otitis media and laryngotracheobronchitis (measles croup) are other respiratory symptoms that practitioners should be aware of when suspecting measles infection. Diarrhea is the primary gastrointestinal symptom and may cause severe dehydration. As mentioned, conjunctivitis is frequently seen in patients with measles and usually heals without long-term effects. In malnourished or immunocompromised patients, conjunctivitis and keratitis can lead to severe consequences such as blindness.[9]

Treatment and Management

Measles vaccination is the key method of prevention in countries that are able to attain high immunization rates. Patients who present with rising fever and a maculopapular rash should be suspected for measles infection. Confirmatory diagnosis is done through plaque reduction neutralization assay to detect for measles-specific antibodies. There are no specific or targeted methods to eliminate measles infection. Thus, supportive therapy is the primary method of treatment. Patients are usually given vitamin A supplements and antibiotic therapy to manage nutritive levels and secondary infection risks.[7]

GINGIVAL CYST OF THE NEWBORN (DENTAL LAMINAR CYSTS)
Frequency and Prevalence

Gingival cyst of the newborn occurs in approximately 13% of infants. They are rarely seen after 3 months of age.[10]

Etiology and Genetics

Dental laminar fragments can remain in the alveolar mucosa after tooth formation. These fragments then proliferate into small keratinized cysts.

Description

Gingival cyst of the newborn occurs on alveolar ridges of newborns and young infants. They are white or yellow cystic lesions, measuring approximately 2 to 3 mm in diameter. They are asymptomatic and do not cause the newborn any discomfort. They can be subdivided into palatal or alveolar depending on location. Radiographs are not indicated for these lesions.

Treatment and Management

These lesions are usually self-limiting and only require observation. If the cysts persist or interfere with feeding, they can be surgically opened to drain.

EPSTEIN'S PEARL
Frequency and Prevalence

Epstein's pearls occur in 60% to 85% of newborns.[11]

Etiology and Genetics

These keratin-filled cysts are found at the juncture of the hard and soft palates. They are possibly derived from epithelial remnants that arise during the formation of minor palatal salivary glands.

Description

Epstein's pearls are small white-yellow cysts near the mid-palatine raphe. They are usually found in clusters of 2 to 6 lesions but can occur as isolated lesions. Their size ranges from 1 to 4 mm. Radiographs are not indicated for these lesions.

Treatment and Management

These lesions are self-limiting and do not require treatment.

BOHN'S NODULE
Frequency and Prevalence

Bohn's nodules occur in 65% to 85% of neonates.

Etiology and Genetics

Bohn's nodules are remnants of mucous gland tissue.

Description

Bohn's nodules are white lesions found on the buccal and lingual aspects of the dental ridges. They are usually found in clusters of 2 to 6 lesions and are less than 3 mm in diameter. Radiographs are not indicated for these lesions.

Treatment and Management

Bohn's nodules are self-limiting and do not require treatment.

NATAL AND NEONATAL TEETH
Frequency and Prevalence

The primary difference between neonatal and natal teeth is timing of eruption (**Fig. 3**). Neonatal teeth erupt during the first 30 days of life, whereas natal teeth are present during birth. Natal teeth occur in 1 in 2000 to 3000 live births annually.[12]

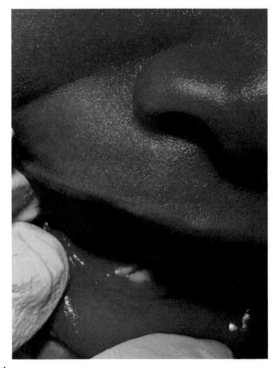

Fig. 3. Natal teeth.

Etiology and Genetics

Natal and neonatal teeth are most frequently a premature eruption of deciduous mandibular central incisors. Fewer than 10% of natal teeth are supernumerary teeth.

Description

Natal and neonatal teeth most commonly present in pairs in the anterior mandible. They can occur as normal teeth, or can be small with a yellowish color owing to poor enamel calcification. They can be blunt and conical, with poor root formation. Sublingual ulceration can be present owing to sharp edges of the natal teeth. Repeated traumatic ulceration is known as Riga-Fede disease. Radiographs should be taken to determine whether the tooth is supernumerary or a prematurely erupted deciduous tooth.

Treatment and Management

If the teeth are supernumerary, excessively mobile, or interfere with feeding, extraction is indicated. If they are not mobile and do not interfered with feeding, no treatment is necessary.

ERUPTION CYST (ERUPTION HEMATOMA)
Frequency and Prevalence

The frequency and prevalence of eruption cyst (eruption hematoma) is unknown.[13]

Etiology and Genetics

Eruption cysts occur owing to an accumulation of fluid in the follicular space once the tooth has erupted over alveolar bone.

Description

Clinically, eruptions cysts present as a swelling above an erupting tooth. They may be a normal mucosal color or purple to blue owing to trauma-induced bleeding into cystic space from mastication. Eruption cysts most often involves first permanent molars and maxillary incisors. They are soft or fluctuant to palpation. Radiographs are not indicated for these lesions.

Treatment and Management

No treatment is required. These lesions resolve with eruption of tooth. If they are symptomatic or interfering with the ability to eat, they can be opened surgically.

EPIDERMOID CYSTS (INFUNDIBULAR CYST, EPIDERMAL INCLUSION CYST)
Frequency and Prevalence

Epidermoid cysts are one of the most common cysts of the skin.[14]

Etiology and Genetics

Epidermoid cysts are likely to occur after inflammation of a hair follicle. The cavity of the cyst is lined with stratified squamous epithelium with a granular layer, abundant keratin, and no adnexal structures on the cyst cell wall.

Description

Epidermoid cysts are subcutaneous nodules that are firm to palpation. They are common on the face in the teenage cohort. Radiographs not indicated for these lesions.

Treatment and Management

Excision is the definitive treatment for an epidermoid cysts. Recurrence is rare.

DERMOID CYST
Frequency and Prevalence

Dermoid cyst is one of the most common cysts of the head and neck region.[15]

Etiology and Genetics

Dermoid cysts are developmental cysts, similar to a teratoma in that it contains specialized developmental structures. They are histologically similar to skin, with adnexal structures such as sebaceous glands, hair follicles, and sweat glands found in the cystic walls.

Description

Dermoid cysts can occur anywhere on the body, but intraorally are most frequently found on the floor of the mouth. If a dermoid cyst occurs above the mylohyoid muscle, it causes elevation of the tongue; if it occurs below the mylohyoid muscle, it causes submandibular swelling. The cyst feels rubbery or doughy to palpation. Radiographs are not indicated for this lesion.

Treatment and Management

Surgical excision is the definitive treatment. Recurrence is rare.

OROPHARYNGEAL CANDIDIASIS
Frequency and Prevalence

Roughly 5% to 7% of infants develop oropharyngeal candidiasis.[16]

Etiology and Genetics

Candidiasis is an opportunistic infection commonly caused by Candida albicans. Oral candidiasis is seen in children with weakened immune systems caused by illnesses or medications. The listed causes of oral candidiasis in adult are antibiotics, immunodeficiency, xerostomia, diabetes mellitus, oral appliances, and/or smoking. Few cases of pediatric oral candidiasis are of idiopathic origin.[16]

Clinical Description

Candidiasis can have a pseudomembranous or erythematous appearance. The pseudomembranous appears as white to yellow plaques that can be wiped off to reveal underlying erythematous mucosa. The erythematous form presents as a red macule(s) on the palate and dorsum of the tongue. No radiographs are indicated for this lesion.

Treatment and Management

Candidiasis is treated with topical antifungal agents (clotrimazole suspension, nystatin oral suspension), or systemic antifungals (fluconazole, ketoconazole).

ANKYLOGLOSSIA (TONGUE TIE)
Frequency and Prevalence

Ankyloglossia, commonly called tongue tie, is estimated to occur in 4% of newborns.[17]

Etiology and Genetics

Currently, the cause of ankyglossia is unknown. Some studies of ankyloglossia suggest an X-linked inheritance as a possible genetic cause.

Description

Clinically, ankyloglossia presents as a restrictive lingual frenum that limits normal tongue mobility. If this condition leads to difficulty with nursing or speaking, a frenectomy may be performed to relieve the attachment. Radiographs are not indicated for this condition.

Treatment and Management

If necessary, ankyloglossia can be relieved with a simple surgical frenectomy.

PARULIS
Frequency and Prevalence

Parulis (intraoral dental sinus) are extremely common because they are the result of chronic dental infection. Because they are a symptom of more widespread disease, data are not available of the prevalence of parulis.

Description

A parulis is a common gingival lesion composed of inflamed granulation tissue that results from chronic periapical dental abscesses (**Fig. 4**). Parulis are seen periapical to the nonvital tooth and present as an inflamed yellow swelling.[18] Parulis appear on radiographs as unilocular radiolucent lesions extending from the apex of a tooth. Sometimes the parulis tract may be located little away from the tooth, and in such cases tooth associated with parulis can be identified by inserting gutta-percha into the abscess tract and periapical radiograph should be taken to identify the offending tooth.

Etiology and Genetics

Parulis result from dental abscesses that have created a communication to the oral cavity by way of a fistula. A parulis can be identified during a dental examination. Parulis can be symptomatic but often times are not. A draining parulis is often painless. To differentiate a parulis from other lesions, the source of the infection must be identified.[18]

Radiographically, a parulis is a radiolucency at the apex of a tooth.

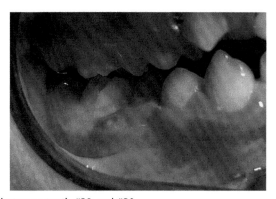

Fig. 4. Parulis in between teeth #29 and #30.

Treatment and Management

Treatment consists of removing the root cause of the infection. This generally means treating the infected tooth with either an extraction or endodontic treatment. A discussion between the patient and provider determines what course of treatment is most appropriate. Once the infected tooth is dealt with, the parulis resolves on its own.[19,20]

HERPES SIMPLEX VIRUS INFECTIONS
Frequency and Genetics

Herpes simplex virus (HSV) infections are extremely common. Ninety percent of all people are infected with some form of HSV, with the vast majority living without symptoms. HSV is classified into 2 types: HSV type 1 (HSV-1) and HSV type 2 (HSV-2). HSV-1 is the oral variant and HSV-2 is the genital variant, although each can occur throughout the body (CDC Fact Sheet 2014).

Description

The initial presentation of symptoms from HSV is called primary herpetic gingivostomatitis. This initial bout of symptoms is more severe than future recurrences. Patients can experience a myriad of systemic symptoms, including fever, an inability to eat, irritability, lymphadenopathy, malaise, and headache. Oral and perioral lesions present as small inflamed vesicles that rupture into ulcers with erythematous borders. Gingivitis also is present and causes bleeding and swelling of the gingiva. This combination of symptoms is quite debilitating and can make feeding very difficult for young patients. Dehydration and subsequent hypovolemic shock is of great concern for patients who are experiencing primary herpetic gingivostomatitis. Monitoring patients for dehydration is of utmost importance. Subsequent recurrences are not nearly as severe in presentation, usually presenting as vesicles on the lips or more rarely in the throat or mouth. Recurrences can be triggered by a variety of causes, including sunlight, stress, fever, oral trauma, and dental work to name a few. Most patients can anticipate a recurrence. Prodromal symptoms can occur for a few hours to a few days before vesicles can be seen clinically. Early treatment during this prodromal period can prevent and shorten a recurrence.[22]

Etiology and Genetics

HSV is spread by direct contact with either an active lesion or the bodily fluid of an infected person. Some examples of bodily fluids that can cause the contraction of HSV are infected saliva, vaginal fluid, seminal fluid, and the fluid found within herpetic blisters. HSV enters the body through breaks in the skin and the mucous membranes in the mouth or genital areas. Spread by asymptomatic carriers occurs most frequently during the first 12 months after initial infection but can also occur for a week leading up to a breakout and for the week after.[21]

Treatment and Management

There is no cure for HSV, and treatment is largely palliative. Treatment and management of HSV varies depending on whether the patient presents with primary herpetic gingivostomatitis or a recurrent herpes outbreak. Both types of outbreaks are self-limiting. Primary herpetic gingivostomatitis will self-resolve in 7 to 14 days and a recurrent outbreak will self-resolve in 5 to 10 days. Primary herpetic gingivostomatitis requires maintenance of whatever systemic symptoms occur, fluids for dehydration, antipyretics for fever, and pain medications for body aches. Cool, bland foods are also advised owing to pain from inflamed and ulcerated soft tissue present in the mouth. Oral acyclovir can be prescribed for immunocompetent patients with a more aggressive and prolonged presentation. Intravenous acyclovir is only used for severely immunocompromised patients. Topical anesthetics should be avoided because there is a risk of overdose and little added benefit from their use. A recurrent outbreak does not require any treatment once vesicles are present. However, various topical and oral antiviral medications can be used to shorten the duration of the outbreak. The use of oral medications during the prodromal stage has been shown to prevent and shorten outbreaks.[22]

SUMMARY

This article emphasized clinical and management aspects of pediatric oral pathologies found in routine general dental practice. It is imperative for general dentists to be aware of pediatric oral lesions and diseases that may influence the course of treatment for these patients. In many of these cases, the patient could be suffering from infection, pain, and severe spacing or occlusion issues. Treatment modalities of pediatric oral pathology include both medical and minimal surgical intervention.

REFERENCES

1. Jones AV, Franklin CD. An analysis of oral and maxillofacial pathology found in children over a 30-year period. Available at: https://onlinelibrary.wiley.com/doi/full/10.1111/j.1365-263X.2006.00683.x.
2. Dummett CO, Thikkurissy S. Abnormalities of the developing dentition. In: Nowak AJ, Casamassimo PS, editors. The handbook of pediatric dentistry. 5th edition. Chicago: American Academy of Pediatric Dentistry; 2018.
3. Parolia A, Kundabala M, Dahal M, et al. Management of supernumerary teeth. 2011. Available at: https://www.ncbi.nlm.nih.gov/pmc/articles/PMC3198547/. Accessed May 05, 2019.
4. Al-Ani AH, Antoun JS, Thomson WM, et al. Hypodontia: an update on its etiology, classification, and clinical management. Biomed Res Int 2017;2017:9378325.
5. Galluccio G, Pilotto A. Genetics of dental agenesis: anterior and posterior area of the arch. Eur Arch Paediatr Dent 2008;9:41–5.
6. CDC Media Statement: measles cases in the U.S. are highest since measles was eliminated in 2000 | CDC Online Newsroom | CDC. 2019. Available at: https://www.cdc.gov/media/releases/2019/s0424-highest-measles-cases-since-elimination.html. Accessed May 04, 2019.
7. Kondamudi NP. Measles. 2019. Available at: https://www.ncbi.nlm.nih.gov/books/NBK448068/. Accessed May 03, 2019.
8. Laksono BM, De Vries RD, McQuaid S, et al. Measles virus host invasion and pathogenesis. 2016. Available at: https://www.ncbi.nlm.nih.gov/pmc/articles/PMC4997572/. Accessed May 07, 2019.
9. Perry T,R, Halsey A,N. Clinical significance of measles: a review. 2004. Available at: https://academic.oup.com/jid/article/189/Supplement_1/S4/823958. Accessed May 03, 2019.
10. Singh RK, Kumar R, Pandey RK, et al. Dental lamina cysts in a newborn infant. BMJ Case Rep 2012;2012 [pii:bcr2012007061].
11. Diaz de Ortiz LE, Mendez MD. Epstein pearls. In: StatPearls. Treasure Island (FL): StatPearls Publishing; 2019. Available at: https://www.ncbi.nlm.nih.gov/books/NBK493177/.
12. Leung AK, Robson WLM. Natal teeth: a review. J Natl Med Assoc 2006;98(2):226.

13. Şen-Tunç E, Açikel H, Şaroğlu-Sönmez I, et al. Eruption cysts: a series of 66 cases with clinical features. Med Oral Patol Oral Cir Bucal 2017;22(2):e228.
14. Zito PM, Scharf R. Cyst, epidermoid (Sebaceous Cyst). In: StatPearls. Treasure Island (FL): StatPearls Publishing; 2019. Available at: https://www.ncbi.nlm.nih.gov/books/NBK499974/.
15. Al-Khateeb TH, Al-Masri NM, Al-Zoubi F. Cutaneous cysts of the head and neck. J Oral Maxillofac Surg 2009;67(1):52–7.
16. Singh A, Verma R, Murari A, et al. Oral candidiasis: an overview. J Oral Maxillofac Pathol 2014;18(Suppl 1):S81–5.
17. Becker S, Mendez MD. Ankyloglossia. In: StatPearls. Treasure Island (FL): StatPearls Publishing; 2019.
18. Glick M. Burket's oral medicine. 12th edition. People's medical publishing house; 2015. 147-172, 175-188, 236-237.
19. Eversole LR. Clinical outline of oral pathology: diagnosis and treatment. PMPH-USA; 2001.
20. "Genital Herpes – CDC Fact Sheet". cdc.gov. December 8, 2014. Archived from the original on 31 December 2014.
21. CDC fact sheet – herpes. Available at: https://www.cdc.gov/std/herpes/stdfact-herpes-detailed.htm. Accessed May 04, 2019.
22. M. Kaye, Kenneth. "Herpes Simplex Virus (HSV) Infections". MSD Manuals.

Referral and Management Considerations for a Biopsy
Why Choose the Oral and Maxillofacial Surgeon

Keith H. Kaner, DDS[a,b,*]

KEYWORDS

- Oral cancer • Odontogenic neoplasms • OMS office practice • Biopsy
- Anesthesia surgical treatment planning

KEY POINTS

- Current trends in the diagnosis and treatment of oropharyngeal neoplasms.
- Coordinating comprehensive anesthesia and surgical treatment planning.
- Choosing an oral and maxillofacial surgeon based on training for place of service (office, outpatient, inpatient).
- Coordinating benefits for a combined dental and medical treatment plan.

GENERAL PATIENT EVALUATION

Patients referred to the oral and maxillofacial surgeon (OMS) are divided into the pediatric and adult categories for purposes of discussing a general overview of incidence and prevalence of disease. Children referred by pediatricians typically require care that can be assessed by the pediatric dentist, general dentist, or in some cases directly by the OMS. In contrast, many adult patient referrals may come from the general dentist, dental specialist (periodontist, endodontist, orthodontist), or a medical provider such as the primary care physician, nurse practitioner, or a medical specialist such as an otolaryngologist, ophthalmologist, neurologist, and dermatologist. The training and education of the OMS allows for the formulation of a focused and coordinated plan to recognize, assess, and manage the pathology and needs of the patient.

AERODIGESTIVE LESION GENERAL CONSIDERATIONS

Oropharyngeal neoplasia can be described primarily as benign or malignant. They can arise as a primary lesion related to disorders of amelogenesis, odontogenesis,

Disclosure Statement: The author has no financial or commercial interests to disclose.
[a] Private Practice, 9250 Glades Road Suite 207, Boca Raton, FL 33434, USA; [b] Department of Oral and Maxillofacial Surgery, Nova Southeastern University, College of Dental Medicine, 3301 College Avenue, Ft Lauderdale, FL 33314, USA
* Private Practice, 9250 Glades Road Suite 207, Boca Raton, FL 33434.
E-mail address: keithkaner@kaneroms.com

inflammatory, developmental, and metastatic disease. Their biologic behavior of local and distant destruction has been well-documented in the medical literature.

The epidemiology of neoplasia has been followed by the American Cancer Society for decades. The statistical analysis of the rate of cancer is a complex formula. Oral cancer malignancy survival rates are generally reported in developed countries approximating a 5-year survival rate of 50%.[1] Delays in diagnosis and subsequent treatment can contribute to advanced stage tumors to be encountered. Treatment modalities for oral cancer include combinations of surgical, chemotherapeutic and radiotherapy. Traditional medical and radiation oncology practice uses a team approach to coordinate surgical intervention as indicated. Comorbid conditions can ultimately guide the care of the patient in a palliative nature.

Odontogenic oral cavity lesions can be categorized based on the rates of incidence and prevalence.[2] Pediatric or growing individuals and adults have differing trends or patterns of disease. Typically, an odontogenic neoplastic lesion is diagnosed radiographically by a dentist (**Box 1**). In addition to radiographic investigation, a soft tissue incision or excision biopsy allows for a histopathologic examination and diagnosis. Odontogenic malignancy is exceedingly rare and often complex and confusing. Odontogenic benign lesions are more common and can also create confusion related to differentiation between a hamartoma or a true neoplasm.

Nonodontogenic oral cavity lesions, which include inflammatory, developmental, and neoplastic lesions, can also be categorized into generally accepted rates of incidence and prevalence and have specific biologic behavior.[3] These lesions can be discovered and diagnosed by dentists and physicians alike (**Table 1**).

DEMOGRAPHICS OF HEALTH CARE AND ORAL PHARYNGEAL CANCER

A review of the 2017 US census statistics estimate the current civilian population to be roughly 320,775,000. Population growth from 2009 to 2017 rate was roughly 1%. Health insurance coverage analysis of these statistical demographics 2009 to 2017 demonstrates a decrease in the uninsured health care rate of 91% to 85%. In 2009, roughly 45 million individuals were uninsured in contrast with 2017, where it is estimated that 28 million individuals were uninsured.[4] A review of these statistics presents a general numerical consideration to access for health care. Access to health care can be further discussed with regard to limitations, such as geographic distances, wait time to office visits, coordination in benefits, and primary care considerations.

Statistical analysis of oral pharyngeal cancer shows the incidence and prevalence to account for 3% of all cancers. The oral cancer locations include the lip, tongue, salivary glands and other sites in the mouth; whereas pharyngeal cancer includes the nasopharynx, oropharynx and hypopharynx. The overwhelming majority of cancers are squamous neoplasms, accounting for more than 90% in total.[5,6]

Early detection of oral pharyngeal cancer presents a dilemma to the general population. The choice of who is the appropriate health care provider to assess the oral

---

Box 1
Odontogenic neoplasms

Child
   Odontoma, ameloblastoma, ameloblastic fibroma, cementoma, odontogenic myxoma

Adult
   Ameloblastoma, calcifying odontogenic cysts/tumors, cementoma, odontogenic myxoma

Table 1 Nonodontogenic oropharyngeal neoplasms		
	Benign	**Malignant**
Child		
Mucosal	Traumatic fibroma, papilloma	Rhabdomyosarcoma, squamous cell carcinoma
Salivary	Vascular tumors, neural tumors, pleomorphic adenoma	Mucoepidermoid carcinoma, adenoid cystic carcinoma
Bony	Giant cell, fibro-osseous,	Osteogenic sarcoma, chondrosarcoma, fibrosarcoma
Adult		
Mucosal	Fibroma, papilloma	Squamous cell carcinoma
Salivary	Pleomorphic adenoma	Mucoepidermoid carcinoma
Bony	Fibrous-osseous lesions	Osteogenic sarcoma

cavity is a topic of debate. The roles of the health care professionals who are not physicians or dentists in oral cancer screening remains poorly defined. Participants such as dental hygienists, physician's assistants, and nurses can contribute to delays in the diagnosis of oral cancers. Patient education to self-examination techniques requires knowledge, experience, and an understanding of the limitations. Self-examination is reasonable and practical for breast cancer; however, for the oral cavity self-examination is complex and requires manipulations of structures with illumination for visual inspection, which cannot be accomplished.

The general population receives information about cancer through various methods. Few individuals can identify 1 sign of oral cancer.[7,8] The dangers of tobacco and alcohol related to lung cancer and cardiovascular disease dominate patient education from health care providers and the media. Less of an emphasis exists related to aerodigestive cancer. Smokeless tobacco with its risks, along with human papilloma virus, remain topics that are often discussed minimally or not at all.

The public has little interest in considering their risk of oral cancer. As the lay public receives health care, it is assumed that the history taking and examination techniques are provided by educated and trained health care providers. The assumption is that the examination will adequately screen for all types of disease, cancer included. Often, an office visit to a primary care physician excludes an examination of the mouth. Oral cancer screening requires a head, neck, and oral cavity examination, and many patients are unclear who should be responsible for screening them for oral cancer.

DISCUSSION OF THE BIOPSY

During the training of a surgeon, a multitude of management scenarios can occur. The variety of oncologic care varies from training programs owing to patient demographics and geography; however, the core elements of diagnosis and treatment remain the same. The principles of physiology and the pathologic basis of disease are integral during training of the OMS. Months to years of training dedicated to the OMS provide a wealth of critical decision-making experience. These skills acquired during rotations through the anesthesia, general surgery, plastic surgery, otolaryngology, critical care, and emergency room services provide a substantial portion of the overall education and training of the OMS. These skills acquired are essential to incorporate into the initial encounter when discussing the indications for a biopsy. Empathy and compassion during the initial discussion cannot be overstated. Many patients feel embarrassed and vulnerable during the consultation and do not provide a true historical account of the problem. Regardless of the circumstance, it is both recognized and accepted that patient responses can be unpredictable. Again, the ability of the OMS to provide comfort and sympathy cannot be overstated. The act of sharing a potential life-altering or life-threatening treatment plan is a learned skill.

OFFICE-BASED ANESTHESIA CARE

The universally accepted concept *time is of the essence* remains essential in many health care scenarios. This rings dramatically true in the context of an impending airway obstruction and also for the diagnosis of a potential malignant lesion with its local destruction of peripheral hard and soft tissues and a potential for distant metastasis. When the need arises, the functionally equipped OMS office can provide the full scope of safe and effective anesthesia in conjunction with precise surgical management. This service can minimize delays in care often related to the coordination of medical benefits and conflicts with busy hospital operating room schedules. OMS office practice can provide prompt and timely patient evaluation and coordinate rapid access to the appropriate anesthesia and surgical treatment plan.

In addition, most OMS practices have established relationships with general pathology service providers (medically trained pathologists) and frequently have the need for a lesion to be diagnosed by an oral pathologist.

HOSPITAL-BASED ANESTHESIA CARE: AMBULATORY SURGERY UNIT OR INPATIENT

The OMS residency training is hospital-based surgical training. OMS residents are dentists who receive graduate medical education and supervision ranging from 36 to 72 months. The training consists of inpatient care in the areas of internal medicine, emergency medicine, critical care medicine, anesthesia, general surgery and head and neck surgery. The objective of this training is to provide the resident with comprehensive experience that will translate to private practice care. Upon completion of training, the OMS can elect to acquire hospital privileges. The core privileges generally provide operating room access for outpatient or ambulatory care and inpatient care. These privileges must be maintained in accordance with the individual hospital bylaws and require ongoing clinical competency.

From time to time, patients with indications for a biopsy present with a comorbidity that requires hospitalization. The OMS with operating room privileges can coordinate the admission to efficiently manage the medical, anesthesia, and surgical needs of the patient. Surgical pathology as an inpatient can be coordinated if the need arises for frozen section–guided excisions, fine needle aspiration, and specialized staining and cytology techniques.

OBSTACLES TO PATIENT CARE FOR PROVIDERS

A lack of national prevalence data related to oral cancer creates a barrier to educating the public of its occurrence. A review of the current literature demonstrates a void in studies directed to the topic of oral cancer symptoms and risk factors.

Currently, 2018 worldwide cancer data statistics rank lip and oral cancer as 11 in men and 19 in women for newly diagnosed cases. When including laryngeal and pharyngeal cancers, the rate increases to a rank of the seventh in the most frequent anatomic sites worldwide.[9,10]

Current medical and dental school education provides the student the fundamental principles of physiology and the pathologic basis of disease. The course of study ranges from the molecular basis of disease to the clinical management of the patient. The educational process in pathology allows for an initial understanding of neoplasia. The foundation for understanding neoplasia and its behavior is acquired during primary care medical training in addition to specialty medical and surgical training.[11] Each area of training has specific considerations and concerns related to neoplasia. The recognition of risk factors by history, problem-focused physical examination, and decision making for additional diagnostic methods such as imaging and chemistry are essential for an accurate assessment of the patient. This concept of recognition and assessment guides the overall management of the patient.

Common Administrative and Clinical Areas of Misinformation

When the adult patient or parents of a minor are informed of a diagnosis of a possible lesion, a number of predictable intellectual thoughts and behaviors typically occur. Shock, anger, denial, and fear occur to different degrees initially, which can lead to acceptance. Depression can develop as a consequence of being informed of a potentially life-threatening illness. Ultimately, hope is the target thought or emotion that can allow for the process of a cure to be attempted.[12] The patient, parent, legal guardian, and/or caregivers often do not have a clear understanding of the coordination of benefits for a recommended surgical anesthesia treatment plan. OMS office practice is uniquely designed to be the practice or specialty model of choice for the management and detailed explanation of the dental and medical plans, as well as their associated coverage guidelines.

The following topics are essential to consider for patient care by the OMS and the supporting practice ancillary staff. **Box 2** provides a list commonly encountered scenarios that can contribute to a delay in care.[13] Additional areas of management that can delay care may occur less frequently, but need to be appreciated by the patient and OMS alike. They are essential when considering initial and ongoing surgical diagnostic therapy. **Box 3** provides important secondary and/or more involved issues to be discussed with the patient.

Strategy: Introduction of the Oral Cancer Foundation to Dentists, Physicians, and the Public

The Oral Cancer Foundation (oralcancerfoundation.org) was established as a nonprofit public service charity serving as a resource for patients and dental and

---

Box 2
Commonly encountered delay of care discussion points

1. Lack of access to medical care owing to insurance terms, limitations, and exclusions

2. Many patients seek care from a dentist more frequently than a primary care physician, or do not have a primary care physician

3. Pediatrician and ancillary staff's reluctance to coordinate odontogenic tumors as important or medical in nature

4. Explanation to the patient for the following question: "Why doesn't my dental insurance cover my biopsy?"

5. Coordination of benefits such as anesthesia plan and place of service

---

Box 3
Discussion of specific factors related to previous oral lesion management

1. Understanding the factors involved in the previously biopsied patient
2. Understanding the factors of the multiply operated patient
3. Understanding the previous radiation therapy history
4. Extraction of teeth for access to a lesion
5. The need, indications, or medical necessity for preradiation extractions and alveoplasty
6. Comorbidities, diet and life style, and nutritional considerations
7. Understanding the factors involved in the patient surviving the 5-year date and a new primary lesion occurs
8. Staging consideration for future reconstruction

---

medical professionals.[14] Its published agenda promotes annual oral cancer screenings along with community awareness and outreach programs.

April has been designated as oral head and neck cancer awareness month. The Oral Cancer Foundation encourages professionals to engage the public through scheduled office screening, office events and out-of-office events such as walk and run events and sponsoring charity campaigns.

The treatment of oral cancer benefits from a team approach, ranging from surgical subspecialists, medical subspecialists, to family and friends. The Oral Cancer Foundation provides the patient and their supporting caregivers a wealth of knowledge and information in combating their disease.

REFERRALS

The general dentist should determine and document the reason for referring the patient to the oral surgeon. They should explain to the patient why the referral is necessary and possibly that a biopsy may be needed. After deciding to refer, the general practitioner's office should make the appointment with the surgeon before the patient leaves the office. The patient should be given a referral slip with the reason for referral along with the surgeons address, telephone number, and directions.

Other than for routine dentoalveolar referrals, the dentist should personally contact the surgeon directly to discuss the referral. He or she should provide information on the patient's current situation along with available radiographs. When the surgeon report arrives, the results should be reviewed and recommendations adhered to. Failure to read and follow specialist advice could be grounds for a malpractice claim. Patients are not obligated to go see the oral surgeon and so they may not go. If the patient does not keep the referral appointment, the referring dentist should speak with the patient to find out why, and document the response. This would medicolegally close the case, although the patient can still be encouraged to see the surgeon.

SUMMARY

Maxillofacial mucosal and skeletal neoplasia occurs with a diverse array of presentations and is often diagnosed by dentists and physicians alike. Decades of education to the lay public and dental and medical professionals have demonstrated a relative steady rate of diagnosis. Continual and continuous emphasis on public awareness, patient education and profession examination remain as the primary methods to an early diagnosis and curative treatment.

REFERENCES

1. Sllverman S Jr, Eversole LR, Truelove E. Essentials of Oral Medicine; Oral Premalignancies and Squamous Cell Carcinoma. Hamilton, (ON): BC Decker Inc; 2002. p. 186.
2. Kaban LB, Troulis MJ. Pediatric oral and maxillofacial surgery: jaw tumors in children. Philadelphia: Saunders; 2004. p. 213.
3. Kaban LB, Troulis MJ. Pediatric oral and maxillofacial surgery: salivary gland tumors in children. Philadelphia: Saunders; 2004. p. 202–11.
4. US Census Bureau, 2008 to 2017, American Community Surveys.
5. The Oral Cancer Foundation. Early detection, diagnosis and staging; website CDC oral cancer background papers.
6. Shahrokh B, Bryan BR, Husain AK. Current therapy in oral and maxillofacial surgery; oral squamous cell carcinoma: epidemiology, clinical and radiographic evaluation, and staging. St. Louis, (MO): Elsevier Saunders; 2012. p. 414–22.
7. Horowitz AM, Nourjah P, Gift HC. US adult knowledge of risk factors and signs of oral cancer: 1990. J Am Dent Assoc 1995;126:39–45.
8. Referral patterns, lesion prevalence, and patient care parameters in a clinical oral pathology practice. Oral Surg Oral Med Oral Pathol Oral Radiol Endod 1999; 87(5):583–8.
9. World Cancer Research Fund International; World Cancer Data, Bray F, Ferlay J, Soerjomataram I, et al. Global Cancer Statistics 2018: GLOBOCAN estimates of incidence and mortality worldwide for 36 cancers in 185 countries. CA Cancer J Clin 2018;68(6):394–424. The online GLOBOCAN 2018 database is Available at: http://gco.iarc.fr/, as part of IARC's Global Cancer Observatory.
10. World Cancer Research Fund International; Mouth, pharynx and larynx Cancer report 2018; Diet, Nutrition, Physical Activity and cancers of the mouth, pharynx and larynx.
11. Carter Lachlan M, Ogden Graham R. Oral cancer awareness of undergraduate medical and dental students. BMC Med Educ 2007;7:44.
12. Kübler-Ross E, Kessler D. On grief & grieving: finding the meaning of grief through the five stages of loss. New York: Scribner; 2014.
13. Dang-Tan T, Franc EL. Diagnosis delays in childhood cancer: a review. Cancer 2007;110(4):703–13.
14. Oral Cancer Foundation website. 2019. Available at: oralcancerfoundation.org. Accessed April 28, 2019.

Atypical Facial Pain

Earl Clarkson, DDS, Eunsu Jung, DDS

KEYWORDS

- Atypical facial pain • AFP • Persistent idiopathic facial pain • PIFP

KEY POINTS

- Atypical facial pain (also known as persistent idiopathic facial pain) is chronic facial pain without clear etiology.
- The condition is challenging to diagnose and diagnosis is made by excluding other causes of facial pain.
- Currently, no clear guideline for diagnosing the disease is available.
- Pharmacotherapy, especially tricyclic antidepressants, is proved to be effective and considered the treatment choice for the condition.

INTRODUCTION

Atypical facial pain (AFP), otherwise known as persistent idiopathic facial pain (PIFP), is a chronic and diffuse distribution of facial pain along the territory of the trigeminal nerve.[1,2] This condition is unique in that it occurs in the absence of any neurologic deficit or any other obvious etiology. AFP is one of the most challenging conditions to diagnose due to the lack of clear diagnostic criteria. As a result, AFP is a diagnosis by exclusion of other known etiologies of facial pain and have no distinguishable lab markers or abnormalities.

In 1924, the first known diagnosis of AFP was recorded by Frazier and Russell who determined that 10% to 15% of patients who presented with chronic facial pain had symptoms that differed from the characteristic clinical pattern of trigeminal neuralgia, leading them to coin the term, *atypical neuralgia*. The diagnosis and terminology for this condition are surrounded by controversy and disagreement, with a wide variation in names adopted by different organizations and societies. The World Health Organization has adopted the term *AFP* whilst the International Headache Society and the International Association of the Study of Pain use the terminology, *persistent idiopathic facial pain*. Owing to the fact that patients with this disorder experience pain that neither follows the distribution of the peripheral nerve nor responds to antiepileptic agents, labeling this condition as atypical has served to distinguish it from the

Disclosure Statement: The author has nothing to disclose.
Department of Dentistry/Oral and Maxillofacial Surgery, Woodhull Medical Center, 2c320, Brooklyn, NY 11203, USA
E-mail address: eicddsoms@yahoo.com

typical trigeminal neuralgia. Although this provides a means of categorizing patients with similar pain history and profiles, the basis on which this disorder is distinguished can be considered to have diagnostic limitations because the condition is defined by exclusion rather than inclusion.

CLINICAL PRESENTATION

Clinical presentation of AFP is largely variable and depends on the patient. Generally, patients suffering from this disorder experience pain that presents as poorly localized, deep, dull, aching, burning, pulling, and involving diffuse areas of trigeminal nerve distribution in the face. Additionally, the pain is long in duration, presents daily, and tends to last most of the day. Pain can be continuous or intermittent with periods of no pain. Stress and fatigue may elicit symptoms. At onset, pain can be confined to a limited area, which usually is unilateral and then may spread to a diffuse, larger area. In some cases, pain can present as sharp, shooting, and bilateral. Patients with AFP often report that analgesics are ineffective and this pain has been present for several years. This condition seems to have a predilection for the maxilla, women, and the middle aged–elderly, with most ages 30 years to 50 years.

EPIDEMIOLOGY

The estimated incidence and prevalence of AFP diverge significantly. In a study of Dutch primary care patients, the incidence was 39.5 per 100,000 person-years. In an epidemiologic study conducted in Germany, Mueller and colleagues[3–5] estimated the prevalence of AFP as 0.03%, whereas other studies suggested it can be more than 1%.[6–12] This large discrepancy in estimates of incidence and prevalence is owing to the absence of clear diagnostic guidelines. An inability to distinctly evaluate and diagnose this condition has likely contributed to both underestimates and overestimates in the various studies. As such, there are insufficient data providing evidence of the incidence, prevalence and predilection of this condition.

ETIOLOGY

The etiology attributable to AFP is not well understood. Researchers have suggested that the underlying causes of AFP are associated with injury to the trigeminal nerve, peripheral central demyelination, or minor trauma, such as a dental extraction. Some literature suggests that it is possible that an abnormal sensitization of the trigeminal nociceptive system may play a crucial role in the onset of AFP, whereas other researchers have suggested that AFP is a centrally mediated pain and may even be psychological in origin because they have found associations with underlying psychological disorders, such as depression and anxiety. Research has not provided clarity as to whether these psychological disorders are responsible for AFP or whether AFP plays a role in the onset of these conditions because other conditions of chronic pain are commonly associated with these psychological disturbances. Altogether, research thus far has yielded suggestion of associations and possible etiologies of AFP; however, the associations are weak and the suggested etiologies lack a scientifically evident justification.

DIAGNOSIS

Given the unclear etiology of AFP and high variability in presentation of symptoms, there are no clear studies or tests that can confirm an accurate diagnosis of AFP. Currently, AFP is a diagnosis made based on a good clinical assessment by an experienced oral surgeon who can eliminate all other causes of facial pain; it is diagnosed by means of exclusion. Some guidelines have been put in place to offer a diagnostic criterion. The International Headache Society has offered diagnostic criteria of AFP. These criteria were evaluated by Zebenholzer and colleagues,[13] who, using these criteria, suggested that most patients could be classified with accuracy and comparisons of management made easier. Their classification and definition are as follows.

INTERNATIONAL CLASSIFICATION OF HEADACHE DISORDERS

AFP: persistent facial and/or oral pain, with varying representations but recurring daily for more than 2 hours per day over more than 3 months, in the absence of clinical neurologic deficit.[14]

Diagnostic criteria
A. Facial and/or oral pain fulfilling criteria B and C
B. Recurring daily for greater than 2 h/d for greater than 3 months
C. Pain has both of the following characteristics:
   1. Poorly localized and not following the distribution of a peripheral nerve
   2. Dull, aching, or nagging quality
D. Clinical neurologic examination normal
E. A dental cause excluded by appropriate investigations
F. Not better accounted for by another *International Classification of Headache Disorders*, *3rd Edition*, diagnosis.

Although the IHS classification aids in diagnosing AFPT, the diagnostic criteria is still based on symptoms that are nonspecific. The symptoms are commonly present in other diseases and not required for diagnosis of AFP. Most studies hence will continue to support AFP (or PIFP) as a diagnosis of exclusion, with patient who present that do not fulfill any criteria of other known disease. As such, it is pertinent that patients receive a thorough clinical examination to rule out any other possible cause of their chronic pain, including but not limited to dental infection, sinusitis, vascular causes, craniofacial tumors, temporomandibular disorder, trigeminal neuralgia, glossopharyngeal neuralgia, central poststroke pain, complex regional pain syndrome, migraine, and multiple sclerosis. Clinical examination should be supplemented by radiographic imaging, such as computed tomography or magnetic resonance imaging, of the craniofacial region, when a patient's history and clinical examination suggest other causes.

MANAGEMENT

The precise etiology of AFP is unknown; hence, specific disease modalities cannot be targeted, resulting in a deficiency of clear treatment protocol. More aggressive attempts in the form of surgical intervention with procedures ranging from local neurectomies to motor cortex stimulation and cerebral ablative procedures have had limited to no success. Surgical intervention for treatment of AFP is supported by limited literature, which lacks consistency and scientific justification. Although there are no clear guidelines, some successful pain management has been evident with the use of antidepressants, anticonvulsant medications, conventional analgesic medications, and opioids. Pharmacotherapy can be effective with select individuals and often can be accompanied by a comprehensive cognitive-behavioral therapy (CBT).[15–17] Because AFP is a diagnosis based on the exclusion of other diseases processes, pharmacotherapy should be initiated in coordination with a primary physician and other specialties.

There are only a few randomized controlled trials that assess and prove effective treatment modalities for AFP. Among those trials, tricyclic antidepressants (TCAs) have most strongly shown evidence in treating AFP. TCAs, such as amitriptyline (50–100 mg/d) or nortriptyline (20–50 mg), can be effective if used for at least 6 months. In the study of Sharav and colleagues,[18] they have demonstrated the effectiveness of low-dose or high-dose amitriptyline (25 mg or 100 mg). Although this study is useful, these results are limited in their application for patients with isolated AFP, because the patients treated in this study had a mixture of chronic idiopathic facial pain, temporomandibular disorder pain, and other neuropathic pain. Despite the limitations of evidence-based literature available, TCAs are considered the choice of pharmacotherapy for patients with AFP.

When TCAs are contraindicated or poorly tolerated, gabapentin or pregabalin has been found an appropriate alternative. Other appropriate medications to consider are selective serotonin reuptake inhibitors: duloxetine, fluoxetine, escitalopram, and venlafaxine often are used because they are more tolerable and associated with fewer side effects. Their efficacy in pain relief, however, is lower. In a study by Forsell and colleagues,[19] venlafaxine versus a placebo was investigated in a double-blind, crossover randomized clinical trial consisting of 30 patients. The study found that there was no difference between placebo and active drug in treatment of pain intensity, anxiety, and depression, but there was a significant improvement in pain relief scores among the active treatment group. Venlafaxine proved to provide only modest pain relief; however, it is likely this result was compromised due to small sample size.

In addition to pharmacotherapy, it is postulated that patients may benefit from simultaneous psychotherapy, which may result in a better quality of life. CBT has proved effective in patients with chronic pain and is commonly combined with use of TCAs. In a study evaluating its efficacy in AFP, however, rather than experience pain relief, patients found that they were better able to control their pain. A study by Harrison and colleagues[20–22] evaluated 178 patients with mixed chronic facial pain by dividing their treatment in 4 groups: fluoxetine, placebo, CBT with placebo, and CBT with fluoxetine, and they were followed-up for 3 months. At the end of the study, fluoxetine effectively reduced pain compared with the placebo whereas CBT provided no pain relief. As opposed to pain relief, CBT provided patients with better control of their lives, effects that were maintained after discontinuation of pharmacotherapy.

REFERENCES

1. Agostoni E, Frigerio R, Santoro P. Atypical facial pain: clinical considerations and differential diagnosis. Neurol Sci 2005;26(S2):s71–4.

2. Cornelissen P, Kleef MV, Mekhail N, et al. Evidence-based interventional pain medicine according to clinical diagnoses. 3. Persistent idiopathic facial pain. Pain Pract 2009;9(6):443–8.

3. Mueller D, Obermann M, Yoon M, et al. Prevalence of trigeminal neuralgia and persistent idiopathic facial pain: a population-based study. Cephalalgia 2011; 31(15):1542–8.

4. Nóbrega JC, Siqueira SR, Siqueira JT, et al. Diferential diagnosis in atypical facial pain: a clinical study. Arq Neuropsiquiatr 2007;65(2A):256–61.

5. Saarto T, Wiffen PJ. Antidepressants for neuropathic pain. Cochrane Database Syst Rev 2007;(4):CD005454.

6. Dieleman JP, Kerklaan J, Huygen FJ, et al. Incidence rates and treatment of neuropathic pain conditions in the general population. Pain 2008;137(3):681–8.
7. Elrasheed A, Worthington H, Ariyaratnam S, et al. Opinions of UK specialists about terminology, diagnosis, and treatment of atypical facial pain: a survey. Br J Oral Maxillofac Surg 2004;42(6):566–71.
8. Feinmann C, Harris M. Psychogenic facial pain. Part 2: management and prognosis. Br Dent J 1984;156(6):205–8.
9. Manzoni GC, Torelli P. Epidemiology of typical and atypical craniofacial neuralgias. Neurol Sci 2005;26(S2):s65–7.
10. Mcquay HJ, Tramér M, Nye BA, et al. A systematic review of antidepressants in neuropathic pain. Pain 1996;68(2):217–27.
11. Melzack R, Terrence C, Fromm G, et al. Trigeminal neuralgia and atypical facial pain: use of the McGill pain questionnaire for discrimination and diagnosis. Pain 1986;27(3):297–302.
12. Mock D, Frydman W, Gordon A. Atypical facial pain: a retrospective study. Oral Surg Oral Med Oral Pathol 1985;59(5):472–4.
13. Zebenholzer K, Wöber C, Vigl M, et al. Facial pain in a neurological tertiary care centre — evaluation of the international classification of headache disorders. Cephalalgia 2005;25(9):689–99.
14. Headache Classification Committee of the International Headache Society (IHS) The international classification of headache disorders, 3rd edition. Cephalalgia 2018;38(1):1–211.
15. Weiss AL, Ehrhardt KP, Tolba R. Atypical facial pain: a comprehensive, evidence-based review. Curr Pain Headache Rep 2017;21(2):8.
16. Zakrzewska J. Differential diagnosis of facial pain and guidelines for management. Br J Anaesth 2013;111(1):95–104.
17. Zakrzewska JM, Jensen TS. History of facial pain diagnosis. Cephalalgia 2017;37(7):604–8.
18. Sharav Y, Singer E, Schmidt E, et al. The analgesic effect of amitriptyline on chronic facial pain. Pain 1987;31(2):199–209.
19. Forsell H, Tasmuth T, Tenovuo O, et al. Venlafaxine in the treatment of atypical facial pain: a randomized controlled trial. J Orofac Pain 2004;18:131–7.
20. Harrison SD, Glover L, Feinmann C, et al. A comparison of antidepressant medication alone and in conjunction with cognitive behavioural therapy for chronic idiopathic facial pain. In: Jensen TS, Turner JA, Wiesenfeld- Hallin Z, editors. Proceedings of the 8th World Congress on pain. Progress in pain research and management. Seattle (WA): IASP Press; 1997. p. 663–72.
21. Lascelles RG. Atypical facial pain and depression. Br J Psychiatry 1966;112(488):651–9.
22. Madland G. Chronic facial pain: a multidisciplinary problem. J Neurol Neurosurg Psychiatry 2001;71(6):716–9.

Neurologic Disorders of the Maxillofacial Region

Mel Mupparapu, DMD, MDS[a],*, Eugene Ko, DMD, MS[a],
Temitope T. Omolehinwa, DMD, DScD[a], Avneesh Chhabra, MD[b]

KEYWORDS

- Trigeminal neuralgia • Facial pain • Headache • Facial paralysis
- Facial movement disorders • Migraine • Magnetic resonance neurography (MRN)

KEY POINTS

- Sensory disturbances of the maxillofacial region include trigeminal neuralgia, glossopharyngeal neuralgia, persistent idiopathic facial pain, burning mouth syndrome, cluster headache, geniculate neuralgia, and temporal arteritis.
- Motor disturbances that are of importance to dentists include Bell palsy, multiple sclerosis, central poststroke pain, syringobulbia, and Tourette syndrome and their association with maxillofacial structures and their management or referral when encountered in dental practice.
- Movement disorders such as cerebral palsy and Parkinson disease, and their maxillofacial manifestations.
- Infections such as neurosyphilis, leprosy, and herpes zoster are discussed with a focus on maxillofacial structures.
- Where possible, imaging of the head and neck region with special focus on magnetic resonance neurography is discussed, with pertinent image sequences.

INTRODUCTION

Diagnosis and management of patients with neurologic disorder in clinical practice remain a challenge to all dentists. A good understanding of the neurologic disorder in all its aspects, including its clinical presentation, examination findings, relevant investigations, and prior management, help clinicians identify the condition when presented as a comorbidity alongside the dental conditions. Once identified

Disclosure: Dr A. Chhabra serves as a consultant to ICON Medical and Treace 3D Medical Inc. Dr A. Chhabra receives book royalties from Jaypee and Wolters. Drs M. Mupparapu, E. Ko, and T.T. Omolehinwa have nothing to disclose.
[a] University of Pennsylvania School of Dental Medicine, 240 S 40th Street, Philadelphia, PA 19104, USA; [b] UT Southwestern Medical Center, Harry Hines Boulevard, Dallas, TX 75390, USA
* Corresponding author. Department of Oral Medicine, Robert Schattner Center, 240 South 40th Street, Philadelphia, PA 19104.
E-mail address: mmd@upenn.edu

or suspected, the patient can be referred for further multidisciplinary work-up and management. This article describes sensory, motor disturbances, and movement disorders of neurologic origin that may be encountered in routine dental practice (**Box 1**) and conditions likely to be seen by dental practitioners in which the initial presenting symptoms could be facial pain, numbness, tingling, or discomfort.

SENSORY DISTURBANCES
Trigeminal Neuralgia (Tic Douloureux)

Definition
According to the International Classification of Headache Disorders, Third Edition (ICHD-3), trigeminal neuralgia, also called tic douloureux, is characterized by sudden onset of recurrent unilateral electric shock–like, stabbing, or shooting pain lasting between a fraction of a second and 2 minutes.[1]

It occurs along the distribution of the trigeminal nerve and has a trigger zone/point, typically in the maxillary (V2) and maxillary (V3) nerve distributions.

Pain is triggered by innocuous stimuli such as facial touch, brushing teeth, talking, or cold air. However, patients have intermittently pain-free periods, with pain occurring sporadically and terminating abruptly. Symptoms occur in the absence of neurologic deficits.

Types of trigeminal neuralgia

1. Classic trigeminal neuralgia[2]
   a. Idiopathic form: no disorder is evident.
   b. Classic form: hypothesized to be related to vascular compression on the trigeminal nerve near the skull base or vasospasm.

Box 1
Neurologic disorders of the maxillofacial region

A. Sensory disturbances
   1. Trigeminal neuralgia
   2. Trigeminal anesthesia dolorosa
   3. Glossopharyngeal neuralgia
   4. Persistent idiopathic facial pain
   5. Burning mouth syndrome
   6. Cluster headache
   7. Nervus intermedius neuralgia (geniculate neuralgia)
   8. Migraine

B. Motor disturbances
   1. Bell palsy
   2. Multiple sclerosis
   3. Central poststroke pain
   4. Syringobulbia
   5. Tourette syndrome

C. Movement disorders
   1. Cerebral palsy
   2. Parkinson disease

D. Infections
   1. Lepromatous neuropathy
   2. Herpes Zoster
   3. Neurosyphilis

2. Secondary (symptomatic) trigeminal neuralgia: occurs from presence of brain tumors, infections, multiple sclerosis, trauma, and so forth. Most commonly, prior dental procedures or anesthetic injections can cause such iatrogenic injuries.

Epidemiology
Most cases of trigeminal neuralgia occur in women more than 40 years of age, peaking between 50 and 60 years.[3] An incidence of 4.3 to 32.1 per 100,000 person years and prevalence of 0.07% to 0.3%[1,2] has been reported.

Clinical presentation
Unilateral sharp, shooting, electric shock–like, paroxysmal or episodic pain symptoms are commonly encountered. Pain is severe enough for the patient to stop any ongoing activity, including cessation of talking midsentence.

In addition to patients with paroxysmal pain, there is another group of patients with trigeminal neuralgia that present with constant burning pain, usually affecting 1 side of the face. It is important to consider this subtype and recognize such atypical presentations, in order not to miss a diagnosis of trigeminal neuralgia.

Diagnosis is based on thorough history and clinical examination (**Boxes 2 and 3**).

Investigations
Imaging Imaging techniques include MRI/magnetic resonance (MR) angiography (MRA)/MR neurography (MRN). Brain MRI is important at the time of diagnosis to differentiate between classic and secondary trigeminal neuralgia. MRI detects lesions such as nerve sheath tumor, compressive vascular disorders, and abnormal enhancement with neuritis.

Electrocardiography is especially important to detect the presence of an atrioventricular (AV) block, because carbamazepine and oxcarbazepine (discussed later) are contraindicated in patients with AV block. More recently, MRN has been used to identify the neurologic abnormalities because the three-dimensional (3D) imaging protocols using MRN have evolved with excellent vascular signal suppression. Trigeminal neuralgia can be diagnosed using MRN[4] (**Fig. 1**). The affected nerve s show increased T2 signal and/or thickening on MRN. MRN aids in identification of neuropathy, confirms the clinical suspicion, and can guide focused treatments, such as rhizotomy. MRN aids in detecting the site of neuropathy, injury, or perineural fibrosis. It is also helpful in grading the nerve injury for future neurolysis or nerve repair procedures[5–7] (**Figs. 2 and 3**).

Box 2
The International Classification of Headache Disorders, Third Edition, criteria for diagnosis of trigeminal neuralgia

Pain from trigeminal neuralgia must have the following characteristics:
1. Lasts from a fraction of a second to 2 minutes
2. Sudden onset and termination
3. Paroxysmal
4. Electric shock–like, stabbing, or shooting pain
5. Severe intensity
6. Precipitated by an innocuous stimulus within the affected trigeminal nerve distribution
7. No neurologic deficits

Data from Maarbjerg S, Di Stefano G, Bendtsen L, et al. Trigeminal neuralgia – diagnosis and treatment. Cephalalgia 2017;37:648–57.

Box 3
Diagnosis, pretreatment work-up, and management of trigeminal neuralgia

Diagnosis:
- Thorough history taking
- Cranial nerve examination
- MRI

Pretreatment work-up
- Electrocardiogram
- Complete blood count
- Complete metabolic panel

Management

Pharmacologic:
- Carbamazepine: first-line treatment
- Oxcarbazepine
- Baclofen
- Gabapentin
- Pregabalin
- Lamotrigine

Surgical:
- Microvascular decompression
- Stereotactic (Gamma knife) therapy
- Balloon decompression
- Glycerol blockade
- Radiofrequency thermoregulation

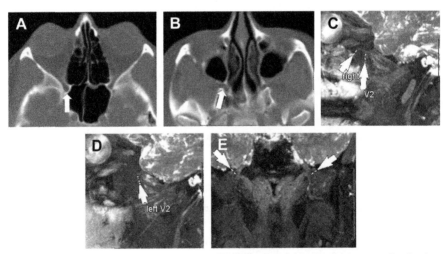

Fig. 1. Young female patient with unrelenting right-sided facial pain in V2/3 distribution. She had multiple imaging studies, including MRI/MRA brain, computed tomography (CT) neck soft tissue, and CT angiography neck. All were reported negative. She was placed on neurontin and started hallucinating as an adverse effect. MRN was performed before prospective rhizotomy. CT images (*A, B*) show widening of the right pterygomaxillary fissure (*arrows*). (*C, D*) MRN images in sagittal reconstructions show thickened right V2 nerve (*C*) compared with left V2 nerve (*D*), confirming the clinical suspicion of right V2 neuropathy. V3 nerve (*white arrows*) was normal (*E*). Final diagnosis of right V2 hypertrophic mononeuropathy.

Laboratory studies
1. Complete metabolic panel, including electrolyte levels, liver function, and renal function, should be assessed before starting the patient on pharmacologic management.
2. Complete blood count (CBC): used in monitoring cell counts during treatment with carbamazepine.

Management
Pharmacologic Sodium channel blockers are the first-line drugs in the management of patients with trigeminal neuralgia. Both carbamazepine and oxcarbazepine are highly effective, with mechanism of action being the blockade of voltage-gated sodium channels.

Patients on carbamazepine require periodic CBC assessment, because this drug is known to cause aplastic anemia in 1% to 2% of users.[8] Oxcarbazepine is better tolerated than carbamazepine and with fewer side effects.

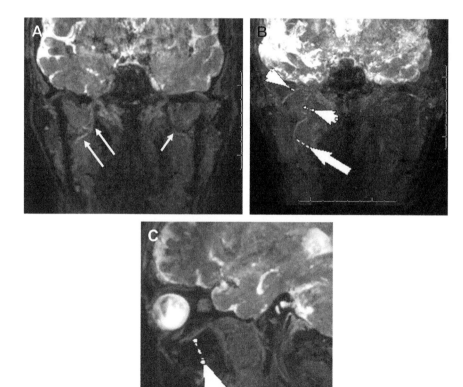

Fig. 2. Middle-aged woman with persistent and increasing right trigeminal neuralgia symptoms following a failed microvascular treatment. (*A*) Coronal 3D MRN image of the maxillofacial area showing abnormally thickened and bright V3 on the right (*large arrows*) and normal left V3 (*small arrow*). (*B*) Also note abnormally enlarged and bright right-sided V3 branch nerves: posterior auricular (*upper arrow*), posterior superior alveolar (*middle arrow*), and inferior alveolar (*lower arrow*). (*C*) Sagittal reconstruction from the 3D MRN. Abnormally thickened and bright V2 nerve (*arrow*). The diagnosis was a presumed idiopathic or autoimmune neuropathy.

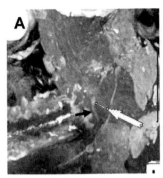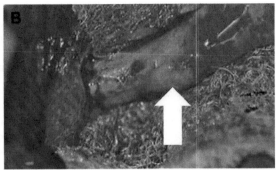

Fig. 3. Young man with 15-month history of right lingual nerve sensory deficit, which started following a molar tooth extraction. Neurosensory testing suggested class II/III injury. (A) Sagittal reconstruction from 3D MRN of maxillofacial area shows a focal 4.9-mm neuroma in continuity in the retroglossal sulcus on the right side (*white arrow*). There is reactive thickening and hyperintensity of the adjacent distal nerve (*black arrow*). (B) The findings of Sunderland class IV injury on MRN were confirmed intraoperatively (*arrow*).

For patients with allergies or drug interactions with carbamazepine, or who have low sodium levels, baclofen or lamotrigine are other beneficial alternatives.

Neuromodulation therapy This technique is explored for the treatment of chronic neuropathic pain. Although certain types of peripheral nerve stimulation procedures are US Food and Drug Administration (FDA) approved for pain in the extremities and back, using this technique for facial pain is still considered an off-label use (**Fig. 4**).

Surgical
1. Microvascular decompression is a common surgical procedure if the condition is nonresponsive to medication
2. Glycerol blockade
3. Radiofrequency thermocoagulation
4. Stereotactic (Gamma Knife) radiosurgery

Trigeminal anesthesia dolorosa Trigeminal anesthesia dolorosa is a chronic central neuropathic pain characterized by severe and debilitating deafferentation pain. It is an

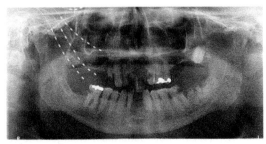

Fig. 4. A panoramic radiograph showing transcutaneous electric nerve stimulators on the right side that were placed to treat trigeminal neuralgia. This procedure is an off-label treatment because FDA did not clear the treatment of facial pain with electric nerve stimulation (it is only approved for extremities and lower back).

uncommon complication after surgical or traumatic injury to the trigeminal nerve. Although rare, it has been reported in patients who underwent trigeminal rhizotomy, a procedure in which heating current is used to destroy nerve fibers sending pain signals to the brain.

Clinical features, investigation, and management
Constant burning or aching pain is noted along the distribution of the affected trigeminal nerve, despite numbness in the area. MRN can show abnormalities of the peripheral trigeminal nerve and/or its branches, confirming the clinical symptoms.[4] This condition is empirically managed by either gabapentin[9] or surgery.

Glossopharyngeal Neuralgia

Definition
Glossopharyngeal neuralgia is an uncommon condition, with pain located in the oropharyngeal area: pharynx, posterior third of tongue, soft palate, ear, and inferior border of mandible.[1,10,11] In addition, patients occasionally present with bradycardia, syncope, or asystole. Pain presents just like in trigeminal neuralgia and is triggered by swallowing, yawning, or talking.

Epidemiology
There is an incidence of 0.2 to 0.8 per 100,00 population per year,[10] with onset noted mostly in patients more than 50 years of age. An equal male to female ratio is reported.[10]

Clinical presentation
Characteristic symptoms of sharp shooting pain in the oropharynx and inner part of the lower mandible aids diagnosis. A thorough history and clinical examination is therefore beneficial.

Types of glossopharyngeal neuralgia

1. Classic glossopharyngeal neuralgia: can be idiopathic or from vascular compression of glossopharyngeal nerve.
2. Secondary glossopharyngeal neuralgia: secondary to trauma, tumor, surgery, or irradiation of the oropharynx.

Investigations
Laboratory
1. Erythrocyte sedimentation rate (ESR)
2. CBC
3. Complete metabolic panel
4. Antinuclear antibody

Imaging
Techniques include MRI, MRA, and MRN. MRI and MRA are used to exclude an organic lesion. MRN aids in direct visualization of neural lesions.

Treatment
Pharmacologic treatment is similar to treatment of trigeminal neuralgia.

Glossopharyngeal nerve block with local anesthesia, with or without the addition of steroids, can be used as an adjunct to pharmacologic management.

Surgical
Treatment modalities are similar to treatment of trigeminal neuralgia. In addition, rhizotomy is an effective surgical treatment option.

Persistent Idiopathic Facial Pain

Persistent idiopathic facial pain (PIFP) is also known as atypical odontalgia, phantom facial pain, and atypical facial pain. According to ICDH-3, PIFP is defined as constant facial and/or oral pain with varying presentations, occurring for at least 2 h/d, and lasting for more than 3 months. Diagnosis is established when the patient presents with the symptoms listed earlier, and with no clinical neurologic deficit.[12] It is unrelated to burning pain in the tongue or oral mucosa, as discussed later in relation to burning mouth syndrome (BMS).

Epidemiology

PIFP is a rare condition with an incidence of 4.4 per 100,000 years and prevalence of 0.03%.[9,13,14]

Eighty percent of patients with this condition attribute onset of symptoms to a dental treatment.[15]

Clinical presentation

Patients describe an aching, throbbing, or burning type of pain. Pain is poorly localized, deep, and usually unilateral, with no evident disorder on the routine imaging studies.

There is an association between the onset of symptoms and a previous dental treatment.[12]

Investigation Diagnosis might involve an inferior alveolar nerve block or local infiltration with local anesthetic agent. However, patients sometimes have an equivocal response to this maneuver, with occasional complete resolution of pain and, at other times, pain persisting.

Imaging

Panoramic or periapical radiographs are used to rule out an odontogenic source of pain. MRN is being increasingly used for such patients. It is common to see entrapment neuropathy or evidence of prior peripheral trigeminal nerve injury, aiding in clarifying the cause in many such cases.

Management

Pharmacologic Use of low-dose antiseizure medications (eg, gabapentin or tricyclic antidepressants) has proved effective in patient management. Topical medications such as capsaicin have also shown some efficacy.

Other treatments Some patients report benefit with low-level laser treatment or behavioral management. Other forms of management with few evidence-based studies include trigeminal ganglion blocks, high-frequency repetitive transcranial magnetic stimulation, and hypnosis. Use of computed tomography (CT)–guided injection and pulsed radiofrequency treatment of sphenopalatine ganglion has been reported in a small number of refractory cases (**Fig. 5**).[9]

Burning Mouth Syndrome

Definition

BMS presents as an unexplained pain, dysesthesia, or burning in a clinically normal and healthy oral mucosa.[16,17] A diagnosis is established if the symptoms discussed earlier recur daily for more than 2 h/d and for at least 3 months as per the definition from the Committee of the International Headache Society.[12] It is a diagnosis of exclusion, and other systemic, local medical or dental sources of pain must be ruled out.[18]

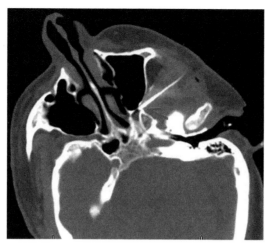

Fig. 5. Older man with persistent left V2 distribution facial pain. Left sphenopalatine ganglion anesthetic and steroid injection under CT guidance. Note the needle in appropriate position (*arrow*).

Epidemiology

The disorder is more common among postmenopausal middle-aged-women, with a male to female ratio of 1:5 to 1:7[19,20] and prevalence of 1%.[21]

Although the cause is unknown, some associated factors, such as stress, hormonal dysfunction, parafunctional habits, anxiety, depression, psychiatric disorders, and neuropathy, might play a role in the syndrome onset and/or excerbation.[18]

Clinical presentation

Patients with BMS describe a spontaneous onset of continuous scalding, rawness, and annoying burning pain. Sensation can vary in intensity during the day, and usually occurs bilaterally. The most common site is the tip of tongue, but it can present on other oral mucosal surfaces.

Some patients report a temporary relief of symptom with food in the mouth, whereas some report aggravation with spicy and acidic foods or alcohol.

Investigation

There is no investigation diagnostic for BMS; however, the following tests can help rule out other systemic or local causes of oral burning:

1. Gram stain and culture to rule out candidiasis.
2. CBC, folate, ferritin, iron, B_{12} to exclude anemia or nutritional deficiency.
3. Salivary flow test to rule out xerostomia.

There are also no positive findings on imaging.

Management

Patients with this condition occasionally present with cancer phobia and typically have been to multiple providers before the diagnosis is established.

The first step in managing these patients is to reassure them that there is no association with cancer and the condition can be managed with conservative means.

Topical or systemic pharmacologic agents have been used successfully to manage or distract some patients with BMS. These agents include alpha lipoic acid, low-dose clonazepam, which should be discontinued with caution as a result of associated withdrawal syndrome (suicidal tendencies); topical capsaicin; gabapentin; amitriptyline; and doxepin. Other treatment strategies used are low-level laser therapy, stress, and behavioral management.

Cluster Headache

Definition

Cluster headache (CH) is classified as a trigeminal autonomic cephalgia by the International Headache Society.[12,22] This form of headache comes in clusters occurring at about the same time each day for a few weeks to several months, after which patients experience pain-free periods.

CHs can be chronic or episodic and have a serious impact on quality of life and the patient's productivity. Patients also have suicidal thoughts and typically present with anxiety and/or depression.[22]

Epidemiology

CH is most common in young men, with a prevalence of 0.1%.[19] The age of onset is, on average, 30 years, with clusters commonly noted in the spring weather.[22–24]

Risk factors include alcohol and nitroglycerine intake.[25]

Clinical presentation

The pain onset is sudden and often severe, and presents unilaterally in the temporal/periorbital area, with about 1 to 8 attacks occurring daily or every other day. Each attack lasts from 15 minutes to 3 hours. The patients also present with the following symptoms on the affected side: tearing in eyes, nasal congestion, runny nose, edema of eyelids, drooping eyelids, and bloodshot eyes.

Investigation

Imaging studies MRI or MRA to rule out brain/pituitary mass. MRN may be used to evaluate supraorbital or occipital nerves. Distention and tortuosity of optic nerve sheaths may be seen in ocular hypertension or intracranial increased pressure.

Laboratory Calcitonin gene–related peptide (CGRP) is being evaluated as a potential biomarker for CH, although its sensitivity and specificity are yet to be established.

Risk factors include alcohol and nitroglycerine intake.[25]

Management The first thing to consider in the management of patients with CH is to prevent acute attacks by preventing triggers, such as tobacco and alcohol, and daily use of pharmacologic agents such as verapamil, topiramate, short-term corticosteroids, and lithium. Triptans are very effective in the treatment of acute episodes of CH, especially when administered subcutaneously or intranasally. One-hundred percent oxygen and sublingual ergotamine have also been used successfully in managing the acute pain. Fremanezumab and galcanezumab are monoclonal CGRP antibodies currently being considered as investigational drugs in the treatment of CH.[22]

Nervus Intermedius Neuralgia (Geniculate Neuralgia)

Nervus intermedius neuralgia is an extremely rare neuralgia arising from the sensory fibers of nervus intermedius, a branch of the facial nerve. It supplies the pinna, external auditory meatus, and retroauricular area.[26] ICH-3 defines nervus intermedius neuralgia as paroxysmal pain episodes presenting deep in the ear and lasting a few seconds to minutes.[12]

There are 2 types of nervus intermedius neuralgia:

1. Classic
2. Secondary

Although there is no specific underlying cause of the classic type, the secondary type is seen after herpes zoster infection (Ramsay Hunt syndrome) involving the nervus intermedius.

Clinical presentation
The classic type presents as recurrent paroxysmal unilateral stabbing, shooting, or sharp pain deep to the auditory canal. It can be triggered by a mechanical or sensory stimulus, with occasional radiation to the parieto-occipital area.

In the secondary type, in addition to the features in classic nervus intermedius neuralgia, the patients further present with ipsilateral facial paralysis and signs of herpetic eruptions on/in the ear on the affected side.

Investigations
On MRI or MRN, the nerve may show thickening, T2 hyperintensity, and enhancement of the facial nerve and its branches.

Management
Management is similar to trigeminal neuralgia.

Migraine

Definition
Migraine is a type of primary headache. It is recurrent and patients usually experience at least 5 episodes before the diagnosis is established. Each episode lasts between 2 hours and 72 hours.[12]

There are 2 subtypes of migraine:

1. Migraine with aura: patients present with neurologic symptoms that are focal and transient. This aura occurs either before or concurrent with the headache. The most prevalent aura is visual aura, with patients experiencing light flashes and photophobia. Other forms of aura include motor weakness and speech disturbance.
2. Migraine without aura: no specific neurologic symptoms that give the patient a premonition of an incipient migraine attack.

Like CH, it presents with autonomic symptoms. The difference between the two conditions is that migraines present with bilateral autonomic features. Recently, new hypothesis of neural compressions has been proposed for migraine attacks: supraorbital or supratrochlear nerve involvement in frontal headaches and occipital nerve compression by posterior skull base muscles in the occipital neuralgia. These conditions have been shown to produce pain improvement with anesthetic and botulinum toxin injections at the trigger points, somewhat validating this hypothesis.[27]

Epidemiology
Migraine is the third most prevalent condition and the seventh leading cause of disability worldwide.[4] It is more common in women, with an incidence of 14.1 to 18.9 per 1000 years and a prevalence of 17% to 33%.[28] A positive family history is present in 26% of cases.[29]

Clinical presentation
The patients present with a sudden onset of unilateral moderate to severe throbbing or pulsating pain in the frontotemporal area. In children and teenagers, the symptoms

can be bilateral. Patients may also present with light and sound sensitivity, nausea, and vomiting.[30]

Investigation The diagnosis is usually clinical. MRN may be performed in doubtful cases or with nonspecific symptoms. Imaging may show abnormal T2 hyperintensity and/or thickening of the greater or lesser occipital nerves (**Fig. 6**).

Management

The initial management is mostly pharmacologic. Triptans (eg, almotriptan, eletriptan, frovatriptan, naratriptan, rizatriptan, sumatriptan, and zolmitriptan) as well as nonsteroidal antiinflammatory drugs are effective medications in the treatment of acute migraine. Also, staying in darkened areas, avoiding bright light, and adequate sleep are useful adjuncts to the medications in patients with acute migraine. Preventive strategies include adequate sleep, regular food intake, exercise, and drugs such as β-blockers, anticonvulsants, and tricyclic antidepressants.

Temporal Arteritis/Giant Cell Arteritis

Although not classified under this category of disorders by the International Headache Society, because of its relevance to this topic, this condition is presented here. According to the American College of Rheumatology, temporal arteritis is a granulomatous inflammation of the temporal artery characterized by a new-onset headache with tenderness to palpation in the temporal area.

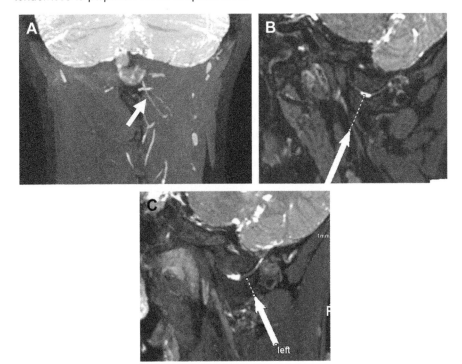

Fig. 6. Young female patient with left-sided migraines in the occipital area with radiation to periauricular area and part of the face. (*A*) Coronal 3D MRN image shows an abnormally thickened left greater occipital nerve (GON; *arrow*). (*B, C*) For comparison, right GON (*arrow in B*) versus left GON (*arrow in C*). The left GON shows persistent thickening and hyperintensity as it travels toward paraspinal muscles distally.

Epidemiology
It is typically present in white women more than 50 years of age, with incidence rates being highest among the people of Scandinavian descent, and a worldwide prevalence of 2.6% to 8.16%.[31,32]

Clinical manifestation
The patients present with jaw claudication and tenderness on palpation of muscles of mastication, especially in the temporal area, localized temporal headache of sudden onset, hyperalgesia of the skin overlying the temples, and double vision.[30]

Investigation Biopsy of the temporal artery, a branch of the carotid artery, aids in the diagnosis of temporal arteritis. Histologic findings of granulomata, multinucleated giant cells, macrophages, lymphocytes, intraluminal thrombosis, and damaged blood vessel wall (including intima thickening) are diagnostic of temporal arteritis.[33]

Laboratory studies
ESR and C-reactive protein levels are increased in patients with temporal arteritis:

Imaging

1. MRI/MRA may show intimal thickening and enhancement of the vessel.
2. Vascular ultrasonography may show altered flows on Doppler examination.

Management
High-dose corticosteroid therapy is the first line of treatment in suspected or proven cases. However, steroid-sparing medications, including biologics, have been introduced as the definitive treatment because of the complications associated with long-term steroid use. One such drug is an FDA-approved immunomodulator, tocilizumab, an interleukin-6 inhibitor. A particularly disabling complication of delayed diagnosis and treatment is loss of vision. Early diagnosis of this condition is therefore very important.

MOTOR DISTURBANCES
Bell Palsy

This condition is named after Sir Charles Bell, a nineteenth century Scottish surgeon who initially described the facial nerve disorder and its connection to this condition. Bell palsy is an acute facial paralysis resulting from damage to the facial nerve (cranial nerve [CN] VII), usually at its exit at the stylomastoid foramen. For most of its course, CN VII travels through a narrow, bony canal called the fallopian canal in the skull and supplies the muscles on each side of the face. The facial nerve has 5 terminal branches that innervate the muscles of facial expression: the temporal branch, the zygomatic branch, the buccal branch, the marginal mandibular branch, and the cervical branch supplying the platysma.

Epidemiology
Bell palsy affects approximately 40,000 Americans each year. Annual incidence has been reported to be around 20 cases per 100,000 people.[34] The cause of Bell palsy is still unclear. Viral infections, hypertension, vascular disease, and diabetes have all been indicated as possible causal agents. Other causes include infections, such as Lyme disease and otitis media; tumors, such as acoustic neuroma, facial neuroma, geniculate hemangioma, and parotid neoplasm; developmental causes, including Mobius syndrome and hemifacial microsomia; and traumatic causes, including temporal bone fracture, forceps delivery, penetrating injuries, dog bites, stab wounds, and gunshot wounds.[34] Adour[35] in 1977 suggested that reactivation of herpes simplex

type 1 may play a major role in the pathogenesis of Bell palsy.[36] Men and women are equally affected, and the peak incidence occurs between the ages of 15 and 45 years.[35]

Clinical presentation

Facial paralysis significantly impairs critical facial functions such as blinking of the eyes, cornea protection, nasal breathing, lip competence, speech, and smiling.

Comprehensive evaluation of the patient determines the extent of facial palsy and the level of functional impairment of the facial nerve. The history should determine the onset, progression, associated symptoms, and the risk factors. The patient is asked to elevate the eyebrow, close eyes, frown, smile, pucker the lips, puff the cheeks, and tense the neck to assess the platysma. Classic symptoms include ipsilateral sagging of the eyebrow, drooping of the face, flattening of the nasolabial fold, and inability to fully close the eye, pucker the lips, or raise the corner of the mouth. It is also known that the symptoms develop within hours to 3 days. Around 70% of cases have associated ipsilateral pain around the ear.[34,37] Bilateral cases of Bell palsy have been reported but are rare.[38]

Investigations

In Bell palsy, wrinkling of the forehead on the affected side when raising the eyebrows is absent or asymmetrical. If the forehead muscles are spared, and the lower face is weak, it represents a central lesion, such as stroke, and not a peripheral lesion of the facial nerve (Bell palsy). Auditory testing may be needed if the hearing is impaired. Several facial reflexes can be tested, including the activation of orbicularis oculi, palpebral oculogyric muscles, and the corneal reflex.[32] Bell palsy is graded (I–VI) using the House-Brackmann scale[39] for the diagnosis as well as prediction of recovery. Grade I is normal and grade VI represents complete paralysis.

CBC with differential is usually ordered to rule out infection or a lymphoproliferative disorder. Hemoglobin A_1C may be helpful to exclude diabetic neuropathy. The patients are also screened for Lyme disease by enzyme-linked immunosorbent assay and Western blot tests. If vesicles are noted, the patient should be tested for herpes zoster. Human immunodeficiency virus (HIV) disease should be ruled out. Cerebrospinal fluid (CSF) analysis rules out Guillain-Barré syndrome.

Imaging is not routinely recommended in the initial evaluation. Because 5% to 7% cases of facial palsy are caused by a tumor such as facial neuroma, hemangioma, cholesteatoma, or meningioma, the patients with sudden onset of symptoms should be imaged with CT or contrast-enhanced MRI of the internal auditory canal and the face.[34] MRI and MRN show abnormal asymmetrical thickening and T2 hyperintensity of the ipsilateral facial nerve with abnormal enhancement (**Fig. 7**).

Management

Bell palsy is a diagnosis of exclusion because, in 30% to 60% of cases of facial palsy, there is an underlying cause, such as stroke, parotid gland tumor, Lyme diseases, Ramsay Hunt syndrome, granulomatous disease, otitis media, cholesteatoma, diabetes, trauma, and Guillain-Barrésyndrome.[39]

Corticosteroids are recommended in the first 72 hours after the onset of symptoms for patients who are 16 years of age or older. The recommendation is prednisolone 50 mg by mouth daily for 10 days or 60 mg by mouth daily for 5 days, followed by a 5-day taper. Antiviral therapy has been shown to offer modest benefit. Surgical decompression remains controversial and there is insufficient evidence for both

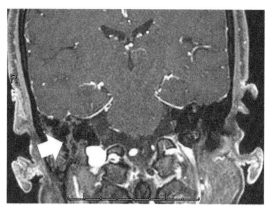

Fig. 7. Middle-aged woman with symptoms and clinical findings of right-sided Bell palsy. Coronal postcontrast T1-weighted MRI shows abnormal thickening and enhancement of the right facial nerve in the temporal segments in the stylomastoid canal consistent with active neuritis (*arrow*). No organic mass lesion noted.

physical therapy and acupuncture. Eye protective gear is of paramount importance, especially if the paralysis is bilateral.[39]

Multiple Sclerosis

Definition
Multiple sclerosis (MS), an autoimmune condition that results in reversible demyelination at various sites in the central nervous system (white matter more than gray matter). Scarring (gliosis) results following chronic inflammatory episodes.[40,41]

Epidemiology
In September 2008, the Multiple Sclerosis International Federation (MSIF) and the World Health Organization (WHO) published, the Atlas: Multiple Sclerosis Resources in the World 2008, and developed the first Atlas of MS Web site, enabling users to search the online data. In 2012 to 2013, MSIF performed a second survey and the data were added to the 2008 atlas.[35] The estimated numbers of people with MS increased from 2.1 million in 2008 to 2.3 million in 2013. The global median prevalence increased from 30 per 100,000 to 33 per 100,000. MS is 2 to 3 times more common in women, especially between the ages of 15 and 45 years. The average onset of MS in patients is usually at age 30 years.[42]

Clinical features
Common presentations include visual loss; sensory symptoms in 1 side of the face or limbs, including tingling or numbness of extremities; motor weakness; gait changes; spasticity; diplopia; optic neuritis; fatigue; and heat sensitivity. Various categories of MS exist, such as relapsing-remitting MS (RRMS), primary progressive MS, secondary progressive MS, and progressive-relapsing MS. RRMS is the most common form, and is observed in 85% to 90% of patients. Although the clinical outcomes vary in each patient, about 50% of all patients with MS require the use of a walking aid within 10 years after the clinical onset.[43,44]

Trigeminal neuralgia associated with MS (TNMS) differs from the other varieties of trigeminal neuralgia in that TNMS occurs in younger patients and is more frequently bilateral. In addition, in patients with MS, carbamazepine is not well tolerated, and microvascular decompression is contraindicated.[45]

Presentations that are of concern to dentists include speech problems, dysphagia, and tremors that may be suspicious of early MS apart from breathing problems, seizures, and hearing loss. A prompt referral to a medical specialist is needed.

Investigations
MR imaging shows MS plaques as alterations with high T2 signal intensity, especially in periventricular areas and corpus callosum (Dawson fingers). Enhancement or diffusion restriction is associated with activity of the lesions, whereas T1 hypointensity and diffusion enhancement are associated with chronicity of the lesions. Additional diagnostic aid is provided by the presence of oligoclonal bands (protein) in the spinal fluid.

Management
MS is not a curable disease but there are several disease-modifying therapies available with medications for relapsing MS and also for primary MS. Ocrelizumab, natalizumab, alemtuzumab, and mitoxantrone are available for intravenous infusion, whereas dimethyl fumerate, teriflunomide, and fingolimod are available as oral agents, and glatiramer acetate, pegylated interferon beta-1a, and interferon beta-1a are available as injectable agents. The other important aspects of management include functional rehabilitation and provision of emotional support.[46]

Central Poststroke Pain

Central poststroke pain (CPSP) was previously known as Dejerine-Roussy syndrome or thalamic pain syndrome. This condition is a dreaded complication of cerebrovascular accidents affecting approximately 8% of patients after stroke. If the stroke involves the lateral medulla, the prevalence of CPSP is around 25% and, if it involves the inferior thalamus, the prevalence is around 17% to 18%.[47]

Epidemiology
Cerebrovascular events are among the most common causes of morbidity and mortality in the United States, with an occurrence of nearly 800,000 new strokes each year and a prevalence of 6.6 million in patients more than 20 years of age.[48]

Clinical presentation
The patients complain of pain within the distribution of the body affected by stroke. Almost all patients have allodynia. The pain typically fluctuates in intensity as well as distribution throughout the day.[49]

Investigations
The diagnosis of CPSP is accomplished based on the history and physical examination. Imaging (especially MRI) can be done to rule out other diagnoses and mostly to confirm the previous history of stroke. The differential diagnosis is very broad and includes conditions such as MS, syringomyelia, peripheral neuropathy, complex regional pain syndrome, poststroke headache, spasticity, herpes zoster, and deep venous thrombosis.

Management
Tricyclic antidepressants, specifically amitriptyline, are useful. Anticonvulsants, specifically lamotrigine, gabapentin, pregabalin, carbamazepine, and phenytoin are all used with varying success rates.

Syringobulbia

Syringobulbia is a neurologic disorder characterized by a fluid-filled cavity called a syrinx within the spinal cord extending to involve the brainstem (medulla). It usually involves 1 or more lower CNs, causing facial paralysis (CN VII), tongue weakness (CN XII), sternocleidomastoid and trapezius weakness (CN XI), dysphagia (CN IX), and dysarthria (CN X). In addition, both sensory and motor nerve pathways may be affected by either compression or interruption. This condition is also closely associated with syringomyelia, in which the syrinx is limited to the spinal cord and to the Chiari I malformation (tonsillar herniation).

Epidemiology
This condition affects men and women equally and is seen before the age of 30 years.

Clinical presentation
This is a slow, progressive disorder that can cause vertigo, nystagmus, and loss of pain and temperature sensations of the face. Atrophy and small involuntary contractions of tongue can occur (fibrillation). There might be dysphonia (stuttering). Other symptoms may include impaired vision, numbness, altered gait, and scoliosis.[50] It has been reported that, sometimes, orofacial pain is the only manifestation of this condition, associated with syringomyelia and Arnold-Chiari malformation.[51]

Investigations
The diagnosis of syringobulbia is made by means of neuroimaging, typically sagittal plane MRI.

Management
The management is always surgical in symptomatic cases and diversion of CSF via diversion tubes or shunts is attempted. All surgical approaches for syringobulbia must be combined with the treatment of syringomyelia. Procedures may include decompression of the craniovertebral junction; posterior fossa decompression, including suboccipital craniectomy; C1 laminectomy; and duraplasty.

Tourette Syndrome

Tourette syndrome (TS) is a neurologic disorder in which repetitive, involuntary movements and vocalizations called tics are noted. This syndrome was first described by a French neurologist named Dr Georges Gilles de la Tourette in 1885.

Epidemiology
Based on parents' reports (65,540 US children aged 6–17 years from the National Survey of Children's health), 0.9% of US children had TS.[52,53]

Clinical presentation
The early symptoms of TS begin between the ages of 3 and 9 years. There is no predilection for any specific ethnic or racial group, but boys are affected about 3 to 4 times than girls. Among children who have a diagnosis of TS, most (86%) also have at least 1 additional mental, behavioral, or developmental disorder, such as attention-deficit/hyperactivity disorder, depression, autism spectrum disorder, learning disability, intellectual disability, and developmental delay leading to learning difficulties. A third of the people with TS have obsessive-compulsive disorder.[54]

Investigations No laboratory or imaging tests are needed for the diagnosis of TS. If MRI, CT, or electroencephalogram testing is done, it is merely to rule out other organic diseases that might mimic TS when the history is not definitive.

Management Most people with TS do not need any medication for tic suppression. Neuroleptics are the most commonly used medication for tic suppression.[54]

MOVEMENT DISORDERS
Cerebral Palsy

Definition
Cerebral palsy is a spectrum of permanent motor impairments that result from injury to the developing brain.

Epidemiology
It is the most common cause of severe physical disability in childhood. Overall reported prevalence in children aged 3 to 10 years is 2.4 per 100 children.[55] Preterm birth is the most important risk factor for cerebral palsy.[56]

Clinical
Cerebral palsy is associated with various motor defects, which depend on the brain lesion location.[56] Motor disorders range from subtle motor impairment to involvement of the whole body.[56] However, the clinical signs and level of disability may change over time; for example, motor skills of most children with cerebral palsy improve as they grow.[56,57] Other associated disorders can include mental impairment, learning disability, and seizures.[57] Epilepsy episodes are more frequent in children and adults with cerebral palsy than in the general population.[57]

Investigations
Routine laboratory tests are not necessary because cerebral palsy is primarily a clinical diagnosis that rests on identifying and classifying the movement disorder through history and physical examination.[57] Neuroimaging such as MRI may be indicated in certain cases to exclude an organic lesion. In addition, because children with cerebral palsy also have associated comorbidities, screening for such conditions should be a part of the initial assessment.[57]

Management
Cerebral palsy has no cure and there are a few disease-modifying interventions. Symptom management and rehabilitation is the mainstay of treatment.[50] Assistive devices such as braces, walkers, or wheelchairs can help develop or maintain mobility.[51] In addition, patients with cerebral palsy may need specialized medical care, educational and social services, and other help throughout their lives from families and communities.[51] If appropriate health care is available, affected children without significant comorbidities have survival similar to that of the general population.[57]

Parkinson Disease

Definition
Parkinson disease is a progressive neurodegenerative disease characterized by movement disorders that result from the loss of dopamine-producing nerve cells.

Epidemiology
The prevalence of the disease is generally from 100 to 200 per 100,000 people and the annual incidence is thought to be 15 per 100,000.[58]

Clinical
Parkinson disease is classically characterized by slowness of movement (bradykinesia), rigidity, and rest tremor that affect the limbs asymmetrically.[59] Parkinson disease is also associated with nonmotor features, such as cognitive defects, mood disturbances, olfactory dysfunction, pain, and fatigue. In addition, dementia is also recognized as a feature in Parkinson disease in the elderly.[60,61] In some

cases, these nonmotor dysfunctions can precede the motor lesions by more than a decade.[62]

Investigations
A reliable and easily applicable diagnostic test or marker for Parkinson disease is not yet available.[61] Routine imaging of the brain is rarely helpful in distinguishing parkinsonism because there are other causes of Parkinson disease, although reduced thickness of substantia nigra has been reported.[61] The gold standard for the diagnosis of Parkinson disease is neuropathologic assessment. Diagnosis is confirmed with the loss of dopaminergic neurons within the pars compacta of the substantia nigra, and Lewy body accumulation (aggregates of abnormally folded protein) at postmortem pathologic examination.[61]

Management
The mainstay of treatment of Parkinson disease is the management of symptoms with drugs that increase dopamine concentrations or directly stimulate dopamine receptors.[62] Motor symptoms are usually well controlled in the early stages on dopamine agonists or levodopa.[62] Furthermore, a good response to levodopa therapy in the setting of asymmetrical motor symptoms and resting tremor can often help confirm the diagnosis of Parkinson disease.[61–63] Anticholinergics may also be tried to counter excessive cholinergic effects.

INFECTIONS
Lepromatous Neuropathy

Definition
Peripheral neural damage can be caused by mycobacterial infection, *Mycobacterium leprae*, characterized by demyelination, intraneural abscess, and fibrosis.

Epidemiology
A global detection rate of 2.8 per 100,000 population was reported in 2017 as per the data from 159 countries. Of the reported patients with leprosy, 95% were from 22 specific countries.[63] Leprosy is rare in the United States.[63]

Clinical presentation
There are 2 forms of leprosy, characterized by presence or absence of inflammatory response. A cell-mediated immune response defines the tuberculoid form, whereas, in the lepromatous form, there seems to be no resistance.[64] *M leprae* infection classically presents with peripheral nerve damage of the upper and lower extremities. However, cranial nerves can also be affected, with the CN V and VII being the most common.[65] The characteristic neuropathy is sensory anesthesia (ie, loss of thermal, nociceptive, and pressure sensations), which can ultimately progress to paralysis and crippling deformities of fingers and toes.[65–68] Clinical presentation reveals palpable painful nerve enlargement and hypopigmented skin lesions.[62] In the tuberculoid form, there may only be a single lesion, whereas, in the lepromatous form, there can be involvement of multiple parts of the body with numerous lesions.[66]

Investigations
The gold standard for the diagnosis of leprosy is a full-thickness skin biopsy sample from an active lesion.[59] Biopsies reveal granulomatous inflammation. In the tuberculoid form, tissues rarely show acid-fast bacilli, whereas, in the lepromatous form, there are very large numbers of bacilli. No serologic tests are available for the routine laboratory diagnosis of leprosy.[67]

Management

Multidrug therapy consisting of dapsone, rifampicin, and clofazimine is the recommended treatment of leprosy. Since 1995, the WHO has provided free multidrug therapy for those affected globally.[63]

Herpes Zoster

Definition

Herpes zoster is reactivation of the varicella zoster virus associated with painful skin eruptions.

Epidemiology

More than a million cases of herpes zoster occur in the United States each year, with an annual rate of 3 to 4 cases per 1000 persons.[69]

Clinical

Herpes zoster (shingles) is usually characterized by a unilateral rash limited to a dermatome that does not cross the midline. The most common sites are along the thoracic nerves and the ophthalmic division of the trigeminal nerve. The rash is preceded by tingling, itching, or pain for 2 to 3 days (prodromal) before the development of the vesicular rashes. In 7 to 10 days, the rashes dry out and crust over. A frequent complication of herpes zoster is postherpetic neuralgia, which is persistent neuropathic pain lasting for more than 3 months after the rash has healed. In immunocompromised patients, herpes zosters can present with systemic dissemination with involvement of the lung, liver, and brain.[70] The neurologic complications of herpes zoster can include myelitis, encephalitis, ventriculitis, and meningitis.[71]

Investigations

Clinical presentation of unilateral dermatomal vesicular rash is characteristic enough for the diagnosis of herpes zoster. However, laboratory diagnostic testing with polymerase chain reaction can help to confirm the diagnosis.[72]

Management

Antiviral agents (acyclovir) aids in the resolution of herpes zoster lesions and decrease the severity of acute pain, but these have not been shown to reduce the risk of postherpetic neuralgia.[69] In older adults, zoster vaccine can reduce the incidence and severity of herpes zoster, including postherpetic neuralgia.[73]

Neurosyphilis

Definition

Neurosyphilis is *Treponema pallidum* infection involving the central nervous system.

Epidemiology

Globally, syphilis continues to affect 36.4 million people, with about 10 million new cases per year.[74] *T pallidum* invades the cerebrospinal fluid early in the course of disease, but immunocompetent individuals tend to clear early central nervous system infection even without therapy. Those who fail to clear infection tend to be at risk for symptomatic neurosyphilis, which is commonly diagnosed in patients who are infected with HIV.[75,76]

Clinical

Early forms of symptomatic neurosyphilis can involve the meninges, cerebrospinal fluid, and cerebral or spinal cord vasculature. The late forms of symptomatic neurosyphilis involve the brain and spinal cord parenchyma.[75] Brain involvement can lead to dementia, psychosis, and cognitive impairment.[76] Involvement of the spinal cord (tabes dorsalis) can give rise to lancinating lightning pains in the legs, loss of proprioception, and progressive ataxia.[75] In addition, otologic and ocular involvement can occur, with common findings being asymmetric sensorineural hearing loss and uveitis, respectively.[76]

Investigations
No single specific and sensitive test exists for the diagnosis of neurosyphilis. However, diagnostic criteria commonly involve the synthesis of clinical presentation, serum and cerebrospinal fluid serologic tests, and HIV status and treatment status.[77]

Management
The mainstay of therapy for all forms of syphilis infection is penicillin treatment. The US Centers for Disease Control and Prevention recommends high-dose intravenous penicillin G as the first-line therapy for neurosyphilis.[78]

REFERENCES

1. Maarbjerg S, Di Stefano G, Bendtsen L, et al. Trigeminal neuralgia – diagnosis and treatment. Cephalalgia 2017;37:648–57.
2. Cruccu G. Trigeminal neuralgia. Continuum 2017;23:396–420.
3. Matwychuk M. Diagnostic challenges of neuropathic tooth pain. J Can Dent Assoc 2004;70:542–6.
4. Chhabra A, Bajaj G, Wadhwa V, et al. MR neurographic evaluation of facial and neck pain: normal and abnormal craniospinal nerves below the skull base. Radiographics 2018;38(5):1498–513.
5. Zuniga JR, Mistry C, Tikhonov I, et al. Magnetic resonance neurography of traumatic and nontraumatic peripheral trigeminal neuropathies. J Oral Maxillofac Surg 2018;76:725–36.
6. Dessouky R, Xi Y, Zuniga J, et al. Role of MR neurography for the diagnosis of peripheral trigeminal nerve injuries in patients with prior molar tooth extraction. AJNR Am J Neuroradiol 2018;39:162–9.
7. Cox B, Zuniga JR, Panchal N, et al. Magnetic resonance neurography in the management of peripheral trigeminal neuropathy: experience in a tertiary care centre. Eur Radiol 2016;26:3392–400.
8. Daughton JM, Padala PR, Gabel TL. Careful monitoring for agranulocytosis during carbamazepine treatment. Prim Care Companion J Clin Psychiatry 2006;8: 310–1.
9. Rozen TD. Relief of anesthesia dolorosa with gabapentin. Headache 1999;39: 761–2.
10. Reddy GD, Viswanathan A. Trigeminal and glossopharyngeal neuralgia. Neurol Clin 2014;32:539–52.
11. Khan M, Nishi S, Hassan S, et al. Trigeminal neuralgia, glossopharyngeal neuralgia, and myofascial pain dysfunction syndrome: an update. Pain Res Manag 2017. https://doi.org/10.1155/2017/7438326.
12. Headache Classification Committee of the International Headache Society (IHS). The international classification of headache disorders, 3rd edition (beta version). Cephalalgia 2013;33:629–808.
13. Benoliel R, Charly G. Persistent idiopathic facial pain. Cephalalgia 2017;37: 680–91.

14. Mueller D, Obermann M, Yoon MS. Prevalence of trigeminal neuralgia and persistent idiopathic facial pain: a population-based study. Cephalalgia 2011;31: 1542–8.

15. Koopman JS, Dieleman JP, Huygen FJ. Incidence of facial pain in the general population. Pain 2009;147:122–7.

16. Zakrzewska JM. Facial pain: an update. Curr Opin Support Palliat Care 2009;3: 125–30.

17. Buchanan J, Zakrzewska J. Burning mouth syndrome. BMJ Clin Evid 2008;1301.

18. Klasser GD, Grushka M, Su N. Burning mouth syndrome. Oral Maxillofac Surg Clin North Am 2016;28:381–96.

19. Kohorst JJ, Bruce AJ, Torgerson RR, et al. A population-based study of the incidence of burning mouth syndrome. Mayo Clin Proc 2014;89:1545–52.

20. Coculescu EC, Tovaru S, Coculescu BI. Epidemiological and etiological aspects of burning mouth syndrome. J Med Life 2014;7:305–9.

21. Jääskeläinen SK, Woda A. Burning mouth syndrome. Cephalalgia 2017;37: 627–47.

22. Hoffmann J, May A. Diagnosis, pathophysiology, and management of cluster headache. Lancet Neurol 2018;17:75–83.

23. Russell M. Epidemiology and genetics of cluster headache. Lancet Neurol 2004; 3:279–83.

24. Weaver-Agostoni J. Cluster headache. Am Fam Physician 2013;88:122–8.

25. Rozen T. Cluster headache as the result of secondhand cigarette smoke exposure during childhood. Headache 2010;50:130–2.

26. Wilhour D, Nahas SJ. The neuralgias. Curr Neurol Neurosci Rep 2018;18:69.

27. Becker D, Amirlak B. Beyond beauty: onobotulinumtoxin A (BOTOX®) and the management of migraine headaches. Anesth Pain Med 2012;2:5–11.

28. Onderwater GLJ, Van Dongen RM, Zielman R, et al. Primary headaches. Handb Clin Neurol 2018;146:267–84.

29. Hwang L, Dessouky R, Xi Y, et al. MR neurography of greater occipital nerve neuropathy: initial experience in patients with migraine. AJNR Am J Neuroradiol 2017;38:2203–9.

30. Mulder E, Van Baal C, Gaist D. Genetic and environmental influences on migraine: a twin study across six countries. Twin Res 2003;6:422–31.

31. Sato H, Inoue M, Muraoka W, et al. Jaw claudication is the only clinical predictor of giant-cell arteritis. J Oral Maxillofac Surg Med Pathol 2017;29:264–9.

32. Salvarani C, Pipitone N, Versari A, et al. Clinical features of polymyalgia rheumatica and giant cell arteritis. Nat Rev Rheumatol 2012;8:509–21.

33. Sammel A, Fraser C. Update on giant cell arteritis. Curr Opin Ophthalmol 2018; 29:520–7.

34. Patel DK, Levin KH. Bell's palsy: clinical examination and management. Cleve Clin J Med 2015;82:419–26.

35. Adour KK. Incidence and management of Bell's palsy. In: Fisch U, editor. Facial nerve surgery. 1st edition. Amstelveen (The Netherlands): Kugler Medical Publications; 1977. p. 319–28.

36. Owusu JA, Stewart M, Boahene K. Facial nerve paralysis. Med Clin North Am 2018;102:1135–43.

37. Peitersen E. Bell's palsy: the spontaneous course of 2,500 peripheral facial nerve palsies of different etiologies. Acta Otolaryngol Suppl 2002;(549):4–30.

38. Muralidhar M, Raghavan MR, Bailoor D, et al. Bilateral Bell's palsy: current concepts in aetiology and treatment. Case report. Aust Dent J 1987;32:412–6.

39. Soldatos T, Batra K, Blitz AM, et al. Lower cranial nerves. Neuroimaging Clin N Am 2014;24:35–47.
40. Hafler DA. Multiple sclerosis. J Clin Invest 2004;113:788–94.
41. Fattahi P, Yeganegi M, Kedzierski K. Neurologic disorders and maxillofacial surgery. In: Ferneini E, Bennett J, editors. Perioperative assessment of the maxillofacial surgery patient. Switzerland: Springer AG; 2018. p. 243–62.
42. Browne P, Chandraratna D, Angood C, et al. Atlas of multiple sclerosis 2013: a growing global problem with widespread inequity. Neurology 2014;83:1022–4.
43. Dendrou C, Fugger L, Friese M. Immunopathology of multiple sclerosis. Nat Rev Immunol 2015;15:545–58.
44. Richards RG, Sampson FC, Beard SM, et al. A review of the natural history and epidemiology of multiple sclerosis: implications for resource allocation and health economic models. Health Technol Assess 2002;6:1–73.
45. Brisman R. Trigeminal neuralgia and multiple sclerosis. In: Brisman R, editor. Neurosurgical and medical management of pain: trigeminal neuralgia, chronic pain, and cancer pain. Topics in neurosurgery, vol. 3. Boston: Springer; 1989. p. 77–81.
46. National Multiple Sclerosis Society. In: Treating MS. 2019. Available at: https://www.nationalmssociety.org/Treating-MS/Comprehensive-Care. Accessed April 30, 2019.
47. Flaster M, Meresh E, Rao M, et al. Central poststroke pain: current diagnosis and treatment. Top Stroke Rehabil 2013;20:116–23.
48. Mozaffarian D, Benjamin EJ, Go AS, et al, On behalf of the American Heart Association Statistics Committee and Stroke Statistics Subcommittee. Heart disease and stroke statistics-2016 update a report from the American Heart Association. Circulation 2016;133(4):e38–60.
49. Keszler M, Gude T, Heckert K. Pain syndromes associated with cerebrovascular accidents. In: Freedman MK, Gehret JA, Young GW, et al, editors. Challenging neuropathic pain syndromes. Philadelphia: Science Direct, Elsevier; 2018. p. 155–65.
50. Greenlee JD, Menezes AH, Bertoglio BA, et al. Syringobulbia in a pediatric population. Neurosurgery 2005;57:1147–53.
51. Penarrocha M, Okeson JP, Penarrocha MS, et al. Orofacial pain as the sole manifestation of syringobulbia-syringomyelia associated with Arnold Chiari malformation. J Orofac Pain 2001;15:170–3.
52. Bitsko RH, Holbrook JR, Visser SN, et al. A national profile of Tourette syndrome, 2011-2012. J Dev Behav Pediatr 2014;35:317–22.
53. Centers for Disease Control and Prevention. Prevalence of diagnosed Tourette syndrome in persons aged 6-17 years – United States, 2007. MMWR Morb Mortal Wkly Rep 2009;58(21):581–5.
54. Lowe TL, Capriotti MR, McBurnett K. Long-term follow-up of patients with Tourette's syndrome. Mov Disord Clin Pract 2018;6:40–5.
55. Koman LA, Smith BP, Shilt JS. Cerebral palsy. Lancet 2004;363:1619–31.
56. Graham HK, Rosenbaum P, Paneth N, et al. Cerebral palsy. Nat Rev Dis Primers 2016;2:1–25.
57. Ashwal S, Russman BS, Blasco PA, et al. Practice parameter: diagnostic assessment of the child with cerebral palsy. Neurology 2004;62:851–63.
58. Tysnes OB, Sorstein A. Epidemiology of Parkinson's disease. J Neural Transm 2017;124:901–5.
59. Williams-Gray CH, Worth PF. Parkinson's disease. Medicine 2016;44:542–6.
60. Lang AE, Lozano AM. Parkinson's disease. N Engl J Med 1998;339:1044–53.

61. Kalia LV, Lang AE. Parkinson's disease. Lancet 2015;386:896–912.
62. De Lau LML, Breteler MMB. Epidemiology of Parkinson's disease. Lancet Neurol 2006;5:525–35.
63. Global Leprosy Program. In: World Health Organization, 2017. Available at: http://www.searo.who.int/entity/global_leprosy_programme/epidemiology/en/. Accessed May 3, 2019.
64. Ooi WW, Srinivasan J. Leprosy and the peripheral nervous system: basic and clinical aspects. Muscle Nerve 2004;30:393–409.
65. Scollard DM, Adams LB, Gillis TP, et al. The continuing challenges of leprosy. Clin Microbiol Rev 2006;19:338–81.
66. Nascimento OJM. Leprosy neuropathy: clinical presentations. Arq Neuropsiquiatr 2013;71:661–6.
67. Raicher I, Stump P, Baccarelli R, et al. Neuropathic pain in leprosy. Clin Dermatol 2016;34:59–65.
68. De Freitas MR, Said G. Leprous neuropathy. Handb Clin Neurol 2013;115:499–514.
69. Cohen JI. Herpes zoster. N Engl J Med 2013;369:255–63.
70. Sampathkumar P, Drage LA, Martin DP. Herpes zoster (shingles) and postherpetic neuralgia. Mayo Clin Proc 2009;84:274–80.
71. Gilden DH, Kleinschmidt-deMasters BK, LaGuardia JJ, et al. Neurologic complications of the reactivation of varicella-zoster virus. N Engl J Med 2000;342:635–45.
72. Schmader K. Herpes zoster. Clin Geriatr Med 2016;32:539–53.
73. Oxman MN, Levin MJ, Johnson MS, et al. A vaccine to prevent herpes zoster and postherpetic neuralgia in older adults. N Engl J Med 2005;352:2271–84.
74. World Health Organization. In: Global incidence and prevalence of selected curable sexually transmitted disease 2008. Available at: http://www.who.int/reproductivehealth/publications/rtis/stisestimates/en/. Accessed May 3, 2019.
75. O'Donnell JA, Emery CL. Neurosyphilis: a current review. Curr Infect Dis Rep 2005;7:277–84.
76. Marra CM. Update on neurosyphilis. Curr Infect Dis Rep 2009;11:127–34.
77. Bhai S, Lyons JL. Neurosyphilis update: atypical is the new typical. Curr Infect Dis Rep 2015;17:1–6.
78. Marra CM. Neurosyphilis. Continuum 2015;21:1714–28.

Moving?

Make sure your subscription moves with you!

To notify us of your new address, find your **Clinics Account Number** (located on your mailing label above your name), and contact customer service at:

Email: journalscustomerservice-usa@elsevier.com

800-654-2452 (subscribers in the U.S. & Canada)
314-447-8871 (subscribers outside of the U.S. & Canada)

Fax number: 314-447-8029

Elsevier Health Sciences Division
Subscription Customer Service
3251 Riverport Lane
Maryland Heights, MO 63043

*To ensure uninterrupted delivery of your subscription, please notify us at least 4 weeks in advance of move.

ELSEVIER

Printed and bound by CPI Group (UK) Ltd, Croydon, CR0 4YY

03/10/2024

01040407-0010